IMAGING BRAIN STRUCTURE AND FUNCTION

EMERGING TECHNOLOGIES IN THE NEUROSCIENCES

ANNALS OF THE NEW YORK ACADEMY OF SCIENCES
Volume 820

IMAGING BRAIN STRUCTURE AND FUNCTION

EMERGING TECHNOLOGIES IN THE NEUROSCIENCES

Edited by David S. Lester, Christian C. Felder, and E. Neil Lewis

The New York Academy of Sciences
New York, New York
1997

⊗ *The paper used in this publication meets the minimum requirements of American National Standard for Information Sciences—Permanence of Paper for Printed Library Materials, ANSI Z39.48-1984.*

The pattern on the paper-bound cover, from FIGURE *4 of Gary Blasdel's paper "Strategies of Visual Perception Suggested by Optically Imaged Patterns of Functional Architecture in Monkey Visual Cortex," represents a map of the geometric relationship between ocular dominance and orientation cortical slabs in the monkey.*

Library of Congress Cataloging-in-Publication Data

Imaging brain structure and function: emerging technologies in the neurosciences / edited by David S. Lester, Christian C. Felder, and E. Neil Lewis.
p. cm. — (Annals of the New York Academy of Sciences, ISSN 0077-8923; v. 820)
Includes bibliographical references and index.
ISBN 1-57331-069-7 (paper: alk. paper). — ISBN 1-57331-068-9 (cloth: alk. paper)
1. Brain—Imaging—Congresses. 2. Neurosciences—Methodology—Congresses. 3. Neurotoxicology—Methodology—Congresses. I. Lester, David S. (David Simon), 1953– . II. Felder, Christian C. III. Lewis, E. Neil. IV. Series.
[DNLM: 1. Brain—cytology—congresses. 2. Diagnostic Imaging—methods—congresses. 3. Brain Diseases—diagnosis—congresses. 4. Microscopy—methods—congresses. 5. Brain—drug effects—congresses. W1 AN626YL v. 820 1997 / WL 101 I31 1997]
Q11.N5 vol. 820
[QP376]
500 s—dc21
[616.8′04754]
DNLM/DLC
for Library of Congress 97-13820
CIP

SP
Printed in the United States of America
ISBN 1-57331-068-9 (cloth)
ISBN 1-57331-069-7 (paper)
ISSN 0077-8923

ANNALS OF THE NEW YORK ACADEMY OF SCIENCES

Volume 820
May 30, 1997

IMAGING BRAIN STRUCTURE AND FUNCTION

EMERGING TECHNOLOGIES IN THE NEUROSCIENCES[a]

Editors and Conference Organizers
DAVID S. LESTER, CHRISTIAN C. FELDER, AND E. NEIL LEWIS
Scientific Advisory Board
JAMES L. OLDS, IRA W. LEVIN, BUDDY HARISSON, PATRICK TREADO, JEFF STUCKEY, AND TONY CELESTE

CONTENTS

[a]This volume is the result of a conference entitled **Current and Emerging Techniques in Monitoring Brain Structure and Function,** which was sponsored by the Center for Drug Evaluation and Research, Food and Drug Administration, and the National Institute of Mental Health and held on March 28–29, 1996 at the National Library of Medicine, Bethesda, Maryland.

Part II. "Cutting-Edge" Technologies in the Neurosciences

Part III. Future Directions in the Neurosciences

Part IV. Panel Discussion on Neurotoxicity

Financial assistance was received from:

- CENTER FOR DRUG EVALUATION AND RESEARCH, FOOD AND DRUG ADMINISTRATION
- NATIONAL INSTITUTE OF MENTAL HEALTH, NATIONAL INSTITUTES OF HEALTH

Preface[a]

DAVID S. LESTER

Center for Drug Evaluation and Research
Food and Drug Administration
Laurel, Maryland 20708

The title of the meeting upon which this volume is based was "Current and Emerging Techniques in Monitoring Brain Structure and Function." The two-day symposium was held at the National Library of Medicine on March 28th and 29th, 1996. The concept of the meeting arose during a plane flight to the Society of Neuroscience meeting that was held in New Orleans in 1991. I was seated next to a fellow neuroscientist who used NMR spectroscopy for analyzing brain tissue from donors suffering from various neurological disorders. We discussed our frustration as to how brain imaging is generally considered to be either MRI, PET, or CT scan. There is a general lack of awareness among neuroscientists that brain imaging extends beyond these technical approaches, and it is important to demonstrate this breadth in an open forum to a diverse audience with a common interest—the need to understand the functioning of the brain at a higher level. The term *imaging* is recognized generally as MRI, PET, etc.; while some biologists, the microscopists, consider that it represents microscopy. This meeting was conceived to show both of these camps that imaging has wide implications that cross between each of these approaches.

Since joining the FDA, I have been exposed to a very important issue in neuroscience, that of neurotoxicity. The difficulty in determining adverse neurotoxic responses due to therapeutic agents is largely due to the nature of the technical approaches that are now being employed. Standard histology, which has been around for all of this century, has progressed with the introduction of immunohistochemistry. Also, advanced imaging technologies have provided an informative window into the brain and are slowly being transferred to the applied sciences.

The plan of this conference was first to present an overview of the present-day approaches to and capabilities of monitoring changes in brain structure and function. This was followed by two sessions: one on "cutting edge" technologies in the neurosciences that could be applied to problems of neuropathology and neurotoxicity, and the other on future technologies that could be applied to the neurosciences. An outstanding collection of 21 speakers made presentations at the meeting. Even the moderators were specifically selected for their in-depth knowledge of the technologies and the

[a]The chapters in this proceedings do not reflect the beliefs of the Food and Drug Administration; they represent the opinions of the authors only.

complexities of the brain. The meeting closed with a panel discussion on the application of these technologies to issues relating to neurotoxicity. The panel was composed of representatives from five centers of the Food and Drug Administration.

Most of the speakers provided chapters for this volume, and the transcribed discussions have been included, as they provide interesting insights and suggest possible future directions. It is hoped that this book will serve as an aid in transferring these fascinating technologies to the applied sciences, where they can aid in the drug development process in providing better means of predicting and detecting possible adverse neurotoxic effects.

I would like to acknowledge the advisory assistance offered by Dr. James J. Olds, of the American Association of Anatomists; Dr. Ira W. Levin, of the National Institute of Diabetes and Digestive and Kidney Diseases, National Institutes of Health; Mr. Buddy Harisson, of Meridian Instruments, Inc.; Dr. Patrick Treado, of Chemicon, Inc.; Dr. Jeff Stuckey, of Universal Imaging, Inc.; and Mr. Tony Celeste, of Silicon Graphics Imaging, Inc.

I would like to express special thanks to Dr. Anita O'Connor of the Office of Science, FDA, and Dr. James Olds for their continued support in ensuring that this was an exciting and successful meeting.

Opening Remarks

B. SCHWETZ

Office of Science
Office of the Commissioner
Food and Drug Administration
5600 Fisher Lane
Rockville, Maryland 20857

I thank and commend the organizers for putting together what I think is a very promising meeting. I strongly support these kinds of meetings on scientific matters, especially between sister agencies, where we can clearly get more done together than either of us does alone. So I was very pleased to be asked to make some opening comments.

As I reflect on meetings that I have attended over the past 25 years, I must admit that I have often seen the words "emerging technologies" in the title. Every time they are used, they seem to make a lot of promises about where we are and where we are going and the exciting things that are ahead; it makes you wonder what we really mean by *emerging*. We make progress, but did we make the kind of progress that we expected. Over the last six months I have been involved in this kind of meeting in a number of different areas, including developmental toxicology, carcinogenesis, indirect mechanisms of carcinogenesis, and genetic toxicology; and I must say that in each of these areas and in the neurosciences we are probably closer to a scientific threshold than I can remember at any time over the past 20 years.

I think there are several reasons for this. One of them is that we clearly have a better understanding today of the biology, physiology, and chemistry of the nervous system and its functioning than we have had at any time in the past. That has permitted us to develop more sensitive and more specific tools to probe the nervous system than we have had before. But there are other reasons as well. Part of it, I think, is a closer integration today between the clinical and nonclinical parts of the neurosciences than we have seen before. Animal models and the human experience are also more closely integrated. I think all of those are very positive contributions, and they make me consider that we are closer to a scientific threshold today than we have been before.

It is pretty clear that there is better support for risk assessment and risk management as well as clinical decisions today than we have had before. This should result, then, in better protection of public health. The public is more cognizant of what negative impact toxicities of the nervous system can have, and people worry more about not only degenerative diseases of the nervous system but other adverse affects on the developing and the functioning adult nervous system. I think that we should expect to see more emphasis on protecting public health in this arena as we go forward.

Clearly there is plenty of evidence that we need to worry about the health of the nervous system and that this is a real concern and not an imaginary one. Consider that 25 percent of Americans suffer from some brain-related disorder during their life and that some 10 percent of school children have some functional deficit. A real concern of mine is the fact that we have a lot more than 10 percent of kids being treated for some, either real or imagined, mental deficits. A large percentage of TLV's are set on the basis of some neurobehavioral or some neurotoxic effect of the chemicals for that TLV. All of this is evidence of the real concern that we should have for neurotoxicity of chemicals.

At a time of tough budgets and decreasing amounts of money to support research, it is also, I think, appropriate to point out that the cost of treatment and rehabilitation is much larger than the collective research budgets for all of us in this area. Meetings of this type should help bring attention to better ways to predict and identify some of these new concerns and new toxicities of the nervous system of humans. We should then have more accurate identification of the lesions and be better able to predict the sequelae of adverse affects in those particular cells or tissues. I would hope also that this will lead us to better and earlier identification of sensitive subpopulations, whether the metabolic differences be age related, gender related, or genetically determined—whatever those subpopulations might be. We tend to think of diseases as occurring in large percentages of the population, but they do not. For the most part the consequences of overexposure that we see manifest as some toxicity occur in a small percent. For some reason that small percent is more sensitivc than the others. We need to help identify those.

I certainly wish you a good meeting and I thank you for inviting me to participate.

Welcome

S. E. SWEDO

National Institute of Mental Health
National Institutes of Health
9000 Rockville Pike
Bethesda, Maryland 20892

On behalf of my colleagues in the National Institute of Mental Health Intramural Program, I want to welcome you. We are extremely excited about the agenda that our organizers have planned for us. I think that it speaks to the importance of structural and functional imaging to all of the brain institutes but particularly to the one closest to my heart, the National Institute of Mental Health. Neuroimaging has actually transformed the way the public thinks about the mental disorders. If you go back nearly 20 years now to the first structural studies of schizophrenia, demonstrating enlarged ventricular size, that was absolutely the turning point at which schizophrenia went from being a curse to being a neurobiologic illness. The progress has been rapid and exciting since that time. The functional studies by two of our scientists, Drs. Sokoloff and Ketty, have been intimately involved in the development of the techniques that have led to the ability to visualize the brain at work. Again, this has tremendous importance as we begin to think about why mental illnesses might occur, and more importantly how to prevent and treat them. The current state of knowledge allows us to do imaging of real time, thought, behavior, emotion; and again, the potential is absolutely tremendous here. The agenda for this meeting shows promise that other questions that will soon be answered by the emerging technologies are even more exciting and more important. For that reason I am not going to take any more of your time. I am just going to thank you again for allowing me to be part of this and wish that you have a very successful meeting.

Brain-Mapping Neurotoxicity and Neuropathology[a]

ARTHUR W. TOGA[b]

Laboratory of Neuro Imaging
Department of Neurology
Division of Brain Mapping
UCLA School of Medicine
710 Westwood Plaza
Los Angeles, California 90024-1769

The papers presented in this part, entitled "Present Techniques for Monitoring Neurotoxicity and Neuropathology," give evidence of a wide range of technologies for monitoring brain structure and function. These include everything from the examination of histological preparations to *in vivo* functional brain activation measurements. All the data collected using these techniques have one thing in common: they reference an anatomic framework against which data from different modalities, experiments, and subjects can be compared and contrasted. The difficulty in accomplishing these comparisons stems from the fact that no common anatomic reference system can accommodate the variability found across individuals and modalities. The purpose of this introductory article is to describe current efforts that are focused on solutions to these problems of comparison.

The lack of suitably accommodating brain atlases has plagued a wide variety of neuroscientific investigations for a long time. However, a number of human brain atlases exist, usually based upon a single person's description of a single view of anatomy, that enable the identification of specific locations in brain for subsequent description and mapping. Unfortunately, these are not extensible and may not even be acceptably representative. What is clear, upon examination of the following articles, is that a statistical and computerized approach is necessary to accomplish multimodal, multisubject brain mapping. Given the fact that most data are, or will soon be, electronic in nature and have inherent numerical indexing in space and intensity and sometimes time, the ability to incorporate this diversity of information is presently available to us. We only need to create an appropriate framework.

The second challenge evidenced by the papers presented in this part has to do with the tremendous volume of information that is being collected in the monitoring of neurotoxicity and neuropathology. In addition to analyses, the

[a]This work was generously supported by research grants from the National Library of Medicine (LM/MH05639), the National Science Foundation (BIR 93-22434), the NCRR (RR05956), and the Human Brain Project, which is funded jointly by NIMH and NIDA (P20 MH/DA52176).

[b]Phone: (310)206-2101; fax: (310)206-5518; e-mail: toga@loni.ucla.edu

ability to communicate these data effectively across laboratories, sometimes at great geographic distances, is crucial to our full utilization of the knowledge gleaned from it. Therefore, the brain-mapping solutions, which must bear upon the practical issues of coordinate systems, nomenclatures, and statistical analyses, must also incorporate appropriate mechanisms for the dissemination of these data. These mechanisms include visualization, communication and data-basing, so portions of this paper are devoted to these aspects of brain mapping as well.

INTRODUCTION

Atlases

Most atlases of the human brain and, other species[26] are derived from one, or at best a few, individual specimens.[6,24,32,36,35] Such atlases may take the form of anatomical references or they may represent a particular feature of the brain,[47] such as a specific neurochemical distribution[23] or cerebral cortical cytoarchitecture.[6] In existing atlases, proportional scaling systems are typically employed to reference a given brain to the atlas brain. Commonly used human atlases include those of Talairach *et al.*[35] and Schaltenbrand and Wahren.[32]

The anatomical variability between individual human brains is well known. Given the still undefined relationship between neuronal structure and function, an atlas based on an unvarying anatomy does not satisfy the need for measuring, mapping or modeling a population. One need only look at the functional and structural specialization of the hemispheres to recognize the depth of this problem.[17,18,21,28,33,34,48] Single-modality atlases (of limited spatial resolution) are also insufficient, because of the need to establish the relationship between different measurements of anatomy and physiology.

Variability

Variance between human brains is becoming better understood. As was noted above, this occurs not only for gyral patterns but also for interhemispheric differences.[33] Microscopic variation in the human brain also exists, as does the boundaries of microscopic (i.e., cytoarchitectural)[28,31] and macroscopic (gyral/sulcal)[2] landmarks. Since both micro- and macroscopic variations between brains, exist, but earlier published atlases represent one or, at best, a few brains, it is impossible to make generalizations about these varying anatomies for the entire species.

Accurate localization of brain structure and function in any modality is improved by correlation with higher-resolution anatomic data placed within an appropriate spatial coordinate system. Recent brain-mapping efforts have begun to explore this approach, yet remain disadvantaged by the lack of readily available, spatially detailed 3-D morphology of the normal human brain.[10] In response to this need, several computerized atlases have been developed for neurosurgical applications or for analysis of metabolic studies such as those using PET and other modalities.[40,11,22,31] These atlases, based on data acquired using magnetic resonance imaging (MRI), have the advantage of intrinsic three-axis registration and spatial coordinates, but have relatively low resolution and lack anatomic contrast in important subregions. High-resolution MR atlases, using up to 100–150 slices, a section thickness of 2 mm, and 256^2 pixel imaging planes[11,22] still result in resolutions lower than that required to appreciate the complexity of many neuroanatomic structures.

Several digital atlases have been developed using photographic images of cryoplaned frozen specimens.[4,19] The use of photographed material, while providing superior anatomic detail, has limitations. For accurate correlations, data must be placed in the equivalent plane as the image of interest. Digital imaging can overcome some of the limitations of conventional film photography methods. Using 1024^2, 24-bits/pixel digital color cameras, spatial resolution can be as high as 100 microns/pixel for whole human head cadaver preparations or higher for isolated brain regions.[41] Cryosectioning in micron increments permits collection of data with high spatial resolution in the axis orthogonal to the sectioning plane. Acquisition of images in series directly from the consistently positioned cryoplaned blockface avoids the need for serial image registration prior to reconstruction. Serial images can be reconstructed to a 3-D anatomic volume that is amenable to various resampling and positioning schemes.

Anatomical Reference

We have created spatially accurate, high-resolution anatomic reference volumes from postmortem cryosectioned whole human brain. We examined the advantages of this approach and determined the value of the data as an anatomic reference for MR, PET and other modalities. First, we examined anatomic image data (1024^2, 24-bits/pixel) to see whether it contained sufficient resolution to improve the ability to delineate neuroanatomic structures. Second, we tested whether 3-D reconstruction, repositioning, scaling and resampling could be performed while preserving accurate spatial relationships. Statistical morphometrics were calculated to determine the degree of precision in anatomic segmentation and placement within the Talairach coordinate system.[35] Meshes describing sulcal ribbons were used to drive deformations for higher-order mappings across subjects. Finally, we evaluated tissue collected from the cryosectioned specimens for compatibility with specific histochemical staining and analysis for cytoarchitectonic delineation. The goal was to produce a series of high-resolution 3-D anatomic volumes with potential to serve as an anatomic reference for comprehensive human brain mapping in a variety of imaging modalities.

DEFORMABLE ATLASES

Mapping and modeling require that the degree of subtle deviations from normal brain structure and function be measured precisely. As was noted above, this is especially difficult in the brain because its internal geometry is highly individual in character. Recent developments in mathematical approaches to brain mapping offer viable solutions to this problem, retaining comprehensive information on inter-subject variations in brain architecture (FIG. 1).

In view of the complex structural variability between individuals, it would be ideal if an atlas could be elastically deformed to fit a new image set from an incoming subject. Transforming individual data sets into the shape of a single reference anatomy, or onto a 3-D digital brain atlas, removes subject-specific shape variations and allows subsequent comparison of brain function between individuals.[7] Conversely, high-dimensional warping algorithms can also be used to transfer all the information in a 3-D digital brain atlas onto the scan of any given patient, while respecting the intricate patterns of structural variation in their anatomy. Such *deformable atlases*[8,12] can be used to carry 3-D maps of functional and vascular territories into the coordinate system of different patients, as well as information on different tissue types and the boundaries of cytoarchitectonic fields and their neurochemical composition.

Already these approaches have been applied to warp one brain onto another.[37–39,43,44] These transformations redefine the spatial relationship between points in image sets. For the purposes of multimodality and multisubject brain comparisons, warping is defined as those geometric transformations that alter brain shape. They do not include simple repositioning. The implementation, whether density- or spatially based, of the warping is dependent on the type of data and their resolution. For example, if anatomic landmarks are easily obtained, spatially based algorithms may be employed. The location and number of landmarks are crucial to the goodness of fit. In other cases, density-based warping algorithms can maximize the cross-correlation coefficients between data sets without the identification of landmarks. Initial work was based on the success of two-dimensional deformations[16] to produce a three-dimensional plastic deformation for the removal of nonlinear variability in brain shape. If one allows elastic deformations in any plane a three-dimensional approach is required.

Equating the relationship between neuroanatomic labels and a Cartesian (or polar) coordinate systems is one of the byproducts of warping to a digital atlas. In addition, segmentation of neuroanatomic structures within three-dimensional data sets using such anatomic templates as Talairach *et al.*'s[35] stereotactic atlas of the human brain helps make functional measurements between subjects comparable. Fitting anatomic templates to data will greatly increase the number of structures that can be identified. It also provides a common reference system[5,49] for multi-subject comparison and, ultimately, the development of a database with normative data.[12b,15] Clinical usefulness has also been tested. Using PET data and these methods, Clark *et al.*[9] presented initially encouraging results for a statistical model that assessed the probability of whether a patient was normal or had Huntington's disease.

Warping a brain to an atlas can be accomplished by sequentially mapping two-dimensional sections through the data set onto an atlas template, assuming the sections are oriented identically. Alternately, the reconstructed three-dimensional volume can be repositioned, warped, and resampled to correspond with atlas templates.[42] Typically, the spatial resolution of the atlas is significantly less than that of the experimental data so that loss of accuracy due to resampling is not a problem. Warping can be performed to any degree and can be either spatially[37–39,45,46] or density-based.[3]

In order to remove the morphometric variability between data sets one can impose density-based local deformations on the three-dimensional volume data set of high-resolution postmortem digital anatomy. First, the data sets are histogram-equalized and filtered to eliminate high-frequency or artifactual contamination of the warpings. Then the volume to be warped is subjected to principal axes and center-of-mass repositioning. Overall scaling and affine transformations are then applied. If a three-dimensional grid (256^3 points) is placed on the volume, then the elastic forces can be computed at each point when derived using the cross-correlation function between the two volume data sets. An image-similarity function can be computed as a least-square polynomial approximation of the image correlation in the spherical region around the grid point.

Other approaches use anatomic or spatial information to control the warp. We have also developed high-dimensional warping algorithms to drive different brains into precise structural correspondence. This algorithm was designed to calculate the high-dimensional deformation field relating the brain anatomies of an arbitrary pair of subjects. The resulting 3-D deformation maps may be used to quantify anatomic differences between subjects or within the same subject over time, and to transfer functional information between subjects or to integrate that information on a single anatomic template. High spatial accuracy is guaranteed by using a large set of corresponding anatomic surfaces to constrain the complex transformation of one subject's anatomy into the shape of another. These surfaces include critical functional interfaces such as the ventricles and cortex, as well as numerous cytoarchitectonic and lobar boundaries in three dimensions. The construction of extremely complex surface deformation maps on the internal cortex is made easier by building a generic surface structure to model it. Connected systems of parametric meshes model several deep internal fissures, or *sulci,* whose trajectories represent critical functional boundaries. These sulci are sufficiently extended inside the brain to reflect subtle and distributed variations in neuroanatomy between subjects. The parametric form of the system of connected surface elements allows us to represent the relation between any pair of anatomies as a family of high-resolution displacement maps carrying the surface system of one individual onto another in stereotaxic space. The

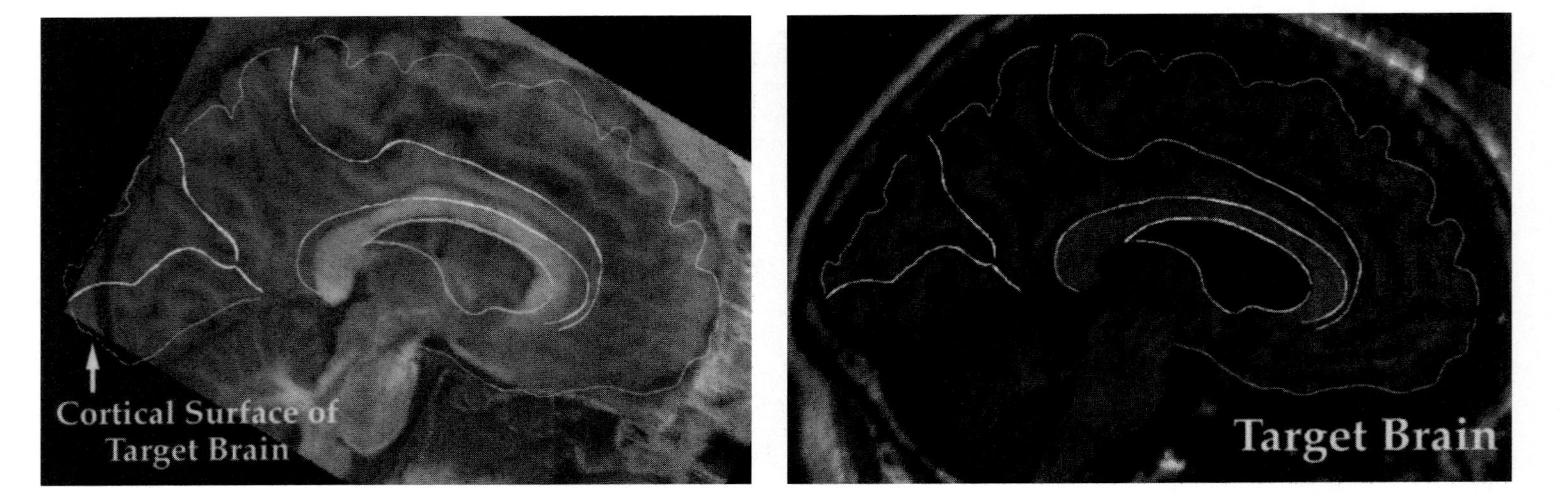
Cortical Surface of
Target Brain
Target Brain

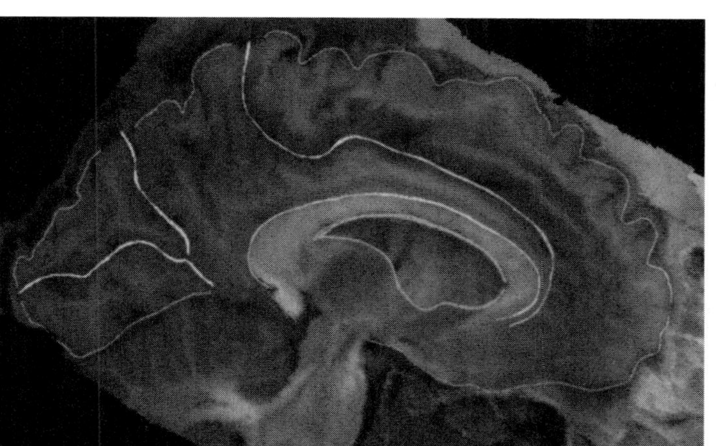

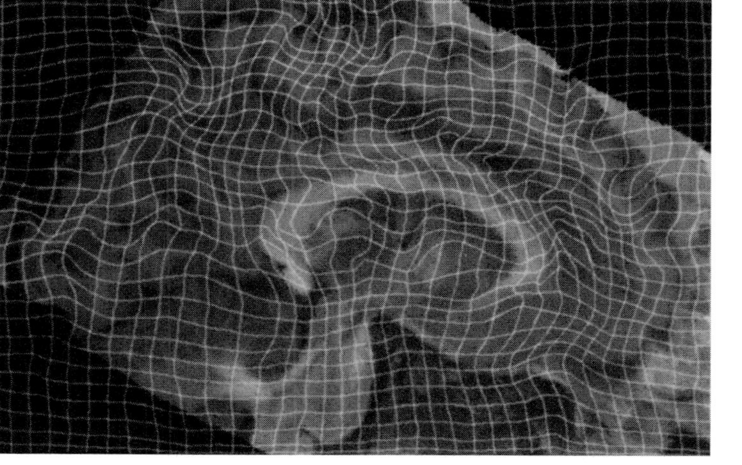

FIGURE 1. Intermodality data fusion: 3-D digital cryosection volumes mapped onto 3D MRI volumes. Sagittal brain slice images from (*top left*) a digitally imaged, cryosectioned whole human head, and (*top right*) a 3-D SPGR T_1-weighted MR target scan. Also shown are the result (*bottom left*) of warping the cryosection image into structural correspondence with the MR scan, and the same transformation (*bottom right*) applied to a regular grid in the reference coordinate system. Note the reconfiguration of the major sulci, and the degree to which the reference *corpus callosum* is transformed into the shape of the target *callosum.* The continuous one-to-one mapping property of the warping transformation preserves the structural integrity of the data, and ensures the smooth continuation of the warping field from the complex anatomic surfaces into the surrounding brain architecture. Recent investigations in our laboratory have involved high-resolution cryosection imaging of whole human heads from subjects whose premortem PET and MR scans are also available.[50] High-dimensional transformation tools enable the integration of cytoarchitectural and molecular maps with functional data obtained from the same individual *in vivo.*

algorithm then calculates the high-dimensional volumetric warp (typically with $384^2 \times 256 \times 3 \approx 0.1$ billion degrees of freedom) deforming one 3-D scan into structural correspondence with the other. Integral distortion functions are used to extend the deformation field required to elastically transform these surface systems into structural correspondence with their counterparts in the target scan.

3-D warping algorithms provide a method for calculating local and global shape changes and give valuable information to scientists studying normal and abnormal growth and development. Deformable atlases not only account for the anatomic variations and idiosyncrasies of each individual patient, but they also offer a powerful strategy for exploring and classifying age-related, developmental or pathologic variations in anatomy. More fundamentally, they also provide a method for spatially normalizing the anatomies of different brains. Such normalization software supplies a basis for comparing data obtained from different subjects or at different research centers.

Probabilistic Atlases

Probabilistic atlasing[14,25,38] is a research strategy whose goal is to generate anatomical templates and expert diagnostic systems which retain quantitative information on inter-subject variations in brain architecture. The recent interest in comprehensive brain mapping also stresses that the comparisons between subjects, both within and across homogeneous populations, are required to understand normal variability and genuine structural and functional differences. Initial attempts to derive average representations of neuroanatomy have underscored the power of this approach in both clinical and research settings.[1,13]

We have developed and implemented an approach for constructing a probabilistic surface atlas of the brain. This method performs a statistical analysis of deep surface structures in the brain (in a reference database of normal scans), and then automatically quantifies and maps distributed patterns of abnormality in the same system of anatomic surfaces in new subjects. Once again, connected systems of parametric meshes model deep fissures in the brain, whose trajectories represent critical functional and lobar boundaries. Additional surface analysis algorithms construct a probability space of random transformations (based on the theory of 3-D Gaussian random fields), reflecting the variability in stereotaxic space of the connected system of anatomic surfaces. Automatic parametrization of the surface anatomy of new subjects has enabled the detection and mapping of subtle shape and volume abnormalities in the brains of patients with metastatic tumors. These shape changes can be visualized in the form of probability maps on a graphical surface model of the subject's anatomy. The resulting surface system can be rotated, magnified and animated interactively for detailed examination and clinical diagnosis.

MORPHOMETRY

Morphometric statistics describing subcortical structures such as anterior commissure, caudate, putamen, globus pallidus, and thalamus as well as cortical sulcal landmarks in image data from postmortem cryosectioned anatomy and MR images were relatively consistent across subjects and in general agreement with the Talairach atlas data. Mean surface area, volume, and center of mass demonstrated significantly less variability between hemispheres in comparison to inter-subject variability. Volume was less susceptible than surface statistics to variance due to complicated geometries; for example, statistics calculated on the ventricular system were highly influenced by slight differences in the lateral extent of this structure and thus unreliable.

The ability to resolve neuroanatomic boundaries is critical for accurate structure delineation. The spatial and densitometric detail provided in high-resolution images of cryosectioned anatomy significantly improved our ability to differentiate structure boundaries. When cryosectioned images were compared to MRI, we found it easier to delineate such structures in the cryosectioned anatomy as the laminar partitions of the basal ganglia and hippocampus. Subsequent histological processing of collected tissue sections proved even more valuable for localization of additional anatomic structure. By correlating digitized histological information with blockface images, it was possible to retain the spatial context of the sections. Histologic sections have previously been used as an anatomic reference to improve interpretation of MR and CT images,[30] but such correlations have primarily been visual. By using digital reconstruction and resampling techniques we were able to display high-resolution anatomy in specified planes to precisely match image data obtained from other modalities.

The differences between tomographic images of *in vivo* human brain and surface imaging of cryoplaned postmortem specimens must be recognized. First, frozen preparation can induce changes in the configuration of anatomic specimens. Previous studies have suggested that alterations in size, shape and attenuation values of specimens may not be significant.[20,27,29] Our own morphometric measurements support this. However, there are certainly many changes that occur postmortem, such as loss of mean arterial pressure and uneven distribution of intracranial fluids, that contribute to differences between *in vivo*– and *ex vivo*–derived data.

The use of postmortem anatomical volumes created from serial cryoplaned heads and brains, in combination with histologically processed tissue from the specimen, provide a detailed high-resolution reference for tomographically acquired images. This approach, in combination with multimodality mapping techniques, will add to the growing database being applied to the goal of mapping the human brain.

Measured and modeled sulci used for deformation proved sufficiently extended inside the brain to reflect subtle and distributed variations in neuroanatomy between subjects. Integral distortion functions were successfully used to extend the deformation field required to elastically transform nested surfaces to their counterparts in the target scan. The algorithm's accuracy was tested by warping 3-D MRI volumes from normal subjects and Alzheimer's patients, full-color 1024^3 digital cryosection volumes of the human head, onto normal MRI volumes and MRI volumes of patients with metastatic tumors causing mechanical distortions of anatomies.

CONCLUSION

In the future, rapid access to digital image archives, as well as to computational tools, will be fundamental to many hypothesis-driven investigations of brain anatomy and function in health and disease. The establishment of powerful brain atlasing approaches, together with methods for guaranteeing the comparability of research findings from different laboratories, is central to the task of comprehensive brain mapping. Internet repositories of software tools, such as those for creating deformable neuroanatomic atlases,[7,12,37] will enable the transfer of multisubject 3-D functional, vascular, and histological maps onto a single anatomic template; the mapping of 3-D brain atlases onto the scans of new subjects; and the rapid detection, quantification, and mapping of local shape changes in 3-D medical images in disease and during normal or abnormal growth and development.

Digital probabilistic atlases based on large populations will also rectify many current atlasing problems since they retain quantitative information on the variability inherent in anatomic populations. As the underlying database of subjects increases in size and content, the digital, electronic form of the atlas will provide efficiency in statistical and computational comparisons between individuals or groups. The atlas will also improve in accuracy over time, achieving better statistics as more information is added. In addition, the digital form of the source data will enable the population on which probabilistic atlases are based to be stratified into subpopulations by age, gender, and stage of development or to represent different disease types. Such archive-based atlasing approaches will therefore allow globally networked sites to benefit directly from vast repositories of image data collected at remote research centers.

ACKNOWLEDGMENTS

Special thanks go to members of my laboratory, Colin Holmes, Paul Thompson and Bradley Payne, without whom none of this could have been done.

REFERENCES

1. ANDREASEN, N. C., S. ARNDT, V. SWAYZE, T. CIZADLO, M. FLAUM, D. O'LEARY, J. C. EHRHARDT & W. T. C. YUH. 1994. Thalamic abnormalities in schizophrenia visualized through magnetic resonance image averaging. Science: 294–298.
2. ARMSTRONG, E., A. SCHLEICHER, H. OMRAN, M. CURTIS & K. ZILLES. 1995. The ontogeny of human gyrification. Cereb. Cortex : 56–63.
3. BAJCSY, R., R. LIEBERSON & M. REIVICH. 1983. A computerized system for the elastic matching of deformed radiographic images to idealized atlas images. J. Comp. Assist. Tomogr. **7**(4): 618–625.
4. BOHM, C., T. GREITZ & L. ERIKSSON. 1989. A computerized adjustable brain atlas. Eur. J. Med. **15:** 687–689.
5. BOHM, C., T. GREITZ, R. SEITZ & L. ERIKSSON. 1991. Specification and selection of regions of interest (ROIs) in a computerized brain atlas. J. Cereb. Blood Flow Metab. **11:** A64–68.
6. BRODMANN, K. 1905. Beitrage zur histologischen lokalisation der grosshirnrinde. Dritte mitteilung: Die rindenfelder der niederen affen. J. Psychol. Neurol. Lpz. **4:** 177–226.
7. CHRISTENSEN, E., M. I. MILLER, J. L. MARSH & M. W. VANNIER. 1995. Automatic analysis of medical images using a deformable textbook. *In* Computer Assisted Radiology: Proceedings of the International Symposium on Computer and Communication Systems for Image-Guided Diagnosis and Therapy. H. U. Lemke *et al.,* Eds. : 146–151. Springer. Berlin.
8. CHRISTENSEN, E., R. D. RABBITT & M. I. MILLER. 1994. 3D brain mapping using a deformable neuroanatomy. Phy. Med. Bio.: 39.
9. CLARK, C. M., C. AMMANN, W. R. MARTIN, P. TY & M. R. HAYDEN. 1991. The FDG/PET methodology for early detection of disease onset: A statistical model. J. Cereb. Blood Flow Metab. **11**(2): A96–102.
10. DAMASIO, H., R. O. KULJIS, W. YUH & J. EHRHARDT. 1991. Magnetic resonance imaging of human intracortical structure *in vivo.* Cereb. Cortex **1**(5): 374–379.
11. EVANS, A., S. MARRET, J. TORRESCORZO, S. KU & L. COLLINS. 1991. MRI-PET correlation in three dimensions using a volume of interest (VOI) atlas. J. Cereb. Blood Flow Metab. **11:** 169–178.
12. EVANS, A. C., W. DAI, L. COLLINS, P. NEELIN & S. MARRETT. 1991. Warping of a computerized 3D atlas to match brain image volumes for quantitative neuroanatomical and functional analysis. Proc. Int. Soc. Opt. Eng. (SPIE): Med. Imag. III: 264–274.
13. EVANS, A. C., D. L. COLLINS & B. MILNER. 1992. An MRI-based stereotactic brain atlas from 300 young normal subjects. Soc. Neuroscience Abs. **22:** 408.
14. EVANS, C., M. KAMBER, D. L. COLLINS & D. MACDONALD. 1994. An MRI-based probabilistic atlas of neuroanatomy. *In* Magnetic Resonance Scanning and Epilepsy. S. D. Shorvon *et al.,* Eds. : 263–274. Plenum. New York, NY.
15. FOX, P. T. & J. L. LANCASTER. 1994. Neuroscience on the net. Science **266**(11): 994–996.
16. FRISTON, K. J., C. D. FRITH, P. F. LIDDLE & R. S. J. FRACKOWIAK. 1991. Plastic transformation of PET images. J. Comp. Assist. Tomogr. **15**(4): 634–639.
17. GALABURDA, A., M. LE MAY, T. KEMPER & N. GESHWIND. 1978. Right-left asymmetries in the brain. Structural differences between the hemispheres may underlie cerebral dominance. Science **199:** 852–856.
18. GESHWIND, N. & W. LEVITSKY. 1968. Human brain: left-right asymmetries in the temporal speech areas. Science **161:** 186–187.
19. GREITZ, T., C. BOHM, S. HOLTE & L. ERIKSSON. 1991. A computerized brain atlas: construction, anatomical content and some applications. J. Comp. Assist. Tomogr. **15**(1): 26–38.
20. HO, P., S. YU, L. CZERVIONKE, L. SETHER, M. WAGNER, P. PECH & V. HAUGHTON. 1988. MR and cryomicrotomy of C1 and C2 roots. Am. J. Neurol. Radiol. **9:** 829–831.
21. LE MAY, M. & D. K. KIDO. 1978. Asymmetries of the cerebral hemispheres on computed tomograms. J. Comp. Assist. Tomogr. **2**(4): 471–476.
22. LEHMANN, E. D., D. HAWKES, D. HIL, C. BIRD, G. ROBINSON, A. COLCHESTER & M. MAISLEY. 1991. Computer aided interpretation of SPECT images of the brain using an MRI derived neuroanatomic atlas. Med. Inf. **16:** 151–166.

23. MANSOUR, A., C. A. FOX, H. AKIL & S. J. WATSON. 1995. Opioid-receptor mRNA expression in the rat CNS: Anatomical and functional implications. TINS **18**(1): 22–29.
24. MATSUI, T. & A. HIRANO. 1978. An Atlas of the Human Brain for Computerized Tomography. Igako-Shoin. New York, NY.
25. MAZZIOTTA, J. C., A. W. TOGA, A. EVANS, P. FOX & J. LANCASTER. 1995. A probabilistic atlas of the human brain: Theory and rationale for its development. NeuroImage **2:** 89–101.
26. PAXINOS, G. & C. WATSON. 1986. The Rat Brain in Stereotaxic Coordinates, 2nd ed. Academic Press. Sydney.
27. PECH, P. 1987. Correlative investigations of craniospinal anatomy and pathology with computed tomography, magnetic resonance imaging, and cryomicrotomy. Uppsala University, Sweden.
28. RADEMACHER, J., A. M. GALABURDA, D. N. KENNEDY, P. A. FILIPEK & V. S. CAVINESS. 1992. Human cerebral cortex: Localization, parcellation and morphometry with magnetic resonance imaging. J. Cognitive Neurosci. **4**(4): 352–374.
29. RAUSCHNING, W., K. BERGSTROM & P. PECH. 1983. Correlative craniospinal anatomy studies by computed tomography and cryomicrotomy. J. Comput. Assist. Tomogr. **7**(1): 9–13.
30. RAUSCHNING, W. 1986. Surface cryoplaning. A technique for clinical anatomical correlations. Uppsala J. Med. Sci. **91:** 251–255.
31. ROLAND, P. & K. ZILLES. 1994. Brain atlases—a new research tool. TINS **17**(11): 458–467.
32. SCHALTENBRAND, G. & W. WAHREN. 1977. Atlas for stereotaxy of the human brain. Yearbook Medical Publishers. Chicago.
33. STEINMETZ, H., A. HERZOG, G. SCHLAUG, Y. HUANG, & L. JANCKE. 1995. Brain (a) symmetry in monozygotic twins. Cereb. Cortex **5:** 296–300.
34. STEINMETZ, H., J. VOLKMAN, L. JANCKE & H. FREUND. 1991. Anatomical left-right asymmetry of language-related temporal cortex is different in left and right handers. Ann. Neurol. **29:** 315–319.
35. TALAIRACH, J. & P. TOURNOUX. 1988. Co-planar Stereotaxic Atlas of the Human Brain. Thieme Medical Publishers. New York, NY.
36. TALAIRACH, J., M. DAVID, P. TOURNOUX, H. CORREDOR & T. KVASINA. 1957. Atlas d'Anatomie Stereotaxique: Reperage Radiologique Indirect des Noyaux Gris Centraux des Regions Mesecephalo-sous-optique et Hypothalamique de l'Homme. Masson Paris.
37. THOMPSON, P. & A. W. TOGA. 1996. A surface-based technique for warping 3-dimensional images of the brain. IEEE Trans. Med. Imag. **15**(4): 402–417.
38. THOMPSON, P. M., C. SCHWARTZ & A. W. TOGA. 1996. High-resolution random mesh algorithms for creating a probabilistic 3D surface atlas of the human brain. NeuroImage. **3:** 19–34.
39. THOMPSON, P., C. SCHWARTZ, R. T. LIN, A. A. KHAN & A. W. TOGA. 1996. 3D statistical analysis of sulcal variability in the human brain. J. Neurosci. **16**(13): 4261–4274.
40. TIEDE, U., M. BOMANS, K. H. HOHNE, A. POMMERT, M. RIEMER, T. SCHIEMANN, R. SCHUBERT & W. LIERSE. 1993. A computerized three-dimensional atlas of the human skull and brain. Am. J. Neurol Radiol. **14**(3): 551–559.
41. TOGA, A. W., K. AMBACH, B. QUINN, M. HUTCHIN & J. S. BURTON. 1994. Postmortem anatomy from cryosectioned whole human brain. J. Neurosci. Meth. **54**(2): 239–252.
42. SANTORI, E. M. & A. W. TOGA. 1994. Superpositioning of three dimensional neuroanatomic data sets. J. Neurosci. Meth. **50:** 187–196.
43. TOGA, A. W. 1991. A digital three-dimensional atlas of structure/function relationships. J. Chem. Neuroanat. **4**(5): 313–318.
44. TOGA, A. W., P. BANERJEE & B. A. PAYNE. 1991. Brain warping and averaging (abst.). Presented at the International Symposium on Cerebral Blood Flow and Metabolism, Miami, Florida. J. Cereb. Blood Flow Metab. **11:** S560.
45. TOGA, A. W., P. K. BANERJEE & E. M. SANTORI. 1990. Warping 3D models for interbrain comparisons. Neurosci. Abs. **16:** 247.
46. TOGA, A. W., B. A. PAYNE & E. M. SANTORI. 1989. Mapping brain function on 3D anatomic models. Presented at the International Symposium on Cerebral Blood Flow and Metabolism, Bologna, Italy J. Cereb. Blood Flow Metab. S243.
47. VAN BUREN, J. M. & D. A. MACCUBIN. 1962. An outline atlas of human basal ganglia and estimation of anatomic variants. J. Neurosurg. **19:** 811–839.

48. WADA, J., R. CLARKE & A. HAMM. 1975. Cerebral hemispheric asymmetry in humans. Arch. Neurol. **32:** 239–246.
49. WILSON, M. W. & J. M. MOUNTZ. 1989. A reference system for neuroanatomical localization on functional reconstructed cerebral images. J. Comp. Assist. Tomogr. **13**(1): 174–178.
50. MEGA, M. S., T. J. KARACA, N. POURATAIN, S. CHEN, C. F. ADAMSON, S. SCHLUENDER & A. W. TOGA. 1995. Premortem-postmortem neuroimaging: A study of brain morphometric changes in man with MRI and cryomacrotome imaging. Soc. Neurosci. Abs. **21:** 154.

Classical and Contemporary Histochemical Approaches for Evaluating Central Nervous System Microanatomy

NATHAN M. APPEL[a]

Division of Applied Pharmacology Research
Office of Testing and Research
Center for Drug Evaluation and Research
Food and Drug Administration
Laurel, Maryland 20708-2476

Laboratory of Neurosciences
National Institute on Aging
National Institutes of Health
10 Center Drive, MSC 1582
Bethesda, Maryland 20892-1582

The gain in brain lies mainly in the stain.
—F. E. BLOOM

INTRODUCTION

For more than a century investigators have been treating brain specimens with chemicals to study its microanatomy, that is, to render visible what is typically invisible (FIG. 1A). In this manner, it has been possible to characterize the different cell types that constitute brain with respect to their cytoarchitecture, organization, and, in some cases, chemical identity. The same techniques are used by pathologists to study adverse effects on brain structure of chemicals, trauma, and disease. In this article I will describe some of the methods used to study the fine structure of the central nervous system (brain and spinal cord) at the light-microscopic level. Information gathered using these neuroanatomical techniques forms the foundation upon which results gathered using emerging technologies to monitor brain structure and function have been validated and interpreted.

The study of anatomy through the microscope is called histology. Histologists consider the minute structure, composition, and function of tissues. Histology encompasses two broad and overlapping disciplines: histochemistry and cytochemistry. Histochemistry focuses on the identification of chemi-

[a]Address for correspondence: FDA Mod 1 Laboratory Facility, 8301 Muirkirk Road, Room 3416, Laurel, Maryland 20708-2476. Phone: (301)594-5027; fax: (301)594-3037; e-mail: appeln@cder.fda.gov

cal components of cells and tissues. It is accomplished using chemicals, dyes and stains which bind to or react with tissue sections so that the final reaction product is visible. Cytochemistry focuses on the locations, structural relationships, and interactions of cellular constituents by means of methods such as electron microscopy, cell fractionation, and immunochemical techniques. A number of the techniques employed by histologists to examine brain fine structure at the light microscopic level are listed alphabetically in TABLE 1. In the following sections some of these techniques are described.

TINCTORIAL STAINING

The most common approach used to study brain histology is tinctorial staining, that is, using dyes. Structures or cytoplasm become stained (dyed) by reacting chemically with the stain, usually as a function of pH. The color of a particular stain or dye is dependent on the presence of certain chemical moieties called chromophores (color bearers). Their fastness, or permanency, is a consequence of other chemical moieties called auxochromes. Stains can be either acids and bases, thereby giving rise to acidic or basic dyes. Chemically, the resultant color is due to the electronic structure and conjugate unsaturated bonding of the dye molecule. The color property of a basic dye is located in its positive-charged ion and for an acid dye in its negative ion. Neutral dyes are produced by mixing acid and basic dye solutions together, the resultant color being a consequence of both the positive and negative moieties. Some dyes have poor staining qualities, but react with heavy metals to form complex structures or coordinate structures. They are called mordants or lakes. The resulting solutions are intensely colored.[1,2]

Probably the most common staining technique employed by pathologists utilizes hematoxylin and eosin (H&E). Hematoxylin is a mordant. On its own, hematoxylin is colorless. It oxidizes to hematein and reacts in the solution with heavy metals, such as aluminum, chromium or iron, to become visible and stains basophilic structures, such as chromatin, blue. Eosin, an acid dye, is tetrabromofluorescein disodium salt. Its color resides in its negative ion. It is used as a counterstain with hematoxylin because it stains cytoplasm pink (FIG. 1C).[3] Hematoxylin stains are useful for detecting neuronal loss. A well-trained pathologist can detect neurotoxicity or disease by closely examining H&E-stained brain sections for subtle changes, but such effects may not be seen at low magnification, making the process time-consuming. For the neuroanatomist, however, H&E-staining is less useful because it provides scant information for resolving brain pathways, that is, where a particular neuron projects to or receives afferents from.[4,5]

Nissl staining has become a generic term to describe tinctorial staining protocols that cause the Nissl substance to become visible. Nissl substance, of which Franz Nissl (1860–1919) was the eponym, is basophilic material in neuronal cytoplasm composed of rough endoplasmic reticulum and polyribosomes.[6] Thus Nissl stains are basic dyes whose color properties are expressed

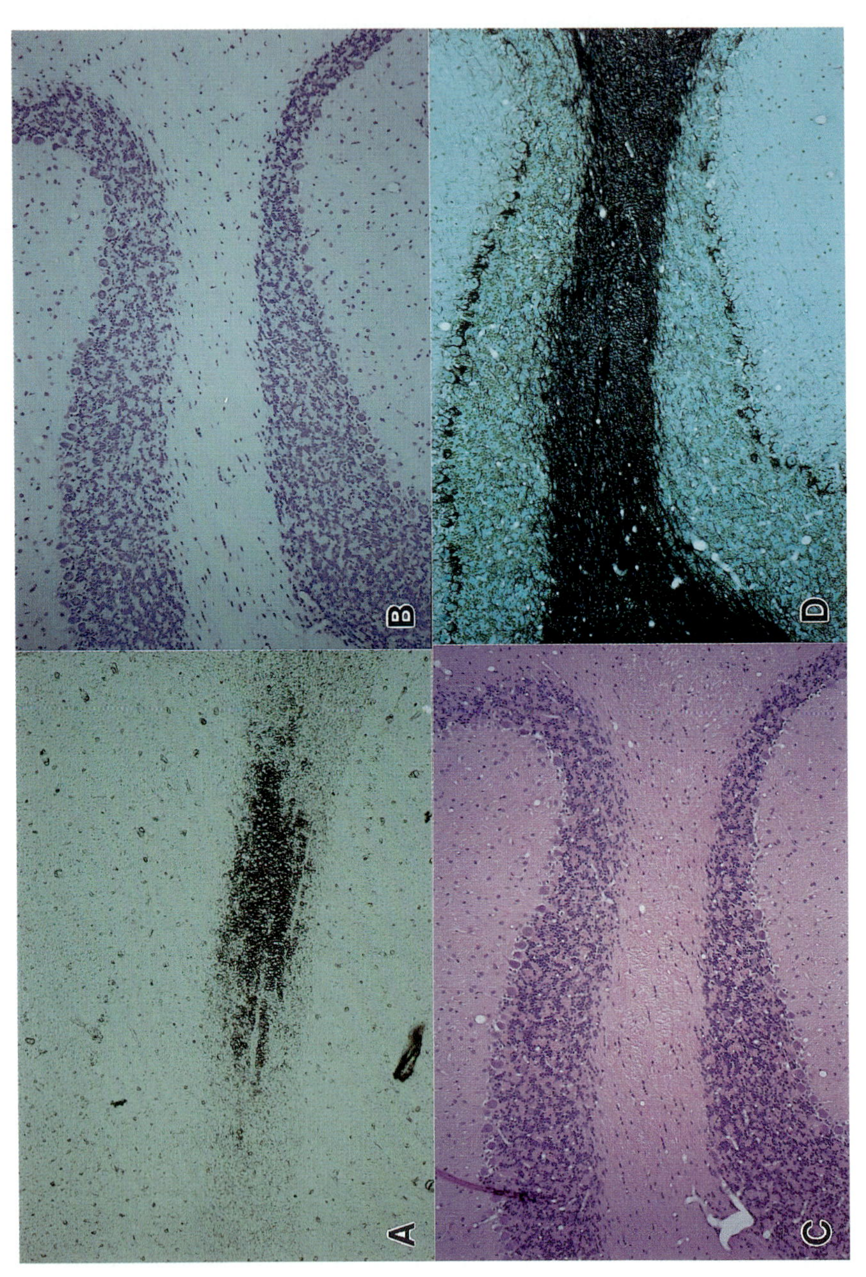

FIGURE 1

TABLE 1. Techniques Used to Study Fine Structure of the Brain at the Light-Microscopic Level

• Enzyme histochemistry	•Lectin histochemistry
• Glia stains	•Receptor localization
• Histofluorescence	•"Special" stains
• Impregnation staining	•Tinctorial staining
• Immunohistochemistry	•Tract-tracing:
• *In situ* hybridization histochemistry	*in vivo*
	in vitro
	transsynaptic

in their positive ions. Examples of Nissl stains are thionin, cresyl violet, neutral red, and toluidine blue.[1,2] Such stains are especially useful to the anatomist for recognizing patterns or the organization of groups of neurons or brain nuclei (FIGS. 1B and 3A). Nissl stains are also useful because the appearance of Nissl substance conveys information about the state of the neuron. The appearance of Nissl substance changes with injury. Chromatolysis, pallor due to loss of Nissl substance, is a response of neuronal somas to damage in their axons. The Nissl reaction refers to a series of stereotyped morphological changes in the soma after injury and, if it occurs, during recovery. Thus, over time one can see chromatolysis and swelling followed by reappearance of Nissl substance in a brain nucleus after peripheral nerve injury. Anatomists use the Nissl reaction to map brain pathways by relating reaction sites to carefully placed distal lesions.[4,7,8]

In addition to staining Nissl substance and chromatin, one can also apply tinctorial techniques to stain nerve processes. Since myelin is an integral component of many neurons, it is a convenient target for staining. By staining myelin, nerve tracts can be revealed. At higher magnification and with "opportunistic" oblique sections through neurons, patterns of nerve processes are also revealed. Moreover, as with Nissl substance, the appearance of myelin (myelinopathy, demyelination) can be used to detect toxic effects of substances and disease. Specific myelin staining protocols have been devel-

FIGURE 1. Series of coronal sections through rat cerebellum. Compare the levels of detail rendered by the different methods. (**A**) Unstained section. The only details visible are a product of the light-refracting characteristics of the tissue. (**B**) Section stained with toluidine blue to reveal Nissl substance. The Nissl substance is basophilic so it is stained blue by the basic toluidine blue dye. The cytoplasm is barely stained. The resultant high contrast makes Nissl staining the method of choice for localizing lesions and mapping brain nuclei. (**C**) Section stained with hematoxylin and eosin. Chromatin is stained blue by the hematoxylin and the cytoplasm pink by the eosin. At higher magnification a pathologist might look for cytoplasmic inclusions and detect injury due to disease, trauma, toxins, or ischemia.[4] (**D**) Section stained using a Bielschowsky stain in combination with Luxol fast blue. The Bielschowsky technique is a silver impregnation method that stains argyrophilic structures. Here the stain reveals the abundant neurofibrils in the axons that make up the cerebellar white matter. In this preparation the Luxol fast blue, which stains myelin, is used as a counterstain.

oped using hematoxylin or Luxol fast blue. Luxol fast blue to stain myelin is often used in combination with cresyl violet to stain Nissl substance so that fiber tracts and neuronal somata are revealed simultaneously.[5,9,10] Standard H&E staining protocols do not reveal the myelin sheaths of fiber tracts well.

IMPREGNATION STAINING

A different approach to studying organization in the nervous system is impregnation or neurofibrillary staining. Neurons are argyrophilic, that is, "silver loving." This property has been exploited to reveal their fine structure. The technique was introduced at the turn of this century by Bielschowsky and Ramón y Cajal.[11,12] Subsequently many other protocols have been developed.[13,14] Essentially, pieces of brain are immersed in silver nitrate–containing solutions. The silver penetrates, or impregnates, the neurons. It is then chemically or physically reduced, making it appear black and revealing the fine structure of the cells the silver has impregnated. The result is striking, but the methodology is nonselective in that it does not differentiate between normal and degenerating fibers. Moreover, with the earliest protocols there could be so much staining that it was difficult to achieve resolution allowing the stained cells to be differentiated from each other. With refinements of the technique, it became possible to stain only a fraction of material (about 10%). Moreover, the silver staining could be maintained in the presence of tinctorial counterstains such as Luxol fast blue to show myelin. Thus, cellular organization and fiber architecture could be revealed simultaneously with fiber tracts and pathways (FIG. 1D).

An important refinement of the impregnation staining approach was the so-called suppressive methodology introduced by Nauta and Gygax.[15] With this technique, and subsequent refinements by others, staining of normal somata and axons is suppressed so that only degenerating axons are rendered argyrophilic and thereby selectively made visible (FIG. 2). Timing of staining with respect to the insult is crucial, however, because different nerve pathways degenerate at different rates. In addition, not all nerve pathways are amenable to detection using argyrophilic methods. The most important caveat, however, when using suppressive techniques to detect dead or dying neurons is to remember that absence of staining cannot be construed as absence of damage. Nevertheless, this approach opened the door for many elegant studies which trace neuronal pathways in a manner analogous to those using the Nissl reaction. That is, carefully placed chemical, electrical or surgical lesions were used to induce argyrophilia and correlate the reaction sites with the lesions.[16]

ENZYME HISTOCHEMISTRY

Another way to appreciate the structure of the brain is to consider its "chemical neuroanatomy," that is, to recognize its structure and organization

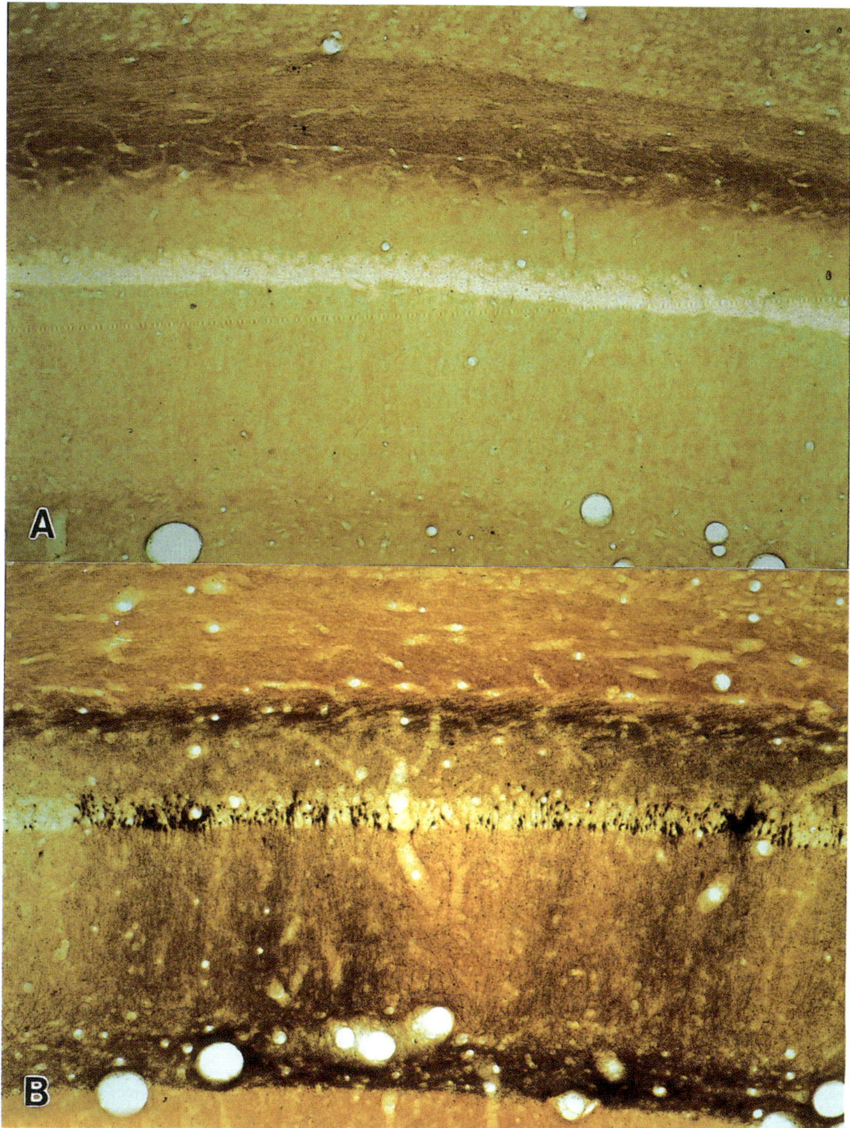

FIGURE 2. Suppressive staining. Coronal sections through rat hippocampus stained using a cupric silver impregnation method.[49] **(A)** CA2 region sampled from the hippocampus of a control rat. There is no staining because the method stains only degenerating neurons; that is, staining in normal tissue is suppressed. **(B)** CA2 region from the hippocampus of a rat treated with domoic acid, a neurotoxin. The degenerating neuronal somata and processes are argyrophilic and so are stained black.

by the "chemicals" individual neurons or populations of neurons make. One way to accomplish this is by detecting enzymes contained in neurons; and one of the methods to detect enzymes in tissues is using enzyme histochemistry. In enzyme histochemistry, one essentially performs an enzyme assay on the tissue and visualizes the reaction product *in situ*. To do this the investigator provides a substrate for the enzyme of interest that results in a visible reaction product. For the results to be meaningful diffusion must be kept to a minimum, that is, the reaction product must remain close to the actual location of the enzyme. Beyond its utility as a mapping tool, enzyme histochemistry is a sensitive diagnostic tool. It can be used to provide a "snapshot" of the functional state of the neurons. Moreover, since the organelles that make certain enzymes are known, changes in enzymatic activity will be indicative of physiological or toxicological effects on those structures in general, and on their metabolic pathways in particular.[17]

A number of enzymes have been localized in brain using histochemical techniques. They include: cytochrome C oxidase; succinate dehydrogenase; γ-aminobutyric acid transaminase; nicotinamide adenine dinucleotide-linked glutamate, isocitrate and malate dehydrogenases; acetylcholinesterase; reduced nicotinamide adenine dinucleotide phosphate diaphorase (nitric oxide synthase or NOS); and alkaline phosphatase.[17,18] For instance, acetylcholine is a major brain neurotransmitter and acetylcholinesterase enzyme terminates acetylcholine activity in cholinergic synapses. Changes in brain acetylcholinesterase enzyme activity occur following exposure to organophosphate and carbamate insecticides or certain nerve gasses.[17] For mapping purposes, localization of acetylcholinesterase enzyme is useful for delineating nuclei and fiber tracts not visible with Nissl staining. In fact, alternating sections stained for Nissl substance and acetylcholinesterase is the basis for a popular rat brain atlas.[19] Acetylcholinesterase is identified in brain by detecting the product of the enzyme's acting on the substrate S-acetylthiolcholine with ethopropazine and sodium sulfide as indicators.[20,21]

HISTOFLUORESCENCE

Studies attempting to understand brain neurochemistry lead to a novel histochemical approach. The technique of histofluorescence histochemistry takes advantage of the property of primary amines, such as dopamine, norepinephrine, serotonin (5-hydroxytryptamine) and histamine, to form fluorescent condensation products with formaldehyde. In this technique sections of freeze-dried nervous tissue are exposed to hot formaldehyde gas generated from solid paraformaldehyde. The treated sections are then examined under a fluorescence microscope at near-ultraviolet excitation (410 nm). Dopamine and norepinephrine form 3,4-dihydroisoquinoline condensation products, which fluoresce green (480 nm). Serotonin forms a 3,4-dihydrocarboline that fluoresces yellow (525 nm).[22,23] By means of this approach the chemical neuroanatomy and pharmacology of brain monoaminergic neurons were first revealed.[24,25]

IMMUNOHISTOCHEMISTRY

Yet another way to examine the chemical neuroanatomy of the brain is by using immunohistochemistry, which employs the principles of immunology to make visible antigens of interest in tissue or cell preparations. This is accomplished by exploiting the binding of specific antibodies to antigens of interest and subsequently detecting that interaction. In the nervous system, immunohistochemistry has been used to identify, localize and map neurotransmitters, biosynthetic and degradative enzymes for neurotransmitters, neurotransmitter receptors, ion channels, growth factors, intracellular organelles, cytoskeleton constituents, and various products of nervous tissue gene expression the function of which remain yet unknown—true chemical neuroanatomy. Theoretically, the only requirements for using immunohistochemistry to detect an antigen in nervous tissue is the availability of a specific antibody directed against the antigen of interest and a reliable means of detecting the resulting antibody–antigen complex in tissue.[26]

Most immunohistochemistry is performed using *indirect* immunohistochemical techniques.[27–29] In this methodology an unlabeled antibody (primary antibody) is allowed to react with tissues to form an antibody–antigen complex with a tissue-bound antigen. The bound primary antibody then serves as antigen for other antibodies (secondary antibodies) which are used to detect the primary antibody. Secondary antibodies may be labeled with indicator molecules or they too may be unlabeled and instead function as an "antigenic bridge" for additional indicator-labeled antibodies applied subsequently (FIG. 3B). A list of commonly used indicator molecules for immunohistochemical study is presented in TABLE 2. Usually the antigen detected by secondary antibodies is a species-specific region (epitope) on the primary antibody. For example, if an anti-serotonin antibody is used that was raised in a rabbit ("rabbit anti-serotonin"), a secondary antibody used to detect it *could* be a goat anti-rabbit antibody. The necessity for appropriate controls to rule out false-positive and false-negative staining cannot be overemphasized.[30–32]

Immunohistochemistry may well be the most powerful tool for studying brain chemical neuroanatomy since theoretically one can raise an antibody to almost any antigen of interest. Moreover, it is extremely versatile. For example, since secondary antibodies are usually directed against a species-specific epitope of the primary antibody one can theoretically apply to tissue a "cocktail" of two or more primary antibodies which are directed against different antigens if they have been raised in different host species. The resultant primary antibody–tissue antigen complexes can then be visualized with different detection systems or, in the case of fluorescence immunohistochemistry, fluorescent secondary antibodies with optically resolvable fluorophores.[30,31] This is the basis of simultaneous immunohistochemical detection

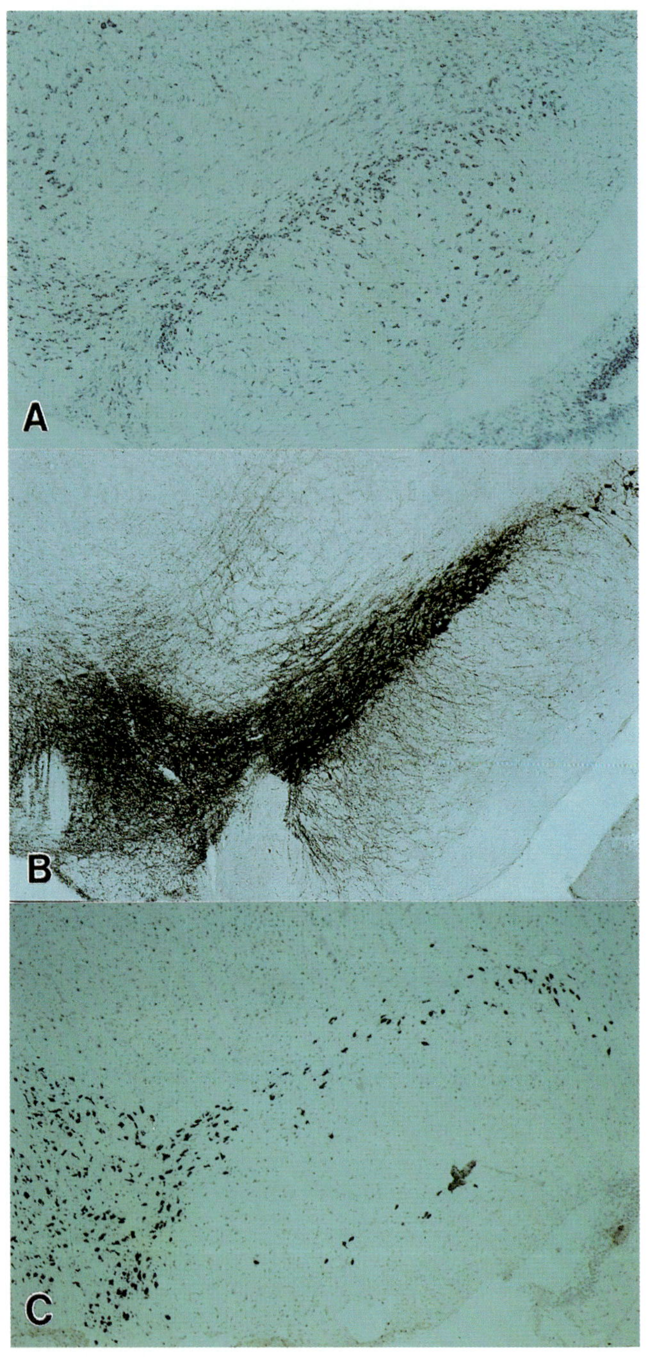

FIGURE 3

TABLE 2. Indicator Molecules That Can Be Associated with Antibodies and Used in Immunohistochemical Detection Systems[26]

Fluorescent molecules
Coumarin derivatives (fluoresce blue with ultraviolet illumination)
Fluorescein derivatives (fluoresce green with blue illumination)
Phycocyanin derivatives (fluoresce red with green illumination)
Phycoerythrin derivatives (fluoresce yellow–orange with blue illumination)
Rhodamine derivatives (fluoresce red with green illumination)
Granular/particulate substances
Alkaline phosphatase enzyme (color depends on substrate chromagen used)
Colloidal gold (black when enhanced with silver)
Ferritin particles (black)
Glucose oxidase enzyme (color depends on substrate chromagen used)
Peroxidase enzyme (color depends on substrate chromagen used)
Radioisotopes
[^{125}]Iodine (black grains of reduced photosensitive silver)
Tritium (black grains of reduced photosensitive silver)

of multiple antigens. In theory the only constraints limiting how many antigens one can detect in a single tissue section are the availability of (1) specific primary antibodies raised in different species, (2) species-specific secondary antibodies to bind each primary antibody individually, (3) truly resolvable indicator molecules to demarcate resulting antibody complexes in tissue, and (4) the imagination of the investigator.[26] Immunohistochemical studies can also be performed quantitatively.[33] In addition, immunohistochemistry can be used in combination with anatomical tract-tracing techniques to allow identification of antigens of interest in structures whose cell bodies of origin or whose projections are unequivocally known (read below).

TRACT-TRACING

Another way to identify neuronal pathways in brain is to take advantage of the fact that neurons can transport substances down their length. If transport

FIGURE 3. Chemical neuroanatomy. Coronal sections through rat substantia nigra. **(A)** Nissl staining with thionin to demonstrate the cellular organization of the substantia nigra. **(B)** Tyrosine hydroxylase–like immunoreactivity revealed using peroxidase anti-peroxidase immunohistochemistry. Tyrosine hydroxylase enzyme catalyzes the rate-limiting step of catecholamine biosynthesis. Somata as well as processes are stained because the enzyme is transported from the soma, where it is synthesized, to axon terminals of catecholaminergic neurons. (Specimen courtesy of Dr. Jan Johannessen, FDA.) **(C)** *In situ* hybridization histochemistry using a digoxegenin-labeled cRNA probe for tyrosine hydroxylase mRNA. Neurons expressing the message of the tyrosine hydroxylase gene (they are presumably dopaminergic) are stained deep blue. These cells should stain for tyrosine hydroxylase-like immunoreactivity in their somata and processes as in **(B)**. Compare also with **(A)** to see that not all cell bodies in the field express this gene message. (Specimen courtesy of Dr. Barbara Wilcox, FDA).

occurs from soma to axon it is called anterograde transport; from axon to soma it is retrograde. A number of substances have been used as tracers, including fluorescent dyes, fluorescent beads, fluorescent dextrans, horseradish peroxidase enzyme, India ink, lectins, toxins, and even viruses. Tract-tracers can be applied *in vitro* in a number of ways and then be detected in tissue sections after animals have been sacrificed. For example, they can be applied to the cut stump of a nerve, pressure-injected into a site of interest, or administered by iontophoresis. Different retrograde tracers can be used simultaneously to determine whether different neurons in a circumscribed region project to more than one distant site. Similarly anterograde and retrograde tracers can be used simultaneously. Moreover (retrograde or anterograde) tract-tracers can be used in combination with immunohistochemical studies to reveal the neurochemical identity of afferents to identified neurons.[34–39]

A novel development in tract-tracing technology is the use of live viruses. A "tracer" virus, such as swine *Herpes simplex* type 1, is applied (inoculated) to the distal end of a pathway under consideration. It replicates, and the virus particles are retrogradely transported to the soma of the inoculated pathway, where they continue to replicate and infect apposing nerve processes. The virus is then detected by immunohistochemical techniques. In this manner second- and third-order neurons in a particular nerve circuit can be identified.[40,41]

Tract-tracing can also be performed *in vitro* in autopsy specimens using fluorescent lipophilic carbocyanine and aminostyryl dyes. These dyes are incorporated into the outer layer of plasma membranes, diffuse laterally within neurons and yield detailed images of neurons and their fine projections.[42,43]

RECEPTOR LOCALIZATION

A different approach to mapping and understanding chemical neuroanatomy is to map neurotransmitter receptors or binding sites, that is, the neuroanatomical targets of action of neurotransmitters. To date, the most-utilized method for localizing neurotransmitter receptors in brain has been receptor autoradiography. This technique is, in essence, an extension of a pharmacological receptor binding assay. In this method, tissues are exposed *in vivo* or *in vitro* to a radioisotope-labeled neurotransmitter or drug which is specifically bound to the receptor of interest. Autoradiographs depicting the distribution of radiolabeled receptors are subsequently generated by exposing isotope-sensitive film or photographic emulsion to the radiolabeled tissues. Using computer-assisted densitometry receptor densities can be easily quantitated. This technique does suffer some deficiencies: Most notably the anatomical resolution possible with autoradiographic methods is limited. Thus, while it is possible to localize receptors to neuronal somata with autoradiography it is difficult to determine whether receptors are localized on cell processes (axons and dendrites) with this technique. Consequently receptor autoradiography in and of itself cannot be used to distinguish between presynaptic and postsynaptic receptors. In addition, determining the neurochemical identity of receptor-bearing structures in conjunction with receptor autoradiography is technically difficult. Moreover, many ligands used to localize receptors bind to more than one receptor site.[44,45]

Recently, advances in cell biology, biochemistry, and genetics have made it possible to extract homogeneous fractions of receptor protein from tissues and to clone, sequence, and express genes for various neurotransmitter and hormone receptors. Such materials have been used as antigens to raise antibodies to individual receptors or portions of receptor molecules. Receptor binding patterns are then mapped by means of immunohistochemical techniques. By using simultaneous techniques to allow identification of neurotransmitters and their receptors and/or combining appropriate tract-tracing protocols, it is possible to obtain detailed neurochemical maps of the brain. There is, however, a major advantage of autoradiographic approaches when compared to immunohistochemical approaches for localizing receptors and drug binding sites. It is much easier to perform quantitative autoradiography than quantitative immunohistochemistry.[26]

IN SITU HYBRIDIZATION HISTOCHEMISTRY

Another way to map brain is by gene expression. This is accomplished using *in situ* hybridization histochemistry. Through this method the distribution and the degree of expression of a particular nucleic acid sequence is studied. The technique is, in essence, the application of a method from molecular biology to answer neuroanatomy and neurochemistry questions. Its theoretical basis is the dissociation–reassociation kinetics of DNA and RNA in solution. One prepares, buys, or receives as a gift single- or double-stranded DNA or single-stranded RNA complementary to the mRNA of interest. They are used as probes to locate the mRNA of interest by hybridizing to it. The probe nucleotide is tagged with a molecule that can be visualized such as fluorescent dyes, antigens that can be bound by labeled antibodies, or radioisotopes that can be detected by autoradiography. The resultant pattern of labeling reflects the pattern of cells expressing the gene, i.e., making protein (FIG. 3C). Changes in gene expression, as reflected in the distribution or density of hybridization, also provide information about how and which populations of neurons respond to drug treatments or hormone stimulation or if they have sustained an adverse effect. The technique is extremely versatile in that it can be combined with immunohistochemical techniques and tract-tracing. This combination approach can offer the investigator simultaneous access to the chemical and functional anatomy of the nervous system by taking advantage of the ability of immunohistochemistry and tract-tracing to provide localization and knowledge of gross changes in neurotransmitter or marker molecules, their release, and uptake, and of *in situ* hybridization histochemistry to provide quantitative data from which biosynthetic activity of relevant molecules can be inferred.[46–48]

CONCLUSION

Classical and contemporary histochemical techniques have helped to define the underlying structure of the central nervous system. It is in light of those findings that all other brain images are interpreted. The emergence of sophisticated imaging technologies will likely contribute greatly towards further clarification of the intricacies of neuronal form and function, as well as knowledge of the effects of trauma, toxins, and disease in the nervous system. Be that as it may, histochemical techniques will also continue to provide meaningful information even as newer technologies emerge for imaging brain structure and function.

ACKNOWLEDGMENTS

I thank my friends and colleagues Drs. Danny A. Brass, Jan N. Johannessen, Martin W. Wessendorf, and Barbara J. Wilcox for their assistance and contributions.

REFERENCES

1. HECHT, B. P. 1983. Dye Powders for Biological Staining No. 103. Rowley Biochemical Institute. Rowley, MA.
2. LILLIE, R. D. 1977. H. J. Conn's Biological Stains, 9th ed. Williams & Wilkins. Baltimore, MD.
3. LILLIE, R. D. 1965. Histopathologic Technique and Practical Histochemistry, 3rd ed. McGraw Hill. New York, NY.
4. JENSEN, K. F. 1995. Neuroanatomical techniques for labeling neurons and their utility in neurotoxicology. *In* Neurotoxicology: Approaches and Methods. L. W. Chang & W. Slikker, Jr., Eds.: 27–66. Academic Press. San Diego, CA.
5. CHANG, L. W. 1979. A Color Atlas and Manual for Applied Histochemistry. Charles C Thomas. Springfield, IL.
6. PETERS, A., S. L. PALAY & H. D. WEBSTER. 1991. The Fine Structure of the Nervous System, 3rd edit. Oxford University Press. New York, NY.
7. BRODAL, A. 1969. Neurological Anatomy in Relation to Clinical Medicine, 2nd ed. Oxford University Press. New York, NY.
8. MCLOON, L. K. & A. LAVELLE. 1981. Dev. Brain Res. **1:** 1–47.
9. KLÜVER, H. & B. E. BARRERA. 1953. J. Neuropath. Exp. Neurol. **12:** 400–403.
10. HECHT, B. P. 1989. Dyes and Stains for Histology and Pathology. No. 101. Rowley Biochemical Institute. Rowley, MA.
11. BIELSCHOWSKY, M. 1904. J. Psychol Neurol. (Lpz.) **3:** 169–188.
12. RAMÓN Y CAJAL, S. 1904. Trav. Lab. Rech. Biol. **3:** 1–7.
13. EBBESSON, S. O. E. 1970. The selective silver-impregnation of degenerating axons and their synaptic endings in nonmammalian species. *In* Contemporary Research Methods in Neuroanatomy. W. J. H. Nauta & S. O. E. Ebbesson, Eds.: 132–161. Springer-Verlag. New York, NY.

14. BELTRAMINO, C. A., J. S. DE OLMOS, F. GALLYAS, L. HEIMER & L. ZÁBORSZKY. 1993. Assessing Neurotoxicity of Drugs of Abuse. NIDA Research Monograph 136. L. Erinoff, Ed.: 101–132. National Institute on Drug Abuse. Rockville, MD.
15. NAUTA, W. J. H. & P. A. GYGAX. 1954. Stain Technol. **29:** 91–93.
16. DE OLMOS, C. A. BELTRAMINO & S. DE OLMOS DE LORENZO. 1994. Neurotoxicol Teratol. **16:** 545–561.
17. DORMAN, D. C., M. BONNEFOI & K. T. MORGAN. 1995. Enzyme histochemical methods. *In* Neurotoxicology: Approaches and Methods. L. W. Chang & W. Slikker, Jr., Eds.: 67–79. Academic Press. San Diego, CA.
18. HUNT, R. D. 1966. Microscopic histochemical methods for the demonstration of enzymes. *In* Selected Histochemical and Histopathological Methods. S. W. Thompson & R. D. Hunt, Eds.: 616–748. Charles C Thomas. Springfield, IL.
19. PAXINOS, G. & C. WATSON. 1986. The Rat Brain in Stereotaxic Coordinates, 2nd ed. Academic Press. San Diego, CA.
20. KOELLE, G. G. & J. S. FRIEDENWALD. 1949. Proc. Soc. Exp. Biol. Med. **70:** 617–622.
21. LEWIS, P. R. 1961. Biblthca. Anat. **2:** 11–20.
22. KIERNAN, J. A. & M. BERRY. 1975. Neuroanatomical methods. *In* Methods in Brain Research. P. B. Bradley, Ed.: 1–77. John Wiley & Sons. London.
23. BJÖRKLUND, A., B. FALCK & O. LINDVALL. 1975. Microspectrofluorometric analysis of cellular monoamines after formaldehyde or glyoxylic acid condensation. *In* Methods in Brain Research. P. B. Bradley, Ed.: 249–294. John Wiley & Sons. London.
24. DAHLSTRÖM, A. & K. FUXE. 1964. Acta Physiol. Scand. **62** Suppl. 232: 1–55.
25. FUXE, K. 1965. Acta Physiol. Scand. **64** Suppl. 247: 39–85.
26. APPEL, N. M. 1993. Immunohistochemistry as a strategy for investigating the functional neuroanatomy of drug actions in the brain. *In* Imaging Drug Action in the Brain. E. D. London, Ed.: 317–336. CRC Press. Boca Raton, FL.
27. CUELLO, A. C. 1983. Immunohistochemistry (IBRO Handbook Series: Methods in Neurosciences, Vol. 3). John Wiley & Sons. Chichester, UK.
28. LARSSON, L.-I. 1988. Immunocytochemistry: Theory and Practice. CRC Press. Boca Raton, FL.
29. CUELLO, A. C. 1993. Immunohistochemistry II (IBRO Handbook Series: Methods in Neurosciences, Vol. 14). John Wiley & Sons. Chichester, UK.
30. WESSENDORF, M. W. 1990. Characterization and use of multi-color fluorescence microscopic techniques. *In* Handbook of Chemical Neuroanatomy. F. Wouterlood, F. & A. van den Pol, Eds. Vol. **8:** 1–45. Elsevier Biomedical Press. Amsterdam.
31. WESSENDORF, M. W. & R. P. ELDE. 1985. J. Histochem. Cytochem. **33:** 984–994.
32. WESSENDORF, M. W., N. M. APPEL, T. W. MOLITOR & R. P. ELDE. 1990. J. Histochem. Cytochem. **38:** 1859–1877.
33. SMOLEN, A. J. 1990. Image analytic techniques for quantification of immunohistochemical staining in the nervous system. *In* Methods in Neurosciences. Vol. 3: Quantitative and Qualitative Microscopy. P. M. Conn, Ed.: 208–229. Academic Press. San Diego, CA.
34. MESULAM, M-M. 1982. Principles of horseradish peroxidase neurohistochemistry and their applications for tracing neural pathways-axonal transport, enzyme histochemistry and light microscopic analysis. *In* Tracing Neuronal Connections with Horseradish Peroxidase. M-M. Mesulam, Ed.: 1–151. John Wiley & Sons. Chichester, UK.
35. BENTIVOGLIO, M. & S. CHEN. 1993. Retrograde neuronal tract tracing combined with immunocytochemistry. *In* Immunohistochemistry II (IBRO Handbook Series: Methods in Neurosciences, Vol. 14). A. C. Cuello, Ed.: 301–328. John Wiley & Sons. Chichester, UK.
36. SAWCHENCKO, P. E., E. T. CUNNINGHAM, JR., M. T. MORTRUD, S. W. PFEIFFER & C. R. GERFEN. 1990. *Phaseolus vulgaris* leukoagglutinin anterograde axonal transport technique. *In* Methods in Neurosciences. Vol. 3: Quantitative and Qulaitative Microscopy. P. M. Conn, Ed.: 247–260. Academic Press. San Diego, CA.
37. APPEL, N. M., M. W. WESSENDORF & R. P. ELDE. 1986. Neurosci. Lett. **65:** 241–246.
38. APPEL, N. M. & R. P. ELDE. 1988. J. Neurosci. **8:** 1767–1775.
39. WESENDORF, M. W., N. M. APPEL & R. ELDE. 1987. Neurosci. Lett. **82:** 121–126.
40. DEHAL, N. S., G. A. DEKABAN, A. V. KRASSIOUKOV, F. J. PICARD & L. C. WEAVER. 1993. Neuroscience **56:** 227–240.

41. MARTIN, X. & M. DOLIVO. 1983. Brain Res. **273:** 253–276.
42. GODEMENT, P., J. VANSELOW, S. THANOS & F. BONHOEFFER. 1987. Development **101:** 697–713.
43. HAUGLAND, R. P. 1996. Handbook of Fluorescent Probes and Research Chemicals, 6th ed.: 344– 350. Molecular Probes. Eugene, OR.
44. KUHAR, M. J., E. B. DESOUZA & J. R. UNNERSTALL. 1986. Annu. Rev. Neurosci. **9:** 27–59.
45. KUHAR, M. J. & J. R. UNNERSTALL. 1996. Receptor autoradiography. *In* Methods in Neurotransmitter Receptor Analysis. H. I. Yamamura, S. J. Enna & M. J. Kuhar, Eds.: 177–218. Raven Press. New York, NY.
46. SHAFER, M. K.-H., J. P. HERMAN & S. J. WATSON. 1993. *In situ* hybridization histochemistry. *In* Imaging Drug Action in the Brain. E. D. London, Ed.: 337–378. CRC Press. Boca Raton, FL.
47. SIMMONS, D. M., J. L. ARRIZA & L. W. SWANSON. 1989. J. Histotechnol. **12:** 169–181.
48. CHIRGWIN, J. M. 1990. Diabetes Care **13:** 188–197.
49. APPEL, N. M., S. I. RAPOPORT & J. P. O'CALLAGHAN. 1997. Synapse. In press.

DISCUSSION

ARTHUR TOGA *(UCLA School of Medicine, Los Angeles, Calif.):* Given the fact that a lot of the anatomic nomenclature has been defined historically prior to the use of the chemo-architectural visions you have shown us, do you think that a lot of the nomenclature and the way in which we catalog or describe brain is going to be influenced by these emerging and lovely ways of looking at brain?

APPEL: I don't know whether they will, but I hope so. It is very hard to sit down with the old anatomy books and the new anatomy books and then go to a meeting and know whether you are talking about the same thing as the presenter. I would like the nomenclature to evolve with the additional information we get.

QUESTION: Do you know of any work where an attempt was made to make better dye? I am thinking of the *in vitro* stain that you alluded to. Has something been made that could be used for analysis of an aldehyde-fixed postmortem tissue, which, of course, would help us understand human neuroanatomy much better.

APPEL: The dye I referred to is called Fluoro-Jade. It is a fluorescent stain used to reveal degenerating neurons and their processes. The staining technique was developed by Dr. Larry Schmued of the FDA National Center for Toxicological Research. The paper is in press in the journal *Brain Research.*

Assessment of Neurotoxicity from Potential Medications for Drug Abuse: Ibogaine Testing and Brain Imaging

FRANK J. VOCCI[a,b] AND EDYTHE D. LONDON[c]

[a]*Medications Development Division*
National Institute on Drug Abuse
Rockville, Maryland 20857

[c]*Brain Imaging Section*
Intramural Research Program
National Institute on Drug Abuse
Baltimore, Maryland 21224

The resistance of drug abuse disorders to existing therapies underscores the need for new medications for treatment. Pharmacological actions of such drugs in the central nervous system (CNS) can be assessed using technologies developed in a variety of disciplines, ranging from anatomy and biochemistry through psychology and medical physics. The development of the hallucinogen ibogaine as a potential therapeutic agent will serve to illustrate the approaches used to elucidate toxic effects in laboratory animals and the proposed assessment of analogous deficits in human subjects.

THE IBOGAINE EXAMPLE

In 1991, the Medications Development Division of the National Institute on Drug Abuse initiated a project to evaluate the toxicity of *Tabernanthe iboga* (ibogaine) as a prerequisite for clinical trials with this agent in cocaine-dependent human volunteers. Ibogaine is extracted from the roots of an *apocynaccous* shrub, which is indigenous to and used in religious rites in west central Africa, mainly Gabon and Zaire.[1] The drug acts as a stimulant at low doses and as a hallucinogen at high doses. In human subjects, the hallucinogenic threshold is approximately 300 mg.[2] Higher doses (6 to 25 mg/kg) reportedly reduced cocaine craving for periods of weeks to months.[1,3]

Preclinical studies have indicated that ibogaine reduced the self-administration of morphine (0.04 mg/kg unit dose)[4] and cocaine (0.4 mg/kg unit dose) in the rat.[5,6] The effects lasted for 24 hours or several days in some animals.[5] Some laboratories have failed to replicate the effect on self-

[b]Address for correspondence: Frank J. Vocci, Ph.D., Acting Director, Medications Development Division, NIDA, Room 11A55, 5600 Fishers Lane, Rockville, Maryland 20857. Phone: (301) 443-6173; fax: (301) 443-2599; e-mail: fv6k@nih.gov

administration of cocaine in the rat,[7] and others could not demonstrate it in the rhesus monkey.[8]

The mechanism of putative anti-addictive properties of ibogaine is unknown, as the drug interacts with several neurotransmitter systems in the CNS. Radioligand binding studies have shown that, at concentrations in the micromolar range, ibogaine binds to the phencyclidine site on the *N*-methyl-D-aspartate (NMDA) receptor complex; to *mu, kappa,* and *delta* opioid receptors;[9–12] to dopamine, norepinephrine and serotonin uptake sites;[11] and to Na^+ channels.[9] Of particular interest, however, is a possible effect of ibogaine on mesocortical and mesolimbic dopaminergic systems, as these systems have been identified as critical to the rewarding properties of drugs of abuse.[13] Cell bodies which originate in the ventral tegmental area project to the medial prefrontal cortex, nucleus accumbens, and amygdala. When administered acutely to rats, most drugs of abuse (amphetamine, cocaine, morphine, nicotine, and ethanol) increase levels of extracellular dopamine in the nucleus accumbens of the brain.[13,14] Amphetamine and cocaine also increase dopamine levels in the prefrontal cortex.[15,16]

Studies using *in vivo* microdialysis have revealed that ibogaine, given alone, increases extracellular levels of dopamine in the prefrontal cortex, but not the nucleus accumbens in rats.[17] Moreover, ibogaine influences the effects of morphine and psychomotor stimulants on extracellular dopamine levels, although the response to ibogaine in this regard is not universal. Whereas ibogaine (40 mg/kg) reduced the morphine-induced increase in extracellular dopamine[18] and blocked increases in motor activity usually produced by morphine (up to 20 mg/kg, i.p.),[19] the drug potentiated the rise in extracellular dopamine levels produced by cocaine (20 mg/kg, i.p.) or amphetamine (1.25 mg/kg, i.p.) in the rat and potentiated the motor response.[19,20]

Standard toxicology studies of ibogaine in the rat revealed that doses above 25 mg/kg produced a constellation of CNS signs, including ataxia, splayed hindlimbs, outstretched forelimbs, Straub tail, and hyperexcitability.[21] In addition to these effects on overt behavior, the drug also had remarkable cerebellar actions. Three doses of ibogaine (100 mg/kg, i.p.) enhanced the expression of glial markers, such as glial fibrillary acidic protein (GFAP), in cerebellar tissue.[22] An increase in GFAP immunoreactivity in narrow radial bands of the cerebellar vermis was likely due to activation of Bergmann glial cells. Astrocytic processes extended through the molecular and Purkinje cell layers and the outer part of the granule cell layer. Microglia labeled with cytochemical markers, such as OX42 (for the CR-3 receptor), OX6 (for the MHC II complex), and W3/25 (for the rat CD4 receptor), were activated in the cerebellar cortex of the vermis of ibogaine-treated rats, with a distribution similar to that seen with GFAP. The increase in astrocytic and microglial markers suggested Purkinje cell loss. Indeed, further work showed that a single dose of ibogaine (100 mg/kg, i.p.) produced losses in Purkinje cells, as demonstrated by the Gallyas reduced silver staining method for degenerating neurons, and reduced binding of molecular markers, such as microtubule-associated protein 2 and calbindin D_{28}.[23] An example of the characteristic neurotoxic effect of ibogaine on Purkinje cells in rat cerebellum is shown in FIGURE 1. Purkinje cells were stained with an antibody to calcium-calmodulin–dependent protein kinase II (Cam KII), a histochemical marker for this cell type in the cerebellar vermis.[23] In this instance, a single dose of 100 mg/kg ibogaine produced Cam KII-negative, parasaggital stripes, indicating neuronal loss. The pattern of damage extended through the Purkinje cell and molecular layers of the vermis and the paravermis, and longitudinal bands reflected cell loss ranging from 1 to 10 cells per band.[24]

Increases in GFAP, measured by an enzyme-linked immunosorbent assay, were noted in several brain regions of female rats after administration of oral ibogaine (25–150 mg/kg) for 14 days.[25] GFAP concentrations were elevated in the hippocampus and brain stem of rats given 25 mg/kg, and in olfactory bulb and cerebral cortex of animals treated with 150 mg/kg. A differential sensitivity to ibogaine was noted between genders, with females showing greater sensitivity.

GFAP levels also were above control values in several brain regions of female dogs following a single dose of ibogaine (100 mg/kg).[26] Involvement at several levels of the neuraxis, from the cerebral cortex to the brainstem, was inferred, suggesting a potentially more widespread phenomenon than that seen in the rat. Histopathological studies were not performed in the dog brain.

Ibogaine neurotoxicity in the rhesus monkey was evaluated following i.p. administration of 50 mg/kg every 3 to 4 hours for 12 hours.[27] Tremor, ataxia, myoclonus, and grand mal seizures were observed 5–10 min after ibogaine administration. Although activated microglia and neuronal cell loss were observed, the degree of both was small compared to that observed in rat cerebellum.

Data generated in preclinical studies are used to assess the relative safety of administration of investigational agents to human subjects. When toxicities are noted, decisions are made either not to begin a clinical study or to proceed and monitor the human subjects for possible similar adverse events. The data summarized above suggested that ibogaine could induce behavioral effects and variable neurotoxicity in rats, dogs, and monkeys. Therefore, the NIDA group designing the proposed clinical study of ibogaine was justifiably concerned about toxicity of ibogaine in the cerebellum and other regions of brain. They devised an approach for evaluating potential neurotoxicity, with baseline measurements of deficits prior to ibogaine administration constituting the initial step. The protocol proposed to evaluate several cerebellar measures, using both clinical and computer-assisted measurements of postural sway. Cognitive measures using standard and computer-driven test batteries were to be assessed at baseline and at specified intervals following a single ibogaine administration.

A related clinical example of drug-induced cerebellar degeneration has been known for almost 40 years, as cerebellar degeneration is a hallmark toxicity of chronic ethanol abuse.[28] Moreover, a recent study showed that

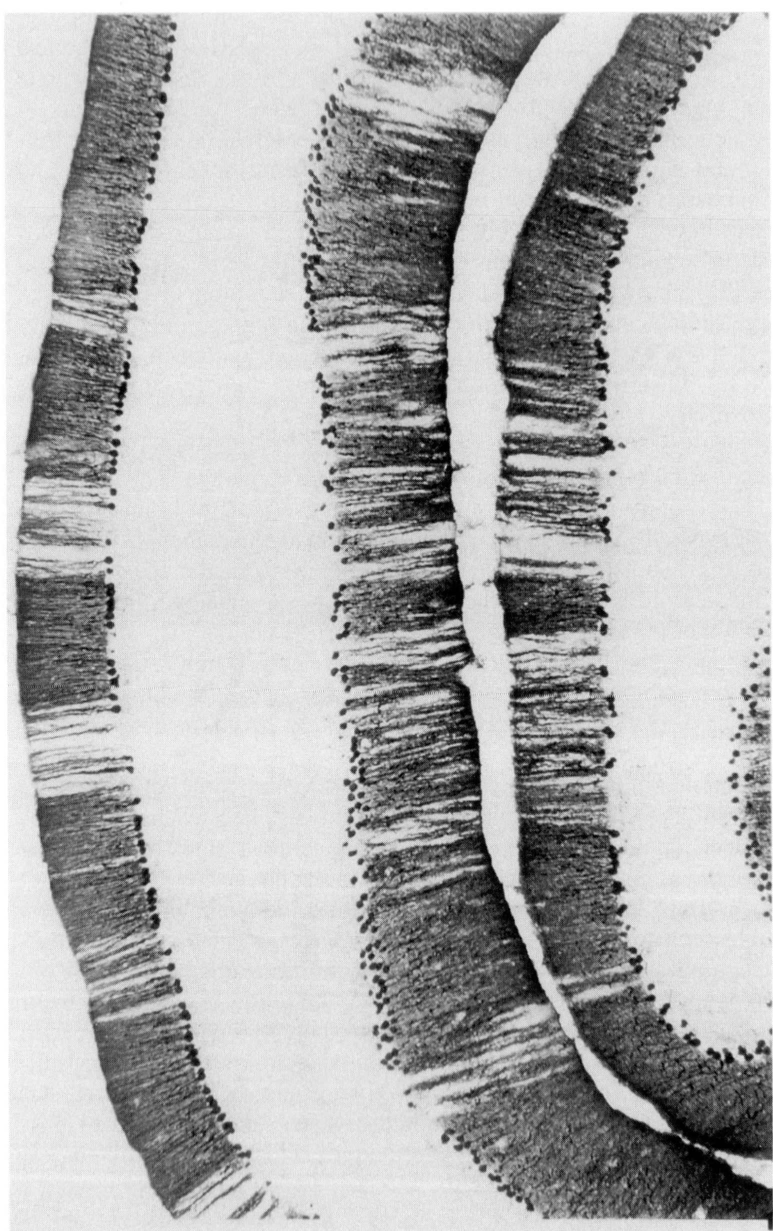

FIGURE 1. Coronal section of the cerebellum of a rat administered a single dose of ibogaine, 100 mg/kg, i.p. Purkinje cells were stained with antibodies to CAM-Kinase II. *Light areas* represent zones of Purkinje cell degeneration resulting from ibogaine treatment. Degeneration occurs in narrow bands in the saggital plane.[23]

long-term alcohol intake (41–80 grams per day for 20–30 years) produced an average loss of 33 percent of Purkinje cells in 66 subjects evaluated at autopsy.[29] Only 4.5 percent of the subjects had macroscopic signs of degeneration. In another clinical series, 78 chronic alcoholics were evaluated neurologically and via posturographic measurements on a force-measuring platform. Clinical signs of cerebellar ataxia were noted in 33 percent of the subjects whereas posturographic abnormalities were seen in 69 percent.[30] Taken together, these results suggest that Purkinje cell damage may occur in heavy drinkers/alcoholics and that posturographic measures may be a more sensitive indicator of damage than clinical examination.

IMAGING PROCEDURES TO ASSESS ACUTE AND CHRONIC TOXICITY DUE TO TREATMENT MEDICATIONS

New technologies utilized for monitoring function can be more sensitive than clinical examination for the assessment of desired or undesired effects. A variety of noninvasive imaging procedures have become available to study the structure and function of the human brain. These procedures have not been used primarily in assessments of potential untoward effects of treatment medications; however, their use in other areas of neuroscience illustrates how they can be applied in the development of new medications for the treatment of drug abuse. These techniques include nuclear medicine procedures, such as positron emission tomography (PET) and single photon emission computed tomography (SPECT) as well as structural and functional magnetic resonance imaging (MRI). In some instances, noninvasive functional imaging can reveal an abnormality years before clinical signs develop. In others, changes seen may be compensated for through system reserves, redundancy, or plasticity.

The technologies used for monitoring may focus on a particular neurotransmitter system (e.g., assay of binding to a specific neurotransmitter receptor) or they may assess structural or functional integrity of a variety of brain regions (e.g., MRI or metabolic mapping with PET). Pharmacological challenges may be used to unmask changes that may be undetected in an unperturbed system. Furthermore, simultaneous application of several assay instruments, including behavioral, electrophysiological and nuclear medicine approaches, may be appropriate and useful for establishing correlations between changes in specific aspects of brain function and amelioration of a disease (drug abuse disorder) or its sequelae. The assay method selected for safety assessment depends on the effect(s) of concern, generated in preclinical testing or observed in patients in previous studies. Similarly, the same types of sophisticated technology can be applied to evaluate proposed changes in brain function, as parameters of efficacy.

One of the most important principles in the evaluation of potential neurotoxicity is the pre-existing condition of the patient/subject. Chronic substance abuse can produce subtle deficits which can be revealed using sophisticated technologies, such as MRI and PET. Studies in polydrug abusers

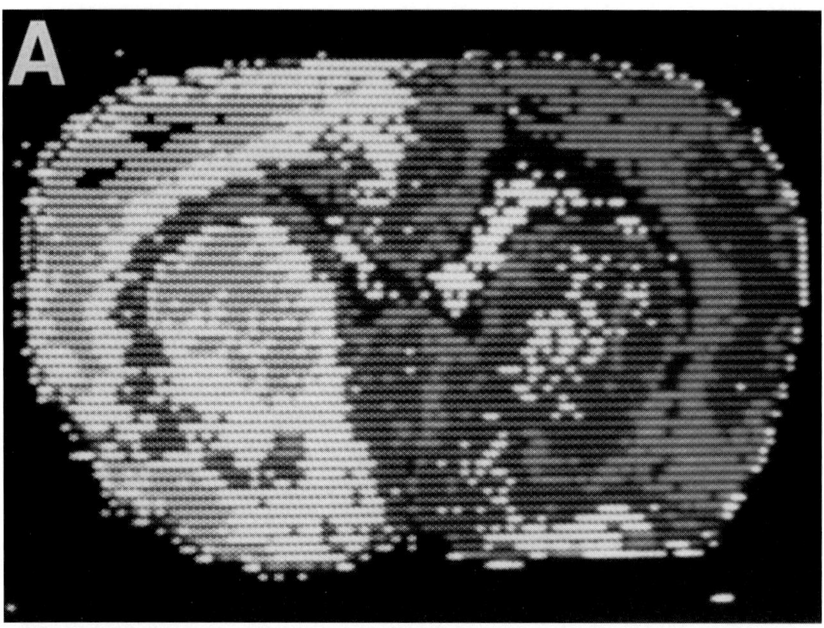

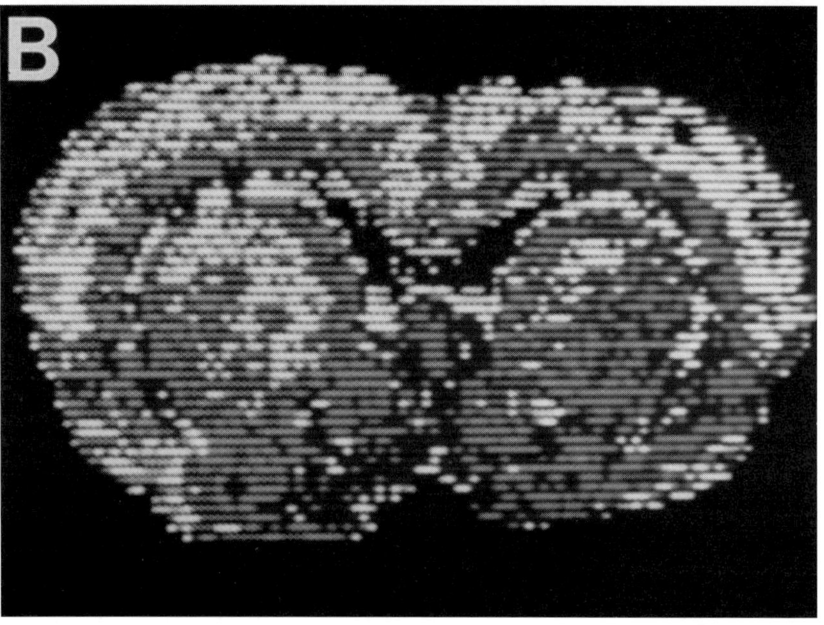

FIGURE 2

have demonstrated the relative to greater sensitivity of functional nuclear medicine procedures as compared with structural imaging in assessing the effects of chronic drug abuse. PET assays of human volunteers using [F-18]fluorodeoxyglucose (FDG) have demonstrated that individuals with histories of polydrug abuse, including intravenous substance abuse, have an abnormal pattern of cerebral glucose metabolism as compared with controls matched for age and socioeconomic status.[30] This abnormality is seen in subjects who have been abstinent from illicit drugs of abuse for up to one month, and consists of a deficit in glucose metabolism in the visual association cortex and abnormally high relative metabolic rate in the orbitofrontal cortex. In addition, deficits in cerebral perfusion have been observed in chronic cocaine abusers, using PET[32] and SPECT.[32] Such differences are not readily apparent when individuals drawn from the same populations are compared with respect to a general measure of structural integrity of the brain, such as the ventricle-to-brain ratio.[34] Volumetric MRI of a group of polydrug abusers revealed no tendency for ventriculomegaly in a group of polysubstance abusers as compared with controls using volumetric MRI scanning. Nonetheless, assays of particular brain regions have revealed differences between polydrug abusers and controls. Substance abusers show significantly smaller volume of the prefrontal lobe, containing the orbitofrontal region,[35] which shows abnormal metabolism on PET scans.[31] Whether or not this difference reflects the effects of chronic drug abuse or hypoplasia, which may have contributed to development of substance abuse disorder, is unknown at this time.

Greater sensitivity of functional measures (e.g., obtained by PET) as compared with structural assays has been documented in the early days of PET scanning. A classic example was presented in the study of Huntington's disease. Serial studies of an individual who ultimately developed the clinical syndrome of Huntington's disease revealed that prior to the manifestation of clinical neurological signs, roentgenographic computerized tomography (CT) scanning revealed no abnormality in the basal ganglia, while glucose metabolism in the basal ganglia was severely reduced.[36]

In addition to assays of brain function, as inferred from rates of glucose metabolism and regional cerebral blood flow, neurochemical integrity has

---

FIGURE 2. Transforms of autoradiograms from 20-μm brain sections from rats subjected to the 2-deoxy-D-[1-^{14}C]-glucose ([^{14}C]DG) procedure. *Dark gray values* represent high levels of grain density; *light values* represent low levels of grain density. **(A)** Autoradiogram of a brain section from a representative rat in which a lesion was induced by ibotenic acid (12 μg) three days prior to the [^{14}C]DG procedure. **(B)** Autoradiogram of a brain section from approximately the same level of a representative rat "lesioned" with ibotenic acid (12 μg) 28 days before being subjected to the [^{14}C]DG procedure. In **(A)**, note the reduction in grain density, representing decreased regional cerebral metabolic rate for glucose in portions of the autoradiogram corresponding with the frontoparietal cortex and striatum of the lesioned hemisphere. In **(B)**, there was virtually no asymmetry in grain density of cortical regions, although the density was somewhat lower in the striatum of the lesioned side.[40]

been assessed primarily by receptor binding assays. Although most receptor binding assays up to this point have attempted to quantitate available receptor number or receptor density in various disease states or in normal physiological conditions, nuclear medicine procedures, such as SPECT and PET, have more recently been considered for assessment of neurotransmitter dynamics and interactions between various neurotransmitter systems.[37] For example, in light of the interaction between cholinergic and dopaminergic systems in brain, assays of ^{11}C-raclopride binding to D2-like dopamine receptors in response to pharmacological perturbation can reflect changes in intrasynaptic dopamine as influenced by the action of an anticholinergic agent.[38] Changes in intrasynaptic dopamine in response to the indirect agonist amphetamine have been observed using SPECT and ^{123}I-iodobenzamide.[39] Given the preclinical findings of cerebellar changes induced by ibogaine, assays of non-dopaminergic systems in cerebellum may be of great interest.

LONG-TERM CONSEQUENCES OF NEUROTOXICITY: ADAPTATION

Studies in animals have suggested that neurochemical changes in brain that might be induced by toxins or potential medications may persist without functional impairment, as the brain adapts to a chronic neurotransmitter deficiency. One example of this type of situation is presented in rats that received unilateral local injection of the glutamatergic neurotoxin, ibotenic acid, into the ventral globus pallidus.[35] In such rats, the neurotoxin causes degeneration of cells of the nucleus basalis magnocellularis, which provides the primary cholinergic innervation to the neocortex. Animals treated with such intracerebral injections showed severe depression in the concentration of choline acetyltransferase, the synthetic enzyme for acetylcholine, and no recovery over a 5-week period.[41] Nonetheless, animals that manifested marked deficits in cortical glucose metabolism within one week of the lesion showed complete recovery and no asymmetry one month after placement of the lesion.[40] Similarly, rats subjected to unilateral nucleus basalis lesions showed a return of choline uptake to control values, with a gradual increase, reaching normal levels after 3 months.[42] These observations indicate that even after substantial neurotoxin-induced lesions, the brain can show significant plasticity over time. The extent to which a history of drug abuse might preclude recovery after treatment with a potentially neurotoxic agent is not known.

SUMMARY

New technologies utilized for monitoring brain function can be more sensitive in the assessment of desired or undesired pharmacological effects than can clinical examination. Nonetheless, careful case-by-case analysis is required to determine to what extent a change detected with a sensitive imaging modality will have clinical significance. Whereas in some instances the technology may suggest a subclinical condition years before clinical signs develop, in other instances changes seen may be compensated for through system reserves, redundancy, or plasticity. Furthermore, simultaneous application of several assay instruments, including behavioral, electrophysiological, and nuclear medicine approaches, may be appropriate and useful for establishing correlations between changes in specific aspects of brain function and amelioration of a disease (drug abuse disorder) or its sequelae. In the example of ibogaine, a testing strategy was developed to assess human subjects for possible changes in cerebellar function (that were suggested by preclinical findings indicating subtle damage). Thus, subjects may be tested for subclinical alterations during and immediately following a clinical trial. This "harbinger of toxicity" approach would provide clinicians the critical data necessary for appropriate follow-up of subjects as well as the propriety of continuance of the clinical trials within the ibogaine project.

REFERENCES

1. Goutarel, R. 1993. Pharmacodynamic and therapeutic applications of iboga and ibogaine. Psychedelic Monographs and Essays. **6:** 71–111.
2. Naranjo, C. 1969. Psychotherapeutic possibilities of new fantasy-enhancing drugs. Clinical Toxicology **2:** 209–224.
3. Lotsof, H. 1986. Rapid method for interrupting the cocaine and amphetamine addiction syndrome. U.S. Patent No. 4,587,243.
4. Glick, S. D., K. Rossman, S. Steindorf & J. N. Carlson. 1991. Effects and after-effects of ibogaine on morphine self-administration in rats. Eur. J. Pharmacol. **195:** 341–345.
5. Glick, S. D., M. E. Keuhnke, J. Raucci, T. E. Wilson, T. D. Larson, R. W. Keller & J. N. Carlson. 1994. Effects of iboga alkaloids on morphine and cocaine self-administration in rats: Relationship to tremorigenic effects and to effects on dopamine release in nucleus accumbens and striatum. Brain Res. **657:** 14–22.
6. Cappendijk, S. L. T. & M. R. Dzoljic. 1993. Inhibitory effects of ibogaine on cocaine self-administration in rats. Eur. J. Pharmacol. **241:** 261–265.
7. Effects of ibogaine on self-administration of cocaine, heroin, and food in rats. 1993. Presented to the Food and Drug Administration's Drug Abuse Advisory Committee #26.
8. Mansbach, R. S., R. L. Balster, M. Gregory & E. Soenghen. 1992. Effects of ibogaine pretreatment on iv cocaine self-administration in rhesus monkey. NIDA Contract Report SA92.16.
9. Deecher, D. C., M. Teitler, D. M. Soderlund, W. G. Bornmann, M. E. Keuhne & S. D. Glick. 1992. Mechanisms of action of ibogaine and harmaline congeners based on radioligand binding studies. Brain Res. **1:** 242–247.
10. Repke, D. B., D. R. Artis, J. T. Nelson & E. H. F. Wong. 1994. Abbreviated ibogaine congeners. Synthesis and reaction of tropan-3-yl-2 and 3-indoles. Investigation of an unusual isomerization of 2-substituted indoles using computational and spectroscopic technique. J Org Chem. **59:** 2164–2171.
11. Sweetnam, P. J., J. Lancaster, A. Snowman, J. Collins, S. Perschke, C. Bauer & J. Ferkany. 1995. Receptor binding profile suggests multiple mechanisms of action are responsible for ibogaine's putative anti-addictive activity. Psychopharmacology (Berl). **118:** 369–376.

12. PEARL, S. M., K. HERRICK-DAVIS, M. TEITILER & S. D. GLICK. 1995. Radioligand-binding study of noribogaine, a likely metabolite of ibogaine. Brain Res. **675:** 342–344.
13. LONDON, E. D., S. J. GRANT, M. J. MORGAN & S. R. ZUKIN. 1996. Neurobiology of drug abuse. *In* Neuropsychiatry. B. S. Fogel, R. B. Schiffer, S. M. Rao, Eds. 635–678. William & Wilkins. Baltimore, MD.
14. DI CHIARA, G. & A. IMPERATO. 1988. Drugs abused by humans preferentially increase synaptic dopamine concentrations in the mesolimbic system of freely moving rats. Proc. Natl. Acad. Sci. USA **85:** 5274–5278.
15. MAISONNEUVE, I. M., R. W. KELLER & S. D. GLICK. 1990. Similar effects of D-amphetamine and cocaine on extracellular dopamine levels in medial prefrontal cortex of rats. Brain Res. **535:** 221–226.
16. MOGHADDAM, B. & B. S. BUNNEY. 1989. Differential effect of cocaine on extracellular dopamine levels in rat medial prefrontal cortex and nucleus accumbens: Comparison to amphetamine. Synapse **4:** 156–161.
17. MAISONNEUVE, I. M., R. W. KELLER & S. D. GLICK. 1991. Interactions between ibogaine, a potential anti-addictive agent, and morphine: an *in vivo* microdialysis study. Eur. J. Pharmacol. **199:** 35–42.
18. MAISONNEUVE, I. M., K. L. ROSSMAN, R. W. KELLER, JR. & S. D. GLICK. 1992. Acute and prolonged effects of ibogaine on brain dopamine metabolism and morphine-induced locomotor activity in rats. Brain Res. **575:** 69–73.
19. MAISONNEUVE, I. M., R. W. KELLER & S. D. GLICK. 1992. Interactions of ibogaine and D-amphetamine: *in vivo* microdialysis and motor behavior in rats. Brain Res. **579:** 87–92.
20. MAISONNEUVE, I. M. & S. D. GLICK. 1992. Interactions between ibogaine and cocaine in rats: *in vivo* microdialysis and motor behavior. Eur. J. Pharmacol. **212:** 263–266.
21. PAGE, J. G., L. E. RODAN, D. R. FARNELL & J. F. MARTIN. 1994. Repeat dose oral toxicity study of ibogaine in rats. NIDA Contract Report SRI-CBE-94-002-7486-LXXII.
22. O'HEARN, E., D. B. LONG & M. E. MOLLIVER. 1993. Ibogaine induces glial activation in parasagittal zones of the cerebellum. NeuroReport **4:** 299–302.
23. O'HEARN, E. & M. E. MOLLIVER. 1993. Degeneration of Purkinje cells in parasagittal zones of the cerebellar vermis after treatment with ibogaine or harmaline. Neuroscience **55:** 303–310.
24. O'HEARN, E. O., P. ZHANG & M. E. MOLLIVER. 1995. Excitotoxic insult due to ibogaine leads to delayed induction of neuronal NOS in Purkinje cells. NeuroReport **6:** 1611–1616.
25. O'CALLAGAHAN, J. P. 1991. Quantification of glial fibrillary acidic protein: Comparison of slot-immunobinding assays with a novel sandwich ELISA. Neurotoxicol. Teratol. **13:** 275–281.
26. PAGE, J. G., T. S. ROGERS, J. P. O'CALLAGAHAN & H. D. GILES. 1994. Acute neurotoxicity study of ibogaine HCl in dogs. NIDA Contract Report SRI-CHM-93-1034-7486-LXX.
27. MOLLIVER, M. E. & E. O'HEARN. 1995. Studies of ibogaine neurotoxicity in rat and monkey. Presented to the NIDA-Sponsored Ibogaine Review Meeting. March 1995.
28. VICTOR, M., R. ADAMS & E. L. MANCALL. 1959. A restricted form of cerebellar cortical degeneration occurring in alcoholic patients. Arch. Neurol. **1:** 579–588.
29. KARHUNEN, P. J., T. ERKINJUNTTI & P. LAIPPALA. 1994. Moderate alcohol consumption and loss of cerebellar Purkinje cells. Br. Med. J. **308:** 1663–1667.
30. SCHOLZ, E., H. C. DIENER, J. DICHGANS, H. D. LANGOHR, W. SCHIED & A. SCHUPMANN. 1986. Incidence of peripheral neuropathy and cerebellar ataxia in chronic alcoholics. J. Neurol. **233:** 212–217.
31. STAPLETON, J. M., M. J. MORGAN, R. L. PHILLIPS, D. F. WONG, B. C. K. YUNG, E. K. SHAYA, R. F. DANNALS, X. LIU, R. L. GRAYSON & E. D. LONDON. 1995. Cerebral glucose utilization in polysubstance abuse. Neuropsychopharmacology **13:** 21–31.
32. VOLKOW, N. D., N. MULLANI, K. L. GOULD, S. ADLER & K. KRAJEWSKI. 1988. Cerebral blood flow in chronic cocaine users: A study with positron emission tomography. Br. J. Psychiatry **152:** 641–648.
33. HOLMAN, B. L., P. A. CARVALHO, J. MENDELSON, S. K. TEOH, R. NARDIN, E. HALLGRING, N. HEBBEN & K. A. JOHNSON. 1991. Brain perfusion is abnormal in cocaine-dependent polydrug users: A study using technetium-99m-HMPAO and ASPECT. J. Nucl. Med. **32:** 1206–1210.

34. Liu, X., R. L. Phillips, S. M. Resnick, D. F. Wong, J. M. Stapleton & E. D. London. 1995. Magnetic resonance imaging reveals no ventriculomegaly in polydrug abusers. Acta Neurol. Scand. **92:** 83–90.

35. Liu, X., J. A. Matochik, J. L. Cadet & E. D. London. Smaller volume of prefrontal lobe in polysubstance abusers: a magnetic resonance imaging study. Unpublished study.

36. Kuhl, D. E., E. J. Metter, W. H. Riege & C. H. Markham. 1984. Patterns of cerebral glucose utilization in Parkinson's disease and Huntington's disease. Ann. Neurol. **15:** S119–S125.

37. Morris, E. D., R. E. Fisher, N. M. Alpert, S. L. Rauch & A. J. Fischman. 1995. *In vivo* imaging of neuromodulation using positron emission tomography: Optimal ligand characteristics and task length for detection of activation. Human Brain Mapping **3:** 35–55.

38. Dewey, S. L., G. S. Smith, J. Logan, J. D. Brodie, P. Simkowitz, R. R. MacGregor, J. S. Fowler, N. D. Volkow & A. P. Wolf. 1993. Effects of central cholinergic blockade on striatal dopamine release measured with positron emission tomography in normal human subjects. Proc. Natl. Acad. Sci. USA **90:** 11816–11820.

39. Innis, R. B., R. T. Malison, M. Al-Tikriti, P. B. Hoffer, E. H. Sybirska, J. P. Seibyl, S. S. Zoghbi, R. M. Baldwin, M. Laruelle & E. O. Smith. 1992. Amphetamine-stimulated dopamine release competes *in vivo* for [^{123}I]IBZM binding to the D_2 receptor in nonhuman primates. Synapse **10:** 177–184.

40. London, E. D., M. McKinney, M. Dam, A. Ellis & J. T. Coyle. 1984. Decreased cortical glucose utilization after ibotenate lesion of the rat ventromedial globus pallidus. J. Cereb. Blood Flow Metab. **4:** 381–390.

41. McKinney, M. & J. T. Coyle. 1982. Regulation of neocortical muscarinic receptors: Effects of drug treatment and lesions. J. Neurosci. **2:** 97–105.

42. Wenk, G. L. & D. S. Olton. 1984. Recovery of neocortical choline acetyltransferase activity following ibotenic acid injection into the nucleus basalis of Meynert in rats. Brain Res. **293:** 184–186.

DISCUSSION

Question: With regard to the ibogaine, do you know whether there is any histopathology in the hippocampal area, given its effects on the excitatory amino acid receptors?

Vocci: Apparently there isn't. There is C-*fos* activation and GFAP elevation at 25 mg/kg in forebrain areas, but no apparent histopathology that we are aware of.

Question: Could you comment on the specificity of effects of drugs that apparently operate via similar mechanisms, such as the glutamate receptors?; because another chemical, domoic acid, has substantial effects on hippocampal areas and rather limited effects on cerebellar regions.

Vocci: That may be because of the fact that the effect on the cerebellum is a transsynaptic one rather than a direct effect. Each drug may have a different mechanism, which may provide the clue to the type of toxicity you see and the region you see it in.

Question: With regard to the nucleus basalis magnocellularis region, although one shows that blood flow or glucose metabolism becomes symmetrical in a chronic lesion, you can see upregulation of postsynaptic M1 regulative signal transduction involving phospholipase A2 *in vivo,* with radiolabeled arachidonic acid. So despite the fact that the M1 receptor density is the same in the cortex after M2 has been removed 2 weeks after a lesion has been made, one can in fact see a neuroblastic response at the level of signal transduction *in vivo* with autoradiography and inference both with PET.

VOCCI: Yes.

QUESTION: What is the neuropharmacopathology of vincristine? Is it the same as oubain? Also, have these same studies been done with cytarabine, which oncologists probably see as a more common cause of ataxia.

VOCCI: I believe that the evidence for neuropathology from vincristine is clinical. I am not sure that anyone has actually looked at whether or not vincristine damages Purkinje cells, but it is an obvious place to look. As for cytarabine, I believe that a generic cytarabine that was on the market several years ago actually produced some cerebellar lesions. All cytarabine will do it. The question is whether this generic compound was more likely to do it than the innovator.

Imaging Studies of Cocaine in the Human Brain and Studies of the Cocaine Addict[a]

NORA D. VOLKOW, GENE-JACK WANG,
AND JOANNA S. FOWLER

Brookhaven National Laboratory
Upton, New York 11973

Positron emission tomography (PET) is a medical imaging modality that measures the regional distribution and kinetics of chemical compounds labeled with short-lived positron-emitting isotopes in the brain and living body.[1] Several radiotracers have been developed that enable the measurement of various aspects of brain neurochemistry and function. Of the PET tracers developed, the one most utilized is 2-deoxy-2-[18F]-fluoro-D-glucose (FDG). FDG is an analogue of glucose that enables the measurement of regional brain glucose metabolism. Because brain regional glucose utilization is tightly associated with brain function,[2] the measurement of FDG with PET has allowed the assessment of brain activity in human subjects.

The availability of PET tracers to monitor specific neurotransmitter systems has made it possible to directly evaluate them *in vivo* in human subjects and provides a tool to investigate their contribution in the pharmacological properties of drugs as well as its disruption with chronic drug use and abuse. Various elements pertaining to neurotransmitter function can be investigated with PET. For example, one can assess receptors subtypes, as has been done with the dopamine D1 and the dopamine D2 receptors. Elements from the presynaptic terminal can be directly evaluated by using tracers that assess metabolism of neurotransmitters, such as is the case for L-DOPA, and/or by monitoring monoamine transporters. The concentration of enzymes in brain that are involved with degradation of monoamines has also been achieved with the development of ligands that bind to MAO-B, MAO-A and COMT.[3]

Since positron emitters can be used to label compounds without affecting their pharmacological behavior, PET can also measure drug pharmacokinetics *in vivo* in brain as well as in various organs throughout the body. Because these studies are done in living subjects, the relation between pharmacokinetics and the temporal course of the behavioral effects of drugs can be investigated.

The relatively short half-life of positron emitters and the relatively benign

[a]This work was supported by Grants DE-ACO2-76CH00016 from the Department of Energy, and ROIDA06891, ROIDA09490 and ROIDA06278 from the National Institute on Drug Abuse.

dosimetry allow the performance of studies with more than one tracer in a given subject. This permits an assessment of the relations between neurochemical parameters and/or the relation between neurochemical and functional parameters. PET can be used to investigate the neurobiology of drug abuse from two perspectives: one that involves an investigation of the pharmacological properties of the drugs themselves and the other that investigates the consequences of these drugs in brain function and neurochemistry. In this paper we illustrate the use of PET in human brain neurochemistry and pharmacology on the investigation of drugs of abuse, taking cocaine as an example since this is the drug that has been most widely investigated.

Cocaine is one of the most reinforcing and addictive of the drugs of abuse[4] and its use is associated with major medical and social problems.[5,6] In spite of the frequency of cocaine abuse, the processes that lead to the uncontrollable patterns of cocaine use and the mechanisms of toxicity are not well understood. PET has provided the opportunity to examine the properties of cocaine that make it such a unique reinforcer and to investigate the mechanisms responsible for its toxicity as well as to study mechanisms that may be involved with the loss of control in the addicted subject. The following questions have been investigated: (1) To what extent do the disposition and pharmacokinetics of cocaine contribute to its reinforcing and toxic properties? (2) Can this knowledge be applied to the development of new treatments? (3) What are the effects of chronic cocaine on the brain dopamine system and on brain function and their relation to toxicity and addiction?

TO WHAT EXTENT DO THE DISPOSITION AND PHARMACOKINETICS OF COCAINE CONTRIBUTE TO ITS REINFORCING AND TOXIC PROPERTIES?

Animal studies have shown that the ability of cocaine to inhibit the dopamine transporter appears to be crucial for its reinforcing properties.[7] We have used PET to investigate the extent to which the same applies to humans and to evaluate the unique properties of cocaine in human brain that may also contribute to its highly reinforcing as well as toxic properties.

Pharmacokinetics of Cocaine in the Human Brain and Body

The amount of drug that gets into the brain, its regional distribution and residence time, and its site of binding are all important factors in understanding its effects. We have directly examined the binding of cocaine in the human brain using [^{11}C]cocaine.[8] PET studies with [^{11}C]cocaine showed that cocaine uptake into the brain is very high (10%) and very fast (peak uptake 4–6 minutes). Cocaine also clears from the brain very rapidly, half-life in striatum corresponds to 20 minutes. In the brain the highest concentration of cocaine occurs in the striatum, where it binds to the dopamine transporter (FIG. 1). The pharmacokinetics of cocaine in the striatum paralleled the time course for the euphoria experienced after intravenous administration of cocaine, supporting the idea that the binding of cocaine into the dopamine transporter is involved with the subjective perception of euphoria in humans. These studies also highlight the importance of the fast pharmacokinetics of cocaine in the human brain that not only enhance its reinforcing effects, but also enable frequent repeated administration.

The distribution and kinetics of cocaine in the human body were also evaluated with [^{11}C]cocaine; this revealed uptake of cocaine in heart, kidneys, liver, gastrointestinal tract, bladder, and adrenals, but not in lungs.[9] The pharmacokinetics of [^{11}C]cocaine in heart were faster than those in brain and probably represent binding to the norepinephrine transporter. Accumulation of cocaine in the heart could enhance its cardiotoxicity, since its local anesthetic properties could directly damage the myocardium.[10] In addition, inhibition of the norepinephrine transporter by cocaine interferes with a protective mechanism of the heart to remove circulating catecholamines.[11]

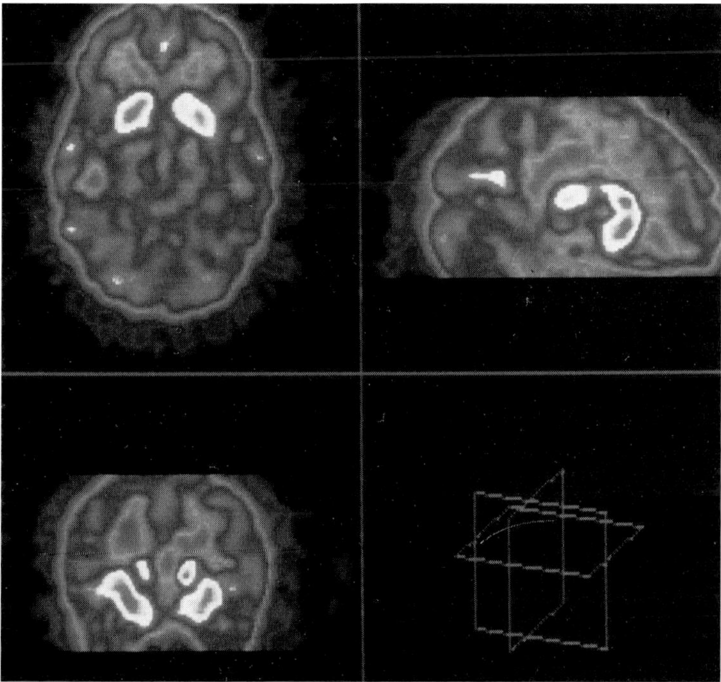

FIGURE 1. Images of cocaine in the human brain obtained with [^{11}C]cocaine and PET. This figure shows an axial, a sagittal, and a coronal plane of the brain for images obtained 15 minutes after administration of [^{11}C]cocaine. Highest uptake of [^{11}C]cocaine occurs in striatum.

The highest accumulation of cocaine was in the adrenals, where uptake was 5 times higher than that in striatum. The high uptake by the adrenals could account in part for the large increases in peripheral catecholamines after acute administration of cocaine,[12] which would further enhance cocaine's cardiotoxicity. Uptake into liver and gastrointestinal tract and bladder was much slower than that for other organs and probably reflects cocaine's metabolism and excretion.

Comparison of Cocaine with Other Psychostimulant Drugs

Cocaine, which is one of the most reinforcing of the abused drugs, has pharmacological properties very similar to those of methylphenidate (MP), another dopamine transporter inhibitor drug which is prescribed in the treatment of attention deficit disorder[13,14] and of narcolepsy.[15] We compared the regional distribution and the pharmacokinetics of these two drugs in the living human brain using PET and [^{11}C]cocaine and [^{11}C]methylphenidate.[16] These two drugs showed essentially identical regional distribution in the human brain and they competed for the same binding sites. They were both taken up rapidly (peak uptake, 4–8 minutes) and in high concentration (7–10% of the injected dose) by the human brain. However, these two drugs differed markedly in their rate of clearance. MP's clearance from striatum (half-life: >90 minutes from peak uptake) was significantly slower than that of cocaine (half-life: 20 minutes from peak uptake) (FIG. 2). For both drugs their fast uptake in striatum paralleled the experience of the "high." For MP the "high" decreased very rapidly despite significant binding of the drug in brain. In contrast, for cocaine the decline in the "high" paralleled the fast rate of clearance of the drug from brain. Because the experience of the "high" is associated with the fast uptake of cocaine and MP in brain, we postulated that the slow clearance of MP from brain would prevent the frequent repeated administration that occurs with cocaine.

Interaction of Cocaine with Other Abused Drugs

The combined use of cocaine and alcohol is very frequent in cocaine abusers,[17] and is associated with increased toxicity and lethality.[18] Part of this toxicity had been ascribed to the formation of cocaethylene, a metabolic byproduct of the interaction between cocaine and alcohol.[19,20] Using PET, we have investigated the characteristics of cocaethylene as labeled with [^{11}C]-cocaethylene and have compared them with those of [^{11}C]cocaine.[21] These studies showed that the distribution, rate of uptake in brain, and pharmacokinetics of these two drugs was almost identical. Thus, altered pharmacokinetics did not explain the increased lethality from the combined use of cocaine and alcohol. We also showed that alcohol intoxication did not change the behavior of [^{11}C]cocaine in human brain. On the basis of these studies, we

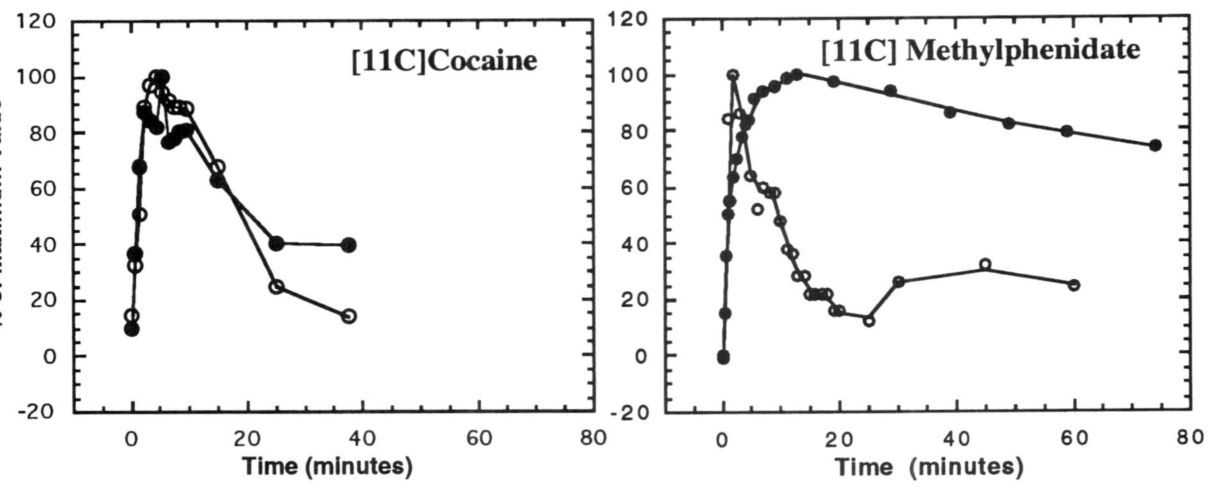

FIGURE 2. Graphs comparing uptake and clearance of [^{11}C]cocaine and [^{11}C]methylphenidate in the human brain vs. values of a "high." Time activity curves for the accumulation of [^{11}C]cocaine and [^{11}C]methylphenidate in striatum are depicted as *solid circles,* and the time course for the high is shown by *open circles.* Note that while cocaine leaves the brain at the same rate that the high diminishes, methylphenidate stays in the brain long past the time that the high has disappeared. (Modified from Volkow *et al.*[16])

postulate that the increased toxicity is probably mediated via the direct effects of the two drugs.

CAN THIS KNOWLEDGE BE APPLIED TO THE DEVELOPMENT OF NEW TREATMENTS?

Because the ability of cocaine to inhibit the dopamine (DA) transporter appears to be crucial for its reinforcing properties, drugs that inhibit the DA transporter for a long time and would interfere with cocaine binding in the brain are being developed as potential treatments for the cocaine addict. Several cocaine analogues have been developed that possess a much higher affinity for the dopamine transporter than does cocaine. These compounds can potentially be used to prevent cocaine's effects.[22–24] Although it could be argued that these drugs could be potentially more reinforcing than cocaine, their slower pharmacokinetics at the dopamine transporter may preclude repeated and frequent self-administration by the addict.

Interaction of Cocaine with Other Dopamine Transporter Inhibitor Drugs

We were particularly interested in the cocaine analogue RTI-55 since human SPECT imaging studies had demonstrated slow uptake in brain and minimal dissociation of the radiotracer from the striatum over a 24-hour period.[25] We therefore conducted a PET study to evaluate the temporal course for the inhibition of cocaine binding in brain after administration of RTI-55.[26] These studies were done in baboons since there are not enough toxicity data about these compounds to perform such studies in humans. Inhibition of cocaine binding at different times after RTI-55 administration in the baboon brain was evaluated with PET and [^{11}C]cocaine. In the baboon brain RTI-55 significantly inhibited [^{11}C]cocaine binding at 90 minutes and 24 hours after administration. The half-life for clearance was estimated to be 2 to 3 days. This study documents complete and long-lasting inhibition of cocaine binding after administration of RTI-55 in baboon brain.

WHAT ARE THE EFFECTS OF CHRONIC COCAINE USE ON THE DOPAMINE SYSTEM AND FUNCTION OF THE BRAIN? HOW DO THESE RELATE TO TOXICITY AND ADDICTION?

The use of PET and specific radiotracers to assess different aspects of brain function provides a sensitive tool to detect damage in brain that can not be assessed with other available techniques as well as a means to investigate functional and neurochemical changes that may be related to the addictive process.

Effects of Chronic Cocaine on Cerebral Blood Flow; Relation to Toxicity

Using PET and [^{15}O]-water, we showed that chronic cocaine abusers had profound defects in cerebral blood flow (FIG. 3).[27] Many studies have

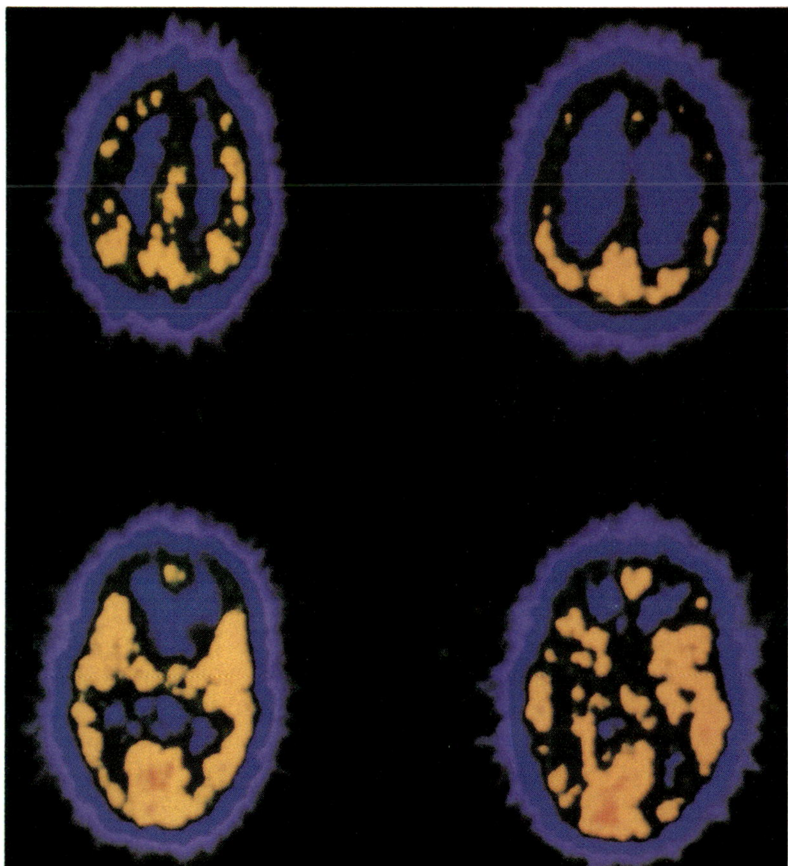

FIGURE 3. Images of cerebral blood flow in a chronic cocaine abuser. Four axial images from the brain of a cocaine abuser obtained with [^{15}O]H_2O to measure cerebral blood flow. For this image cortical flow depicted in *red* and *yellow* correspond to normal values, whereas flow shown in *green* corresponds to reduced values. The cortical flow in this cocaine abuser is significantly reduced throughout the frontal cortex and to a lesser extent in the left temporal cortex.

replicated the widespread abnormalities in cerebral blood flow (CBF) in cocaine abusers.[29,30] These SPECT studies have documented defects in perfusion in moderate as well as heavy cocaine abusers. The defects in CBF seen in the cocaine abusers could reflect the vasoactive properties of cocaine in cerebral vessels.[28] Flow changes from cocaine could result from vasoconstriction, which, if prolonged, could produce vascular damage, tissue ischemia, and necrosis and could also favor the occurrence of cerebral hemorrhages. These findings corroborate the high incidence of cerebral strokes and hemorrhages in cocaine abusers.[31,32] Imaging studies with CBF have also formed the basis to evaluate treatment interventions.[33]

Effects of Acute Cocaine on Regional Brain Glucose Metabolism: Relation to Reinforcement

The effects of acute cocaine administration on regional brain glucose metabolism have also been investigated with PET and FDG. The study was done in cocaine abusers and compared brain glucose metabolism with and without preadministration of 30 mg i.v. cocaine.[34] Cocaine decreased brain metabolism in all brain regions investigated, although to a lesser extent in cerebellum. The magnitude of cocaine-induced decreases in metabolism were correlated with the degree of ventricular enlargement. Subjects with enlarged ventricles were less sensitive to the effects of cocaine on brain metabolism than were those who had less ventricular enlargement. This study postulates that one of the mechanisms of reinforcement of cocaine may involve the reduction of brain metabolic activity.

Effects of Chronic Cocaine on Dopamine Brain Function and Its Relation to Metabolism

The effects of cocaine on the striatal dopamine (DA) system have also been investigated with PET. Dopamine appears to be involved in the reinforcing properties of cocaine[35–39] and it has been postulated the decreased DA activity could underlie cocaine addiction.[40] A multi-tracer approach was used to assess the relation between changes in DA parameters and regional brain metabolism and during different periods of the detoxification.

Regional brain glucose metabolism in recently detoxified cocaine abusers ($<$1 week) was significantly higher in orbitofrontal cortex and in striatum than in healthy non-abusing controls.[41] The metabolic activity in these brain regions was found to be correlated with the days since last use of cocaine. The highest values were observed in subjects tested during the initial 72 hours. Metabolic activity in orbitofrontal cortex and in striatum was also significantly correlated with the intensity of cocaine craving. Cocaine abusers who had the highest subjective ratings for craving were those with the highest metabolic values in orbitofrontal cortex and striatum. Studies done with ^{18}F-NMS on these same cocaine abusers revealed decreases in dopamine D_2 receptor availability.[42]

In contrast to the marked increases in metabolism observed during early cocaine withdrawal, significant reductions in metabolic activity in prefrontal cortex, orbitofrontal cortex, temporal cortex and cingulate gyrus were found in studies done in patients tested between 1 and 4 months of detoxification. (FIG. 4).[43] Measures of dopamine D_2 receptor availability in these patients also showed a significant reduction, as had been observed during early detoxification (FIG. 5). Measures for D_2 receptors correlated significantly with measures of metabolic activity in orbitofrontal cortex, cingulate gyrus, and prefrontal cortex (FIG. 6).[44] Decrements in regional brain metabolism as well

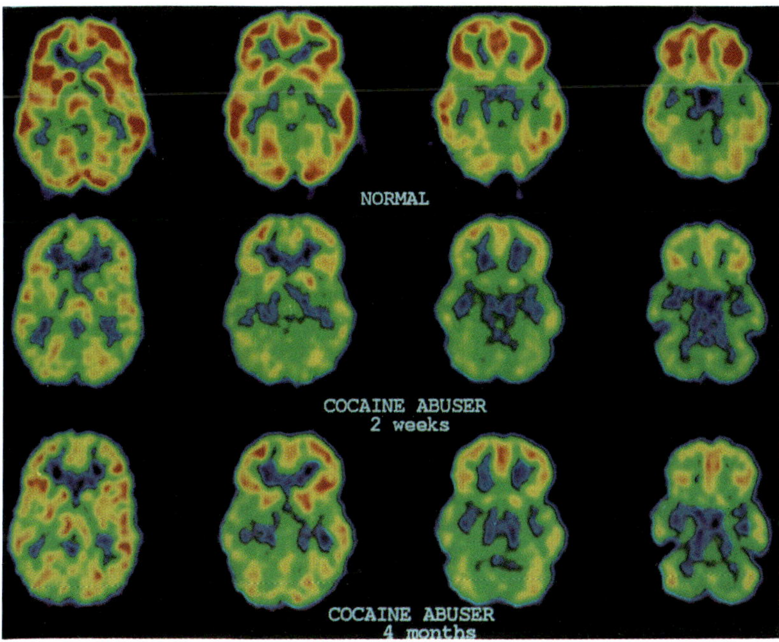

FIGURE 4. Brain metabolism in a normal subject and in a cocaine abuser. PET was used to measure regional brain glucose metabolism using ^{18}FDG in a normal subject **(top row)** and a chronic cocaine user studied at 2 weeks **(middle row)** and at 4 months **(bottom row)** after withdrawal from cocaine. The images of the cocaine abuser show decreased brain metabolism at 2 weeks and at 4 months after the last cocaine dose. Scaling is depicted with highest activity red > yellow > green > blue.

as the reductions in dopamine D_2 receptor availability persisted in the follow-up studies performed 3 months after the inpatient detoxification program was completed. The correlation between dopamine D_2 receptor availability and metabolic activity in orbitofrontal cortex and cingulate gyrus suggests an association between DA activity and the function of these brain regions. Experiments in animals have shown that destruction of the orbitofrontal cortex leads to the emergence of repetitive behaviors that cannot be easily

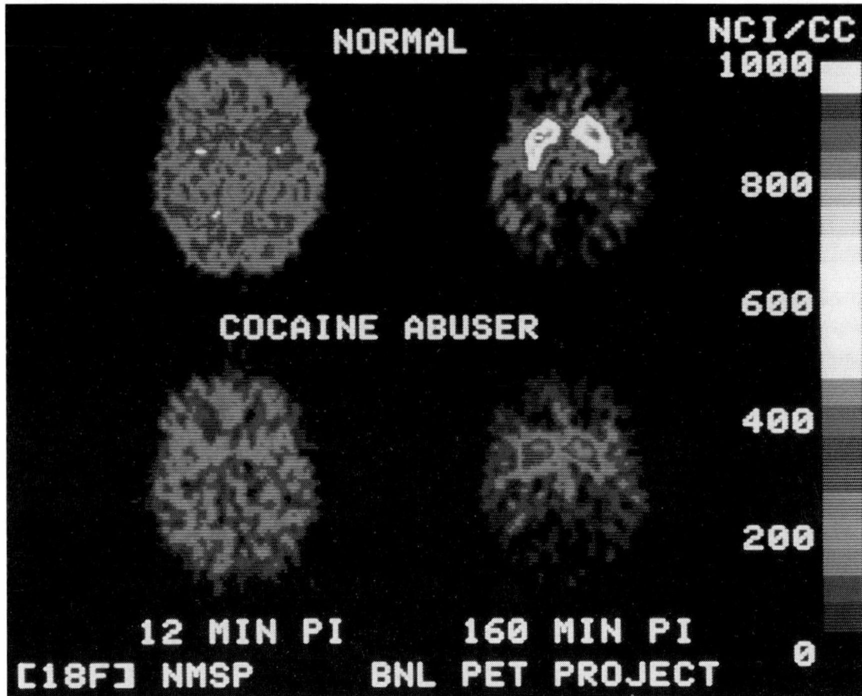

FIGURE 5. Dopamine D_2 receptors in a normal subject and in a cocaine abuser. Images in a normal subject **(top)** and in a cocaine abuser **(bottom)** taken at 12 and at 160 minutes after injection of [^{18}F]*N*-methylspiroperidol to assess dopamine D_2 receptor availability. Notice the marked reduction in the binding of [^{18}F]N-methylspiroperidol in the cocaine abuser at 160 minutes, reflecting the decrease in dopamine D_2 receptors. Scale is to the right.

terminated,[45] and a similar syndrome can be generated by the destruction of the mesocortical DA pathway.[46] Hence we postulate that DA disruption of the orbitofrontal cortex may be one of the mechanisms responsible for the compulsive administration of cocaine during a "binge" and for the loss of control experienced by drug abusers when exposed to cocaine and/or cocaine-related cues. Thus, DA involvement in addiction may be mediated by its interactions with frontal circuits involved in the control of repetitive and impulsive behaviors.

Effects of Chronic Cocaine on Cocaine Binding in Brain

Cocaine's ability to inhibit the dopamine transporters has been linked to its reinforcing properties (see the 1987 work by Ritz *et al.*), yet the involvement of this inhibition in chronic cocaine use is much less clear. Studies in humans to investigate changes in dopamine transporters after chronic administration of cocaine have yielded inconsistent results, with reports documenting increases[47] as well as decreases in DA transporters.[48,49] We used PET and [^{11}C]cocaine to evaluate dopamine transporter availability as well as cocaine uptake in the brain of detoxified cocaine abusers.[50] For this purpose we evaluated 12 cocaine abusers between 3 and 6 weeks of detoxification. Four of these cocaine abusers were rescanned after they completed a 3-month inpatient rehabilitation period. Twenty normal subjects were used as control and 8 of them underwent a second scan 3 to 12 weeks later to assess the reproducibility of repeated measurements. We also evaluated the relationship between DA transporter and DA D_2 receptor availability in those subjects for whom we had also obtained scans with [^{18}F]*N*-methylspiroperidol (NMS). Cocaine abusers had significantly lower uptake of [^{11}C]cocaine in brain (6.2 ± 1% dose/cc tissues) than did controls (7.7 ± 2%). The distribution volumes (DV) for [^{11}C]cocaine were reduced in basal ganglia (BG), cortex, thalamus, and cerebellum (CB) of cocaine abusers. However, there were no differences in the ratio of the distribution volume in basal ganglia to that in cerebellum, which is an estimate of dopamine transporter availability. Values for dopamine D_2 receptor availability were decreased in cocaine abusers and did not correlate with estimates of dopamine transporter availability. In summary, this study showed decreased brain uptake of cocaine as well as decreases in regional DVs for cocaine in the brain of cocaine abusers. However, there was no evidence of changes in DA transporter availability (high-affinity recognition sites) in detoxified cocaine abusers. Future studies are required to determine the extent to which the decrease in binding of

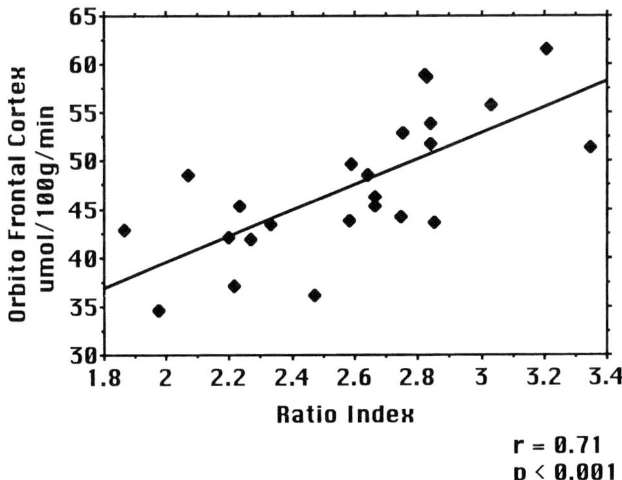

FIGURE 6. Association of glucose metabolism and dopamine D_2 receptors in cocaine abusers. A strong association is shown between low levels of dopamine D_2 receptors (ratio index) and low metabolism in orbitofrontal cortex. (Modified from Volkow *et al.*[34])

cocaine in the cocaine abusers reflects a change in the conformational state of the transporter.

CONCLUSION

In summary, imaging studies in cocaine addicts have started to provide evidence of brain neurochemical and functional changes that may account for their impulsive behavior and loss of control over their intake of drugs. They have also been useful in identifying dynamic parameters that are relevant to the reinforcing properties of psychostimulant drugs in humans. This information can be used in turn to help develop new therapeutic intervention to prevent cocaine's effects as well as to increase the likelihood of recovery of the cocaine addict. It is also hoped that this knowledge will help change the attitude towards the addict as not someone with a "moral fault" but as someone suffering from a disease.

REFERENCES

1. Fowler, J. S., A. P. Wolf & N. D. Volkow. 1990. New directions in positron emission tomography. *In* Annual Reports in Medicinal Chemistry, J. A. Bristol. Ed.: 261–269. Academic Press. San Diego, CA.
2. Sokoloff, L., M. Reivich, C. Kennedy, M. H. Des Rosiers, C. S. Patlak, K. D. Pettigrew, O. Sakurada & M. Shinohara. 1977. The [^{14}C] deoxyglucose method for the measurement of local cerebral glucose utilization: Theory procedure and normal values in the conscious and anesthetized albino rat. J. Neurochem. **28:** 897–916.
3. Volkow, N. D., J. S. Fowler, J. S. Gatley, J. Logan, G.-J. Wang, Y.-S. Ding & S. L. Dewey. Evaluation of the human brain dopamine system with PET: review and update of tracers. J. Nucl. Med. In press.
4. Koob, G. F. & F. E. Bloom. 1988. Cellular and molecular mechanisms of drug dependence. Science **242:** 715–723.
5. Gawin, F. H. & E. H. Ellinwood. 1988. Cocaine and other stimulants. New Eng. J. Med. **318:** 1173–1181.
6. Johanson, C. E. & M. W. Fischman. 1989. The pharmacology of cocaine related to its abuse. Pharm. Rev. **41:** 3–52.
7. Ritz, M. C., R. J. Lamb, S. R. Goldberg & M. J. Kuhar. 1987. Cocaine receptors on dopamine transporters are related to self administration of cocaine. Science **237:** 1219–1223.
8. Fowler, J. S., N. D. Volkow, A. P. Wolf, S. L. Dewey, D. Schlyer & R. R. MacGregor. 1989. Mapping cocaine binding sites in human and baboon brain in vivo. Synapse **4:** 371–377.
9. Volkow, N. D., Fowler, J. S., Wolf, A. P., Wang, G.-J., Logan, J., MacGregor, R., Dewey, S. L., Schlyer, D. J. & R. Hitzemann. 1992. Distribution of ^{11}C-Cocaine in human heart, lungs, liver and adrenals. A dynamic PET study. J. Nucl. Med. **33:** 521–525.
10. Seifen, E., L. M. Plunkett & R. H. Kennedy. 1989. Cardiovascular and lethal effects of cocaine in anesthetized dogs and guinea pigs. Arch. Int. Pharmacodyn. **300:** 241–253.
11. Fowler, J. S., Y. S. Ding, N. D. Volkow, T. Martin, R. MacGregor, S. L. Dewey, P. King, D. Pappas, N. Alexoff, C. Shea, J. Gatley, D. Schlyer & A. P. Wolf. 1994. PET studies of cocaine inhibition of the myocardial norepinephrine uptake. Synapse **16:** 312–317.
12. Chiueh, C. C. & I. J. Kopin. 1978. Endogenous epinephrine and norepinephrine from the sympathoadrenal medullary system of unanesthetized rats. J. Pharmacol. Exp. Ther. **205:** 148–154.

13. WILENS, T. E. & J. BIEDERMAN. 1992. The stimulants. Pediat. Psychopharmacol. **15:** 191–222.
14. BARKLEY, R. A. 1977. A review of stimulant drug research with hyperactive children. J. Child Psychol. Psychiat. **8:** 137–165.
15. MEYER, J. S., F. SAKAI, I. KARACAN, S. DERMAN & M. YAMAMOTO. 1980. Sleep apnea, narcolepsy, and dreaming: Regional cerebral hemodynamics. Ann. Neurol. **7:** 479–485.
16. VOLKOW, N. D., U. DING, J. S. FOWLER, G-J. WANG, J. LOGAN, S. J. GATLEY, S. L. DEWEY, C. ASHBY, J. LIEBERMAN, R. HITZEMANN & A. P. WOLF. 1995. Is methylphenidate like cocaine? Studies on their pharmacokinetics and distribution in human brain. Arch. Gen. Psychiatry **52:** 456–463.
17. GRANT, B. F. & T. C. HARFORD. 1990. Concurrent and simultaneous use of alcohol with cocaine: Results of national survey. Drug & Alcohol Dependence **25:** 97–104.
18. BOAG, F., & C. W. H. HAVARD. 1985. Cardiac arrhythmia and myocardial ischaemia related to cocaine and alcohol consumption. Postgrad. Med. J. **61:** 997–999.
19. HEARN, W. L., D. D. FLYNN, G. W. HIME, S. ROSE, J. C. COFINO, E. MANTERO-ATIENZA, C. V. WETLI & D. C. MASH. 1991. Cocaethylene: a unique cocaine metabolite displays high affinity for the dopamine transporter. J. Neurochem. **56:** 698–701.
20. HEARN, W. L., S. ROSE, J. WAGNER, A. CIARLEGLIO & D. C. MASH. 1991. Cocaethylene is more potent than cocaine in mediating lethality. Pharmacol. Biochem. Behavior **39:** 531–533.
21. FOWLER, J. S., N. D. VOLKOW, R. R. MACGREGOR, J. LOGAN, S. L. DEWEY, S. J. GATLEY & A. P. WOLF. 1992. Comparative PET studies of the kinetics and distribution of cocaine and cocaethylene in baboon brain. Synapse **12:** 220–227.
22. CARROLL, F. I., A. H. LEWIN, J. W. BOJA & M. J. KUHAR. 1992. Cocaine receptor: Biochemical characterization and structure–activity relationships of cocaine analogues at the dopamine transporter. J. Med. Chem. **35:** 969–981.
23. CLARKE, R. L., S. J. DAUM, A. J. GAMBINO, M. D. ACETO, J. PEARL, M. LEVITT, W. R. & E. F. BOGADO. 1973. Compounds affecting the central nervous system 4 3-b-phenyltropane-2-carboxylic esters and analogs. J. Med. Chem. **16:** 1260–1267.
24. MADRAS, B. K., R. D. SPEALMAN, M. A. FAHEY, J. L. NEUMEYER, J. K. SAHA & R. A. MILIUS. 1989. Cocaine receptors labeled by [^{3}H]2b-carbomethoxy-3b-(4-fluorophenyl)tropane. Mol. Pharmacol. **36:** 518–524.
25. INNIS, R. B., J. P. SEIBYL, B. E. SCANLEY, M. LARUELLE, A. ABI-DARGHAM, E. WALLACE, R. M. BALDWIN, Y. ZEA-PONCE, S. S. ZOGHBI, S. WANG, Y. GUO, J. L. NEUMEYER, D. S. CHARNEY, P. B. HOFFER & K. L. MAREK. 1993. Single photon emission computed tomographic imaging demonstrates loss of striatal dopamine transporters in Parkinson disease. Proc. Natl. Acad. Sci. USA **90:** 11965–11969.
26. VOLKOW, N. D., S. J. GATLEY, J. S. FOWLER, J. LOGAN, S. L. DEWEY, Y-S. DING, N. PAPPAS, P. KING, R. R. MACGREGOR, M. J. KUHAR, F. I. CARROLL & A. P. WOLF. 1995. Long-lasting inhibition of in vivo cocaine binding to dopamine transporters by 3β-(4-iodophenyl)tropane-2-carboxylic acid methyl ester; RTI-55 or βCIT. Synapse **19:** 206–211.
27. VOLKOW, N. D., N. MULLANI, L. GOULD, K. KRAJEWSKI, & S. ADLER. 1988. Cerebral blood flow in chronic cocaine users. Br. J. Psychiatry **152:** 641–648.
28. ALTURA, B. M., B. T. ALTURA & A. GEBREWOLD. 1985. Cocaine induces spasms of cerebral blood vessels: Relation to cerebral vascular accidents, strokes and hypertension. Fed. Proc. **44:** 1637.
29. MENA, I., B. MILLER & K. GARRETT. 1989. Neurospect in cocaine abuse: rCBF and HMPAO findings. Clin. Nucl. Med.: 1412.
30. TUMEH, S. S., J. S. NAGEL, R. J. ENGLISH, M. MOORE & B. L. HOLMAN. 1991. Use of SPECT perfusion brain scintigraphy to investigate effects of cocaine in the brain. *In* Physiopathology of Illicit Drugs: Cannabis, Cocaine, Opiates. G. C. Nahas & C. Latur, Eds.: 145–150. Pergamon Press. Oxford.
31. LEVIN, S. R. & K. M. A. WELCH. 1987. Cocaine and stroke: Current concepts of cerebrovascular disease. Stroke **22:** 15.
32. LICHTENFELD, P. J., D. B. RUBIN & R. S. FELDMAN. 1984. Subarachnoid hemorrhage precipitated by cocaine snorting. Arch. Neurol. **41:** 223.

33. LEVIN, J. M., J. H. MENDELSON, L. B. HOLMAN, S. K. TEOH, B. GARADA, R. B. SCHWARTZ & N. K. MELLO. 1995. Improved regional cerebral blood flow in chronic cocaine polydrug users treated with buprenorphine. J. Nucl. Med. **36:** 1211–1215.
34. LONDON, E. D., N. G. CASCELLA, D. F. WONG, R. L. PHILLIPS, R. F. DANNALS, J. M. LINKS, R. HERNING, R. GRAYSON, J. H. JAFFE & H. N. WAGNER. 1990. Cocaine-induced reduction of glucose utilization in human brain. A study using positron emission tomography and [fluorine-18]-fluorodeoxyglucose. Arch General Psychiatry **47:** 567–574.
35. RITZ, M. C., R. J. LAMB, S. R. GOLDBERG & M. J. KUHAR. 1987. Cocaine receptors on dopamine transporters are related to self-administration of cocaine. Science **237:** 1219–1223.
36. DEWIT, H., & R. A. WISE. 1977. Blockade of cocaine reinforcement in rats with the dopamine receptor blockers pimozide but not with the noradrenergic blokers phentolamine or phenoxybenzamine. Can. J. Psychol. **31:** 195–203.
37. ROBERTS, D. C. S., M. E. CORCORAN & H. C. FIBIGER. 1977. On the role of ascending catecholaminergic systems in intravenous self-administration of cocaine. Pharmacol. Biochem. Behav. **6:** 615–620.
38. WOOLVERTON, W. L. & K. M. JOHNSON. 1992. Neurobiology of cocaine abuse. Trends Pharm. Sci. **13:** 193–200.
39. GALLOWAY, M. P. 1988. Neurochemical interactions of cocaine with dopaminergic systems. TIPS **9:** 45.
40. DACHIS, C. A. & M. S. GOLD. 1985. New concepts in cocaine addiction: The dopamine depletion hypothesis. Neurosci. Biobehav. Rev. **9:** 469–477.
41. VOLKOW, N. D., J. S. FOWLER, A. P. WOLF, R. HITZEMANN, S. L. DEWEY, B. BENDRIEM, R. ALPERT & A. HOFF. 1991. Changes in brain glucose metabolism in cocaine dependence and withdrawal. Am. J. Psych. **148:** 621–626.
42. VOLKOW, N. D., J. S. FOWLER, A. P. WOLF, D. SHLYER, CH. Y. SHIUE, R. ALBERT, S. L. DEWEY, J. LOGAN, B. BENDRIEM, D. CHRISTMAN, R. HITZEMANN & F. HENN. 1990. Effects of chronic cocaine abuse on postsynaptic dopamine receptors. Am. J. Psychiatry **147:** 719–724.
43. VOLKOW, N. D., R. HITZEMANN, G. J. WANG, J. S. FOWLER, A. P. WOLF & S. L. DEWEY. 1992. Long-term frontal brain metabolic changes in cocaine abusers. Synapse **11:** 184–190.
44. VOLKOW, N. D., J. S. FOWLER, G.-J. WANG, R. HITZEMANN, J. LOGAN, D. SCHLYER, S. L. DEWEY & A. P. WOLF. 1993. Decreased dopamine D2 receptor availability is associated with reduced frontal metabolism in cocaine abusers. Synapse **14:** 169–177.
45. KOLB, B. 1977. Studies on the caudate putamen and the dorsomedial thalamic nucleus: Implications for mammalian frontal lobe function. Physiol. Behav. **18:** 237–244.
46. LE MOAL, M. & H. SIMON. 1991. Mesocorticolimbic dopaminergic network: Functional and regulatory notes. Physiol. Rev. **71:** 155–234.
47. LITTLE, K. Y., J. A. KIRKMAN, F. I. CARROL, T. B. CLARK & G. E. DUNCAN. 1993. Cocaine use increases [^{3}H]WIN 35428 binding sites in human striatum. Brain Res. **62:** 17–25.
48. HITRI, A., M. F. CASANOVA, J. E. KLEINMAN & R. J. WYATT. 1994. Fewer dopamine transporter receptors in the prefrontal cortex of cocaine users. Am. J. Psychiatry **151:**7: 1074–1076.
49. HURD, Y. L. & M. HERKENHAM. 1993. Molecular alterations in the neostriatum of human cocaine addicts. Synapse **13:** 357–369.
50. VOLKOW, N. D., G.-J. WANG, J. S. FOWLER, J. LOGAN, R. HITZEMANN, S. J. GATLEY, R. R. MACGREGOR & A. P. WOLF. 1996. Cocaine binding is decreased in the brain of detoxified cocaine abusers. J. Neuropsychopharmacol. **14:** 159–168.

DISCUSSION

QUESTION: Concerning the technique and what you see and you know for sure, do you necessarily know that Carbon-11 is associated with the cocaine?

N. D. VOLKOW: That is a very important and crucial question. The majority of the images from PET show carbon-11 or fluorine, so we must ask to what extent the images do reflect the carbon-11 bound to cocaine or whether they correspond to labeled metabolites. In the case of cocaine we labeled the molecule at different positions and compared its regional accumulation and distribution using PET in the baboon brain. We also did experiments in rats in which we directly measured the concentration of carbon-11 that was bound to cocaine versus that which was free or bound to metabolites. When cocaine is labeled on the N-methyl group, which is the way we use it for PET studies, C-11 is mostly bound to cocaine. Thus for a given PET radio tracer one has to do the background binding work to determine that the label is in fact in the parent compound. The same is true, in the case of C-11 methylphenidate. We have measured the fate of C-11 in brain, and what we are observing is predominantly C-11methylphenidate.

QUESTION: A decrease in dopamine receptors is seen in cocaine abuse. Is the same true for repeated administration and dosing with methylphenidate?

VOLKOW: We do not know. We have not investigated repeated users of methylphenidate. There are two possibilities, of course, and one is to work with persons with narcolepsy who are taking methylphenidate, but that is a very different situation because it is given orally, which gives different effects from intravenous administration. There are very few intravenous methylphenidate abusers. Logistically it is a very difficult study to perform.

COMMENT: A recent newspaper article reported an increase in methylphenidate abuse.

VOLKOW: Yes, there has been a reported increase in the use of intravenous methylphenidate in the United States as well as some isolated case reports in Europe. Because of its very slow clearance, methylphenidate has less potential for addiction. Experiments show that repeated methylphenidate administration, with its slow clearance, leads to increased side effects, which in turn make the reinforcing properties less likely. The subjects become much more restless, and their cardiovascular effects are much more long-lasting; so when you repeatedly administer the drug, the side effects become more prominent than with repeated cocaine administration.

In Vivo Imaging of Fatty Acid Incorporation into Brain to Examine Signal Transduction and Neuroplasticity Involving Phospholipids

STANLEY I. RAPOPORT,[a] DAVID PURDON, H. UMESHA SHETTY, ERIC GRANGE, QUENTIN SMITH, COLLINS JONES, AND MICHAEL C. J. CHANG

Laboratory of Neurosciences
National Institute on Aging
National Institutes of Health
Bethesda, Maryland 20892

INTRODUCTION

Phospholipids are major components of neuronal and glial membranes that are involved in membrane synthesis, neuroplasticity, and signal transduction.[1–4] Abnormal phospholipid metabolism occurs in a number of human brain diseases, including malignant brain tumors,[5] Alzheimer's disease,[6] stroke and trauma,[7] and heavy metal or drug toxicity.[8,9] Thus, it would be of interest to have an *in vivo* method to localize and quantify different aspects of phospholipid metabolism in the human brain.

Our laboratory has developed a method and supporting model with this goal in mind.[10] Animal studies show that, following an intravenous injection of a long-chain fatty acid (FA), the method can be used to image and interpret brain phospholipid metabolism when employing quantitative autoradiography or positron emission tomography (PET) to quantify regional brain radioactivity.[11] Additional chemical analysis of brain can provide data for interpreting the imaging observations using operational equations. In this paper, we discuss these studies and their potential clinical applications.

[a] Address for correspondence: Dr. Stanley I. Rapoport, Laboratory of Neurosciences, National Institute on Aging, Bldg. 10, Rm. 6C-103, National Institutes of Health, Bethesda, Maryland 20892; phone: 301/496-1765; fax: 301/402-0074; e-mail: SIR@HELIX.NIH.GOV

ABBREVIATIONS: CBF, cerebral blood flow; CoA, coenzyme A; 1,4,5-IP_3, inositol 1,4,5-trisphosphate; FA, fatty acid; MEP, methyl palmoxirate; MRI, magnetic resonance imaging; NBM, nucleus basalis of Meynert; PC, phosphatidylcholine; PET, positron emission tomography; PLA_2, phospholipase A_2; PLC, phospholipase C; PE, phosphatidylethanolamine; PI, phosphatidylinositol; PS, phosphatidylserine; $rCMR_{glc}$, regional cerebral metabolic rate for glucose; *sn*, stereospecifically numbered position

FATTY ACID MODEL

FIGURE 1 illustrates the two brain compartments that need to be assessed to use the model to evaluate brain phospholipid metabolism: (i) a rapidly turning over precursor FA(acyl)-coenzyme A(CoA) pool whose specific activity equilibrates rapidly with plasma specific activity (<1 min); and (ii) a more "stable" phospholipid/neutral lipid compartment in which FA turnover is comparatively slow.[10] Fluxes J_1, J_2, J_3, J_{oxid} and J_{FA} are defined in the legend

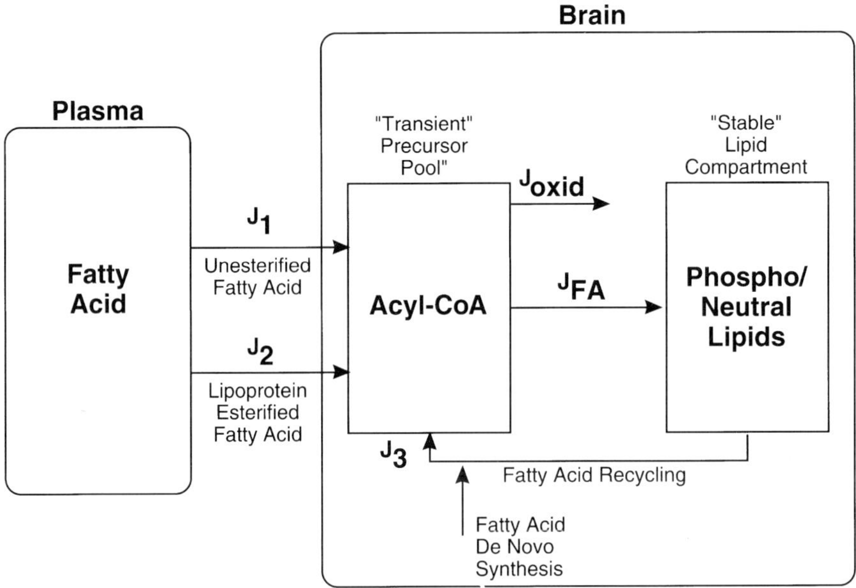

FIGURE 1. Diagram for uptake of a FA from plasma into the brain FA(acyl)–CoA pool and thence into "stable" phospholipids and neutral lipids. J_1, flux of unesterified FA from plasma into FA–CoA; J_2, flux of esterified FA from plasma lipoproteins into FA–CoA; J_3, flux from recycling and *de novo* synthesis from stable lipids into FA–CoA; J_{oxid}, flux of FA from brain FA–CoA into the aqueous compartment, following oxidation in brain mitochondria or microsomes; J_{FA}, net flux of unlabeled FA from FA–CoA to "stable" lipids.

to FIGURE 1. Uptake of a fatty acid from blood into brain and its incorporation into the lipid compartment are independent of cerebral blood flow (CBF) and thus reflect brain metabolism only (TABLE 1).[12,13] Flow-independence arises because >99.99% of plasma FA is bound to plasma albumin, the FA is rapidly released from protein as blood passes through brain (1-sec off-rate), FA permeability at brain capillaries is very high, and unacylated FA in plasma equilibrates very rapidly with brain FA-CoA.

TABLE 1. Effect of Hypercapnia on Incorporation of [9,10-^{3}H]palmitic Acid into Rat Brain

Treatment Group (No.)	P_{CO2} (mm Hg)	Incorporation Coefficient, k* (ml · sec^{-1} per g brain × 10^6) Total Brain	Lipid
Control, awake (6)	41 ± 2	131 ± 7	112.1 ± 6.1
Hypercapnia, awake (3)	66 ± 2[a,b]	131 ± 4	113.3 ± 2.2

NOTE: Mean ± SEM differs significantly from control, [a]$p < 0.001$. k* defined by Equation 2 in text. From Yamazaki *et al.*[12]

[b]CBF increases 2- to 4-fold with this degree of hypercapnia.

Operational Equations for Rates of Incorporation of FAs into and Half-lives within Brain Phospholipids

Rapid equilibration between plasma and the brain FA–CoA pool allows increased neuronal demand for FA to be easily met by the large reservoir of unacylated FA in plasma. As illustrated in FIGURE 2, 2 minutes after a step elevation of [9,10-^{3}H]palmitate in plasma, specific activity of the palmitoyl–CoA pool in brain is at a steady state.[14] At the steady state, the ratio of palmitoyl–CoA-specific activity to plasma palmitate–specific activity (λ, Equation 3 below) is only 0.016, attesting to marked dilution of radioactive palmitoyl–CoA derived from plasma by recycled unlabeled palmitate from brain phospholipids (FIG. 1). Incorporation of palmitic acid into stable brain lipids from palmitoyl–CoA also is very rapid, as 82% of parenchymal brain

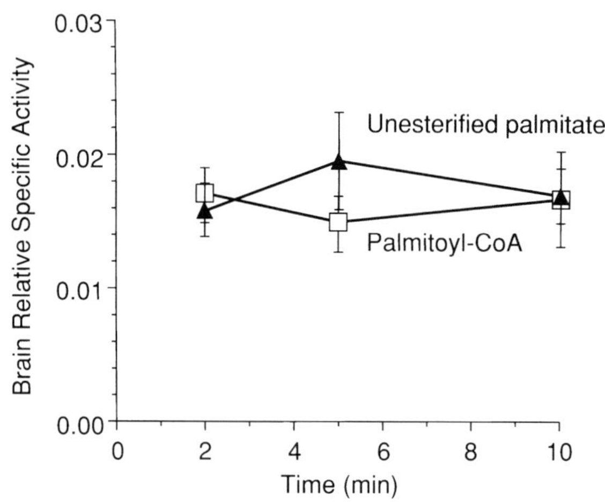

FIGURE 2. Specific activity of brain unacylated palmitic acid and palmitoyl–CoA pools, at different times after step-elevation in plasma [9,10-^{3}H]palmitate in awake rats. Mean ± SEM for 3–6 animals. (From Grange *et al.*[14] Reproduced by permission.)

radioactivity is acylated within stable lipids within only 2 min after a labeled FA infusion (FIG. 3).[14] With regard to arachidonate, steady-state specific activity of brain arachidonoyl–CoA in anesthetized rats is reached within 1 min after infusion is initiated, when 90% of label is incorporated into stable brain lipids.[15]

Operational equations to examine FA flux and turnover within individual brain phospholipids have been derived.[10] Thus, the net rate of incorporation $J_{FA,i}$ ($\Sigma_i J_{FA,i} = J_{FA}$) of an unlabeled FA from the FA–CoA pool into brain phospholipid i (FIG. 1), equals:

$$J_{FA,i} = k_i^* c_{pl}/\lambda \quad (1)$$

where c_{pl} is unlabeled plasma unacylated FA concentration and k_i^*(cm$^3 \cdot$ sec^{-1} per g brain) is the incorporation coefficient of unacylated FA from plasma into

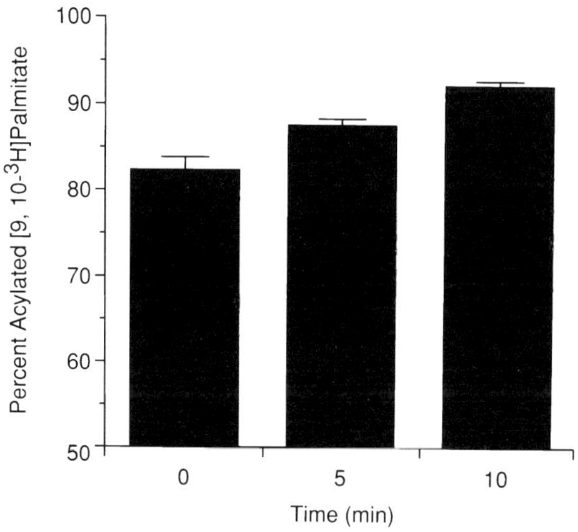

FIGURE 3. Percent acylated [9,10-^{3}H]palmitate in brain parenchyma of anesthetized rat, at various times after establishing a steady state plasma-specific activity by i.v. infusion. Each *bar* represents mean + SEM for 3–6 animals. (From Grange *et al.*[14] Reproduced by permission.)

phospholipid i. k_i^* equals brain radioactivity $c_{br,i}^*(T)$ in phospholipid i at time T of sampling, divided by the integral of plasma unesterified FA radioactivity from the beginning of infusion to time T:

$$k_i^* = c_{br,i}^* \bigg/ \int_0^T c_{pl}^* \, dt \quad (2)$$

where λ is the extent to which brain FA–CoA radioactivity derived from labeled unacylated FA (J_1) in plasma is diluted by unlabeled FA derived from acylated plasma sources (J_2) and from brain recycling and *de novo* synthesis

(J_3). This dilution factor λ equals the ratio of the steady state specific activity of FA–CoA in brain to the specific activity of the unacylated FA in plasma:

$$\lambda = \frac{J_1}{J_1 + J_2 + J_3} \quad (3)$$

As $J_2 \ll J_1$ in adult animals,[16] very low experimentally determined values for λ in awake rats, 0.011 for arachidonate, and 0.016 for palmitate,[14,15,17] reflect extensive recycling (release and reuptake) within brain phospholipids.

At a steady state, turnover (% per unit time) $F_{FA,i}$ of a fatty acid in phospholipid i equals:

$$F_{FA,i} = \frac{J_{FA,i}}{c_{br,i}} = \frac{k_i^* c_{pl}}{\lambda c_{br,i}} \quad (4)$$

TABLE 2. Distribution of Radioactivity within Brain Lipid Fractions in Awake Rats, 15 min after a 5-min i.v. Infusion of Each of Three Labeled Fatty Acids

	Fatty Acid Tracer (% Total Brain Radioactivity)		
Fraction	[9,10-^{3}H]palmitate	[1-^{14}C]arachidonate	[1-^{14}C]docosa-hexaenoate
Lipid fraction	89.2 ± 1.1	89.4 ± 0.5	87.1 ± 1.0
Phospholipids	51.7 ± 0.6	72.9 ± 0.8	64.7 ± 0.9
Sphingomyelin	1.21 ± 0.18	—	—
Phosphatidylcholine	31.7 ± 1.1	27.4 ± 0.2	17.2 ± 0.8
Phosphatidylserine	0.92 ± 0.20	2.09 ± 0.3	2.59 ± 0.30
Phosphatidylinositol	7.34 ± 0.20	35.6 ± 0.4	6.92 ± 0.68
Phosphatidylethanolamine	10.5 ± 0.9	7.14 ± 0.22	37.6 ± 0.8

NOTE: Values are means ± SEM for 3–7 rats. From Nariai *et al.*[5] and Noronha *et al.*[19]

and thus the half-life ($t_{1/2,i}$) of the FA in i equals:

$$t_{1/2,i} = 0.693/F_{FA,i} \quad (5)$$

EXPERIMENTAL APPLICATION OF FA MODEL

Labeling and Half-lives of FAs in Brain Phospholipids

Specificity of Phospholipid Labeling

Following an i.v. bolus injection of a radiolabeled FA, brain labeling peaks within 10 min (FIG. 3) and is mainly in stable lipids (80%–90%),[15,14] particularly phospholipids (TABLES 2 and 3). Regional differences in brain incorporation can be distinguished on autoradiographs (FIG. 5). Regional

TABLE 3. Distribution of Radiolabeled Fatty Acids within *sn*-1 and *sn*-2 Positions of Brain Phospholipids That Receive Most of the Label 15 min after i.v. Injection in Awake Rats

Fatty Acid Tracer	Phospholipid	Percent Distribution of Radiolabel: *sn*-1 Position	*sn*-2 Position
[9,10-^{3}H]palmitate	PC	82.5 ± 1.9	17.5 ± 1.9
	PE	90.7 ± 0.5	9.3 ± 0.5
[1-^{14}C]arachidonate	PC	7.8 ± 1.9	92.2 ± 1.9
	PI	0.0 ± 0.0	100 ± 0
[1-^{14}C]docosahexaenoate	PC	22.9 ± 5.2	77.1 ± 5.2
	PE	0 ± 0	100 ± 0

NOTE: Values are mean ± SEM for 3–7 rats. From Nariai *et al.*[5]

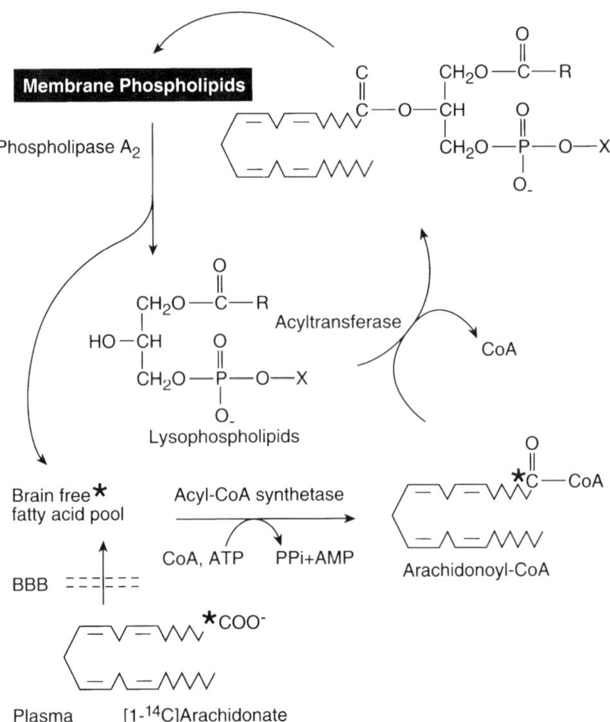

FIGURE 4. Cycling of arachidonate in membrane phospholipid. Following activation of PLA_2, unlabeled arachidonate that is released from a phospholipid (*upper right*) is reacylated into the brain arachidonoyl–CoA pool. The latter has been prelabeled by labeled unacylated [1-^{14}C]arachidonate in plasma (*asterisk*) and provides labeled tracer for reincorporation into resultant lysophospholipids.

differences vary and reflect the tracer employed. Thus, tracer palmitate labels mainly the stereospecifically numbered-1 (*sn*-1) position of phosphatidylcholine (PC), tracer arachidonate enters mainly the *sn*-2 position of phosphatidylinositol (PI) and PC, and tracer docosahexaenoate enters mainly the *sn*-2 position of phosphatidylethanolamine (PE) and PC.[18–20] Combined use of the three FA tracers can provide information about the metabolism of acyl groups at specific *sn* positions of different brain phospholipids.

Half-lives of FAs in Individual Phospholipids

Half-lives (Eq. 5) of arachidonate and palmitate within different phospholipid classes of rat brain have been determined[14,17] using experimental values of λ. Of the four phospholipids studied, TABLE 4 shows that for each of the two FAs, $t_{1/2,i}$ is relatively short in PI, consistent with participation by PI in signal transduction involving phospholipase C (PLC) and/or phospholipase A_2 (PLA_2).[2,3] $t_{1/2,i}$ for palmitate ranges from 2.3 hr in PI to 13.3 hr in phosphatidylserine (PS), compared with some 30- to 50-fold-longer published values of 3–23 days.[1] The published values were obtained by injecting FA tracer intracerebrally and measuring rates of decline of label in brain phospholipids, and likely are erroneous because they ignore dilution of the precursor FA-CoA pool (Eqs. 4 and 5).

TABLE 4. Half-lives of Fatty Acids within Individual Phospholipids of the Cerebral Cortex of Awake Rats

	Phospholipid Class			
	PC	PS	PI	PE
Fatty Acid		$t_{1/2,i}$, hr		
Palmitate (16:0)	11.5	13.3	2.3	12.0
Arachidonate (20:4)	1.7	8.3	0.66	23.8

NOTE: Data calculated as described[10] using λ = 0.011 for arachidonate and 0.016 for palmitate.[13,14,15]

Arachidonate has very short half-lives within PC and PI, reflecting its participation as a second messenger in PLA_2-mediated signal transduction (TABLE 4). The low half-lives are consistent with the very rapid incorporation of labeled arachidonate into brain lipids, suggested in FIGURE 3. Indeed, in two molecular species of PC (16:1–20:4 and 18:2–20:4), $t_{1/2,i}$ of arachidonate is only 5 min,[21] suggesting involvement of these species in dynamic brain phospholipid metabolism, possibly as preferred substrates for PLA_2.

PLA_2 Activity Measured with Labeled Arachidonate or Docosahexaenoate

Imaging PLA_2 Activation during Acute Cholinergic Stimulation

Receptor-mediated signal transduction may involve activation of PLA_2 to release the second messenger arachidonic acid, or activation of PLC to release diacylglycerol and inositol 1,4,5-trisphosphate (1,4,5-IP_3).[2,3] In the latter case, PLA_2 could be stimulated indirectly *via* activation of protein kinase C by diacylglycerol, or by mobilization of intracellular Ca^{2+} by 1,4,5-IP_3. A 14-kDA PLA_2, a 85-kDA cytosolic PLA_2 found in astrocytes, and a 40-kDA cytosolic PLA_2 have been identified in the brain.[22] These forms have different specificities for phospholipids.

Certain neurotransmitters and neurotransmitter agonists, including the M1 cholinergic agonist arecoline, can activate brain PLA_2 directly *via* receptors coupled to membrane-bound GTP-binding proteins, thereby releasing polyunsaturated acyl groups from *sn*-2 positions of phospholipids.[3] In a release–recovery cycle for such a process, illustrated in FIGURE 4 for arachidonate, reincorporation of released FA into newly available lysophospholipid occurs rapidly *via* unacylated FA and arachidonoyl–CoA, to reform the intact phospholipid. By prelabeling the brain FA and FA–CoA pools with an intravenous injection of labeled arachidonate prior to drug administration, increased incorporation of label at sites of PLA_2 activation can be quantified and localized using *in vivo* imaging.

Neurochemical analysis shows that arecoline given to rats increases incorporation of injected [1-^{14}C]arachidonate into the *sn*-2 position of brain PI and PC, and of [1-^{14}C]docosahexaenoate into the *sn*-2 position of PE and PC, without changing [9,10-^{3}H]palmitate incorporation, whereas autoradiography shows that 83% of M1 sites in the brain have increased label (FIG. 5).[20] Increased incorporation of labeled arachidonate can be entirely blocked by the muscarinic antagonist atropine (TABLE 5) or partially blocked by the PLA_2 inhibitor manoalide.[20,23] The increase is found mainly within phospholipids of brain membrane fractions that demonstrate the presynaptic marker synaptophysin (TABLE 6).[24] These results suggest that locally increased labeling is mediated by PLA_2-activated release of polyunsaturated FAs from phospholipids at M1 synaptic sites.

Imaging Reduced FA Incorporation during Acutely Reduced Functional Activity

Incorporation of labeled arachidonate and docosahexaenoate, but not of labeled palmitate, will change in response to acute decreases or increases of brain functional activity, reflecting the fact that PLA_2-mediated signal transduction involving the two polyunsaturated fatty acids is acutely coupled to regional energy consumption. Thus, 1 day after unilateral orbital enucleation in a rat, values of k* for labeled arachidonate and docosahexaenoate, but not for labeled palmitate, are reduced in contralateral visual areas, in proportion to

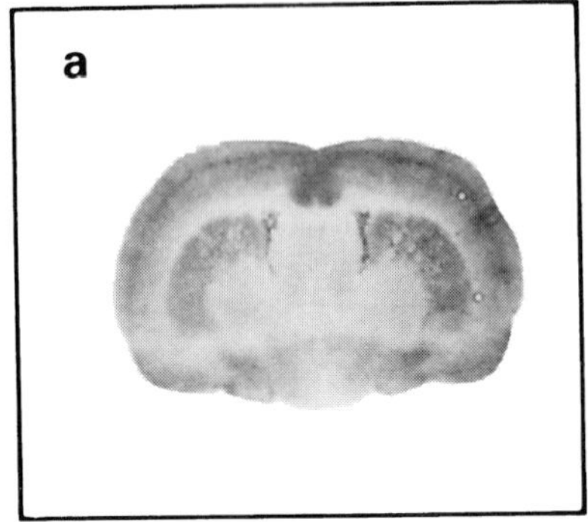

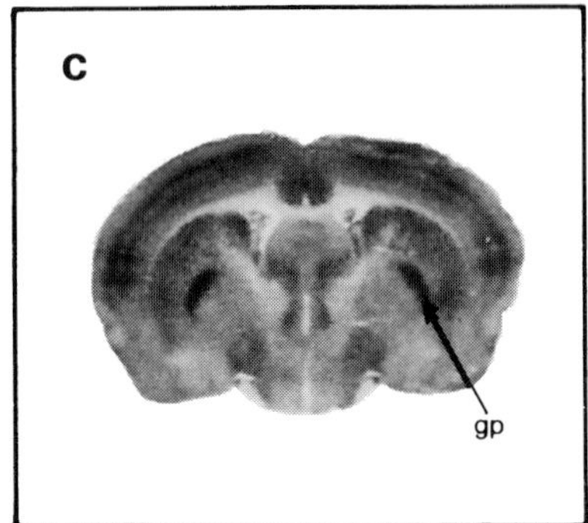

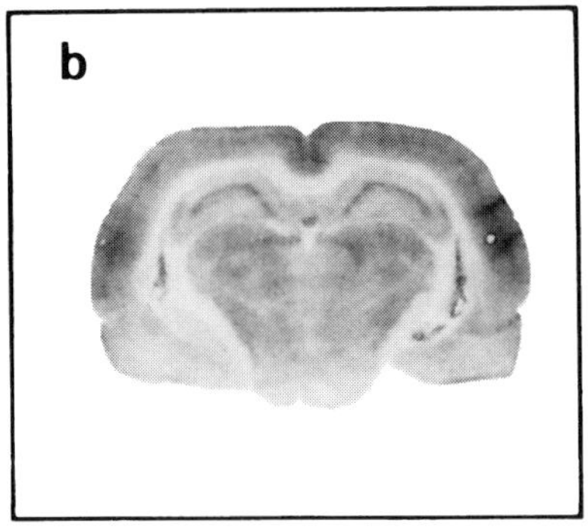

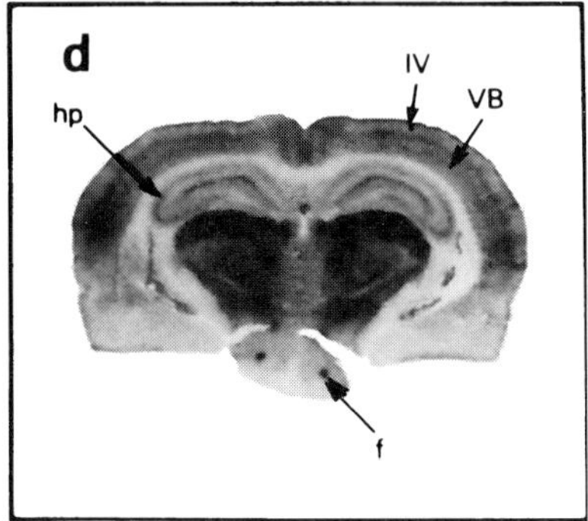

FIGURE 5. Autoradiographs of coronal sections of the brain from a rat given i.p. saline and [1-^{14}C]arachidonate (*left*) or i.p. arecoline and i.v. [1-^{14}C]arachidonate (*right*). *Highlighted areas* (gp = globus pallidus, hp = CA2 region hippocampus; IV and VB = layers IV and VB of cortex; f = mammalothalamic tract) are known to have high densities of M1 cholinergic receptors (unpublished observation).

reduced functional activity measured as the regional cerebral metabolic rate for glucose, $rCMR_{glc}$.[25,26] Similarly, visual stimulation of the intact eye at day 1 increases both $rCMR_{glc}$ and values for k* for labeled arachidonate and docosahexaenoate, but not for palmitate in central visual areas ipsilateral to enucleation.

Imaging Up-regulated PLA_2-Mediated Signal Transduction

Upregulated PLA_2-mediated signal transduction can be imaged. The nucleus basalis of Meynert (NBM) normally provides cholinergic input to the

TABLE 5. Unidirectional Whole-Brain Incorporation Coefficients for Fatty Acid Tracers, Measured 15 min Following 5-min i.v. Infusion of Radiolabel and i.p. Administration of 15 mg · kg^{-1} Arecoline in Awake Rats

	Unidirectional Incorporation Coefficient, k*, $cm^3 \cdot sec^{-1}$ per g brain × 10^{-4}		
Fatty Acid/Treatment[a]	Control	Arecoline	Change
[9,10-^{3}H]palmitate	0.88 ± 0.06	0.94 ± 0.04	+11%
[1-^{14}C]docosahexaenoate	3.08 ± 0.14	4.48 ± 0.26[b]	+48%
[1-^{14}C]arachidonate	3.13 ± 0.18	4.42 ± 0.27[b]	+41%
[1-^{14}C]arachidonate ± 4 mg/kg atropine	3.30 ± 0.15	2.54 ± 0.31	−24%

NOTE: Mean ± SEM for 3–9 animals. From DeGeorge *et al.*[20]

[a]Atropine was given prior to arecoline infusion in one set of experiments, whereas methylatropine was administered routinely to prevent peripheral effects of arecoline.

[b]Differs significantly from control mean, $p < 0.05$.

ipsilateral neocortex and is pathological in Alzheimer's disease.[27] In response to arecoline (see above), rats in which the NBM has been unilaterally lesioned 2 weeks earlier show increased incorporation of labeled arachidonate into denervated cortical regions ipsilateral to the lesion (FIG. 6). These cortical regions demonstrate reduced acetylcholinesterase activity, but likely have a normal M1 receptor density.[28] A similar asymmetric effect has not been noted when measuring $rCMR_{glc}$ or CBF in unilaterally lesioned animals.

Possible Chronic Down-regulation of PLA_2-Mediated Arachidonate Turnover

Lithium, widely used to treat human bipolar disorder, is thought to act by inhibiting the enzyme inositol monophosphatase so as to deplete myoinositol and reduce cycling of PI.[29] The FA model shows, however, that therapeutic levels of lithium in rats also prolong the half-lives by some 5-fold (reduce

TABLE 6. Incorporation Coefficients of [^{3}H] arachidonate in Subcellular Fractions on Rat Brain Following Arecoline (Mean ± SD, $n = 4$)

	Incorporation Coefficient, k* × 10^5, ml · sec^{-1} per g brain		
Subcellular Fraction	Control	Arecoline	Percent Change
Myelin	0.24 ± 0.01	0.41 ± 0.10	171%
Synaptosomal plasma membrane[a]	0.52 ± 0.06	1.39 ± 0.11	267%[c]
Synaptosomes with mitochondria	1.14 ± 0.12	5.09 ± 1.04	446%[c]
Somal mitochondria	0.53 ± 0.12	0.66 ± 0.15	125%
Microsomes	0.94 ± 0.11	3.40 ± 0.28	361%[c]
Cytosol	2.18 ± 0.23	3.46 ± 0.72	159%[b]

NOTE: Animals given 15 mg/kg ip arecoline and 4 mg/kg sc methylatropine before i.v. [^{3}H]arachidonate. Mean differs from control mean, $^bp < 0.05$, $^cp < 0.001$. Values of k* normalized to control plasma integral, 3.7 × 10^9 dpm sec/ml. From Jones *et al.*[24]

[a]*Italicized fractions* demonstrate synaptophysin using specific antibody.

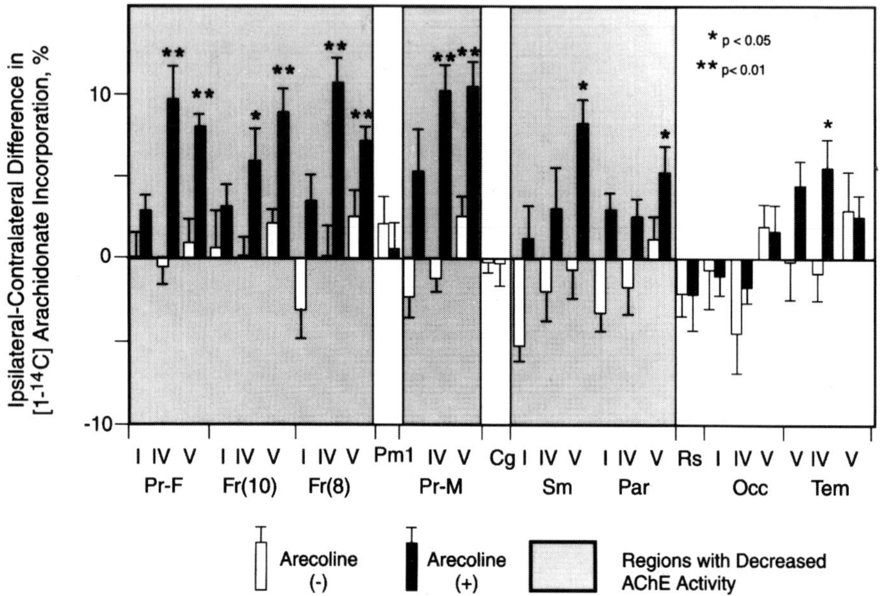

FIGURE 6. Ipsilateral incorporation coefficient k* of [1-^{14}C]arachidonate, as percent contralateral value, in different brain regions 2 weeks after unilateral ablation of the nucleus basalis magnocellularis (NBM) in the rat. Data are for studies with or without prior administration of muscarinic agonist arecoline. *Gray background* identifies regions with decreased acetylcholinesterase (AChE) activity. *Lined bars* are means ± SEM. I, IV, V, layers of neocortex; Pr-F, prefrontal; Fr, frontal; Sm, sensorimotor; M, motor; Par, parietal; Occ, occipital, Tem, temporal. (From Nariai *et al.*[28] Reproduced by permission.)

turnover by some 80%) of arachidonate within the *sn*-2 position of several brain phospholipids, without similarly affecting palmitate half-lives in these phospholipids (TABLE 7).[17] Chronic lithium, by interfering with turnover of PI, may indirectly reduce PLA_2 activity by reducing production of 1,4,5-IP_3 and liberation of intracellular Ca^{2+}, by reducing the production of diacylglycerol and thereby down-regulating protein kinase C activity, or by modifying G proteins.[29,30]

Imaging Membrane Remodeling and Synthesis with Labeled Palmitate

PC is the major phospholipid component of neuronal membranes. Thus, labeled palmitate, which preferentially enters the *sn*-1 position of brain PC, has been used to image changes in membrane remodeling or synthesis, under experimental conditions including Wallerian regeneration, a chronic NBM lesion, chronic unilateral enucleation, and experimental brain tumor.[10] For example, incorporation of [9,10-^{3}H]palmitate is elevated in neocortex ipsilateral to a 2-week-old NBM lesion, when phospholipid synthesis also is changing.[31] Autoradiography shows that Walker 256 carcinosarcoma cells, transplanted intracerebrally in rats, incorporate [9,10-^{3}H]palmitate 3- to 6-fold more than do normal brain cells (FIG. 7; TABLE 8).[28] This change in the signal/background ratio is an order of magnitude higher than found using the $rCMR_{glc}$ method and PET in human brain tumors (tumor radioactivity not more than 40% brain radioactivity). Necrotic areas within a tumor can be distinguished from the tumor by their reduced optical densities in autoradiographs, suggesting another potential clinical application of the FA method.[32]

Potential PET Imaging of Human Brain, Using Labeled FAs

It is hoped that the FA method can be extended when using *in vivo* PET to study brain lipid metabolism in humans with Alzheimer's disease or brain tumors or other disorders, including central nervous system neurotoxicity from drugs or other substances.[8,9] This should be possible, as the positron-emitting isotopes [1-^{11}C]palmitic acid and [1-^{11}C]arachidonate have been synthesized ([^{11}C] has a radioactive half-life of 20.4 min); they have been used successfully to image the monkey brain with PET;[11,13] steady state brain radioactivity is achieved with these isotopes within 5–10 min after their intravenous injection, consistent with rapid incorporation into stable lipids. FIGURE 8 illustrates images of k* for [1-^{11}C]palmitate and of CBF (obtained with PET) in an anesthetized monkey, as well as of brain anatomy obtained with magnetic resonance imaging.[11] An inhibitor of mitochondrial oxidation of [1-^{11}C]palmitate, methyl palmoxirate (MEP) (see below), was administered prior to tracer injection.

Whereas the polyunsaturated carbon-labeled arachidonate and docosahexaenoate are largely incorporated (~89%) into brain lipids after entering the

TABLE 7. Effect of Chronic Therapeutic Levels of Lithium on Half-lives of Arachidonate and Palmitate in Brain Phospholipids of Awake Rats (Mean ± SEM, $n = 5$)

	Phosphatidylinositol		Phosphatidylcholine	
	$t_{1/2,palm}$	$t_{1/2,arach}$	$t_{1/2,palm}$	$t_{1/2,arach}$
	(hours)		(hours)	
Control	2.4 ± 0.2	4.6 ± 0.1	10.0 ± 0.5	3.8 ± 0.1
Lithium	2.7 ± 0.1	26.8 ± 1.3[a]	13.7 ± 0.6	14.0 ± 0.2[a]

NOTE: For palmitate, $\lambda = 0.02 \pm 0.00$ in both control and lithium conditions; for arachidonate, $\lambda = 0.04 \pm 0.00$ in awake controls and 0.18 ± 0.02^a in lithium-treated rats. Mean ± SEM differs significantly from control mean, $^a p < 0.001$; $n = 5$. Data from Chang *et al.*[17]

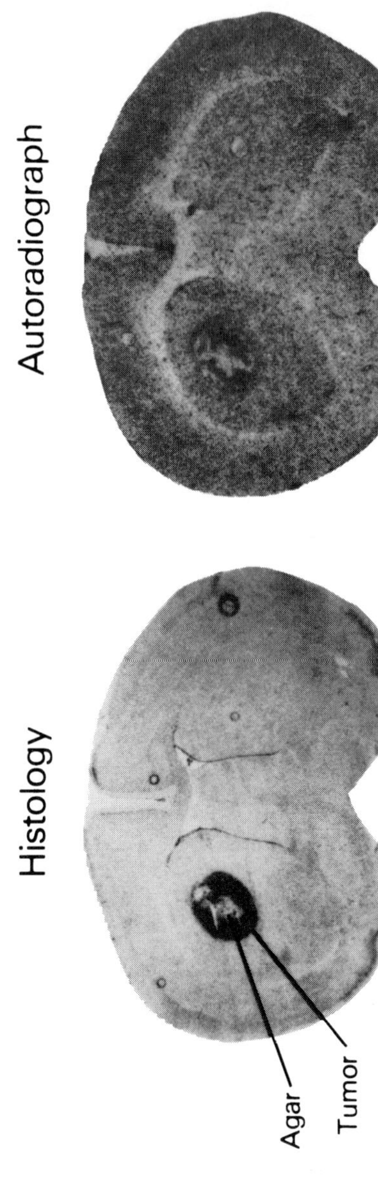

FIGURE 7. Histological section stained with cresyl violet, and corresponding [9,10-^{3}H]palmitate autoradiograph of rat brain, 7 days after implantation of Walker 256 carcinosarcoma in agar solution into caudate nucleus. (From Nariai *et al.*[5] Reproduced by permission.)

TABLE 8. Incorporation of [9,10-^{3}H]palmitate into Intracerebrally Implanted Walker 256 Carcinosarcoma[a]

Tissue Specimen	Incorporation Coefficient k* cm^3 · sec^{-1} per g brain, ×10^{-4}	Ratio to Contralateral Brain
Tumor-bearing rats		
Tumor region[b]		
Highest	11.82 ± 1.76[d]	6.07 ± 0.74[e]
Lowest	6.23 ± 1.02[c]	3.06 ± 0.36[e]
Adjacent to tumor	2.55 ± 0.30	1.28 ± 0.08[e]
Contralateral to tumor	2.03 ± 0.22	—
Control rats		
Control lesion	3.48 ± 0.92	1.33 ± 0.07[e]
Contralateral to lesion	2.63 ± 0.6	—

[a]Means ± SEM for 10 tumor-bearing animals and 6 control-lesioned animals.

[b]Highest and lowest areas of radioactivity in the tumor were measured in each tumor-bearing rat, excluding necrotic areas.

[c]$p < 0.05$; [d]$p < 0.01$, mean different from contralateral brain; [e]$p < 0.01$, different from 1.0.

From Nariai *et al.*[5]

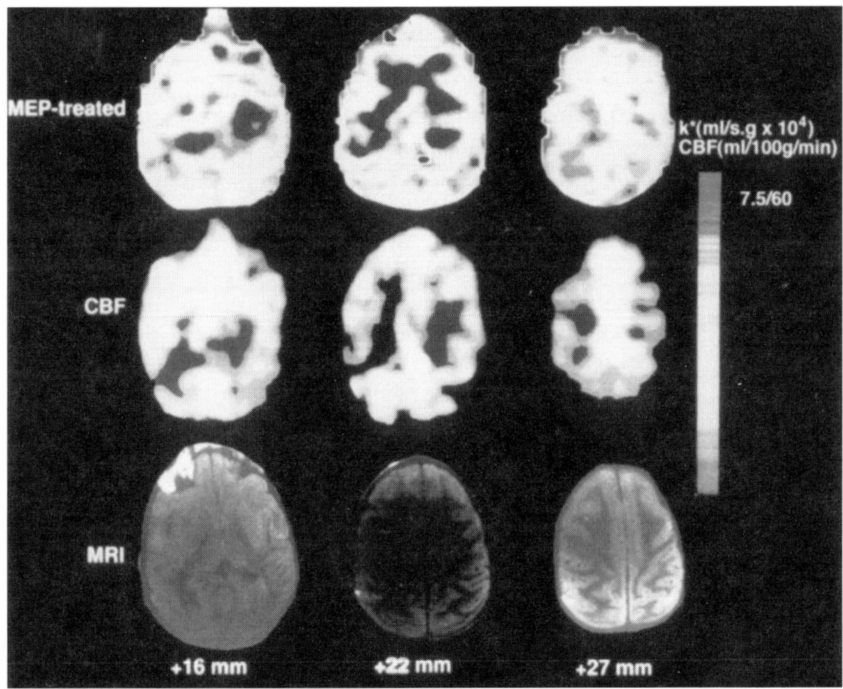

FIGURE 8. PET images of incorporation coefficient k* (**top**) for [1-^{11}C]palmitate in methyl palmoxirate (MEP)-treated anesthetized monkeys. Images of CBF (**center**) measured with $H_2{}^{15}O$ and PET and of brain structure (**bottom**) measured with MRI. Images are horizontal at different levels above the orbitomeatal line. Units for CBF and k* are given in scale. (From Arai *et al.*[11] Reproduced by permission.)

brain, only 40% of carbon-labeled saturated palmitate is incorporated. The remaining carbon label undergoes beta-oxidation after transfer of palmitoyl–CoA to mitochondria *via* carnitine palmitoyl transferase I, to enter the brain aqueous (glutamate and aspartate) pool (J_{oxid} in FIGURE 1).[33] In animal studies using autoradiography, we avoid this problem by using [9,10-^{3}H]palmitate instead of [^{14}C]palmitate. Three of four tritium atoms are converted to [^{3}H]H_2O during beta-oxidation of [9,10-^{3}H]palmitate in brain and can be evaporated during autoradiography to reduce the aqueous signal to only 15% of the total.[19]

On the other hand, to use [1-^{11}C]palmitate in clinical *in vivo* PET studies, we intend to administer methyl-2-tetradecylglycidate (methyl palmoxirate, McNeil Pharmaceuticals, Spring House, PA), an inhibitor of carnitine palmitoyl transferase I, prior to tracer injection.[11,34] At a dose of 2.5 or 10 mg/kg p.o., sufficient methyl palmoxirate enters brain to temporarily inhibit beta-oxidation of carbon-labeled palmitic acid and improve the lipid signal by reducing aqueous background activity (FIG. 9).[35]

DISCUSSION

An experimental method and its associated mathematical model are described to quantitate *in vivo* incorporation rates into and half-lives of FAs within brain phospholipids. Brain uptake and incorporation of labeled FAs are independent of CBF. Different labeled FAs enter different *sn* positions of different brain phospholipids, suggesting that a combination of labels can be used to investigate the metabolism of multiple brain phospholipids. As such, the method has been used to elucidate brain functional activity, cell growth and neuroplasticity in a number of experimental conditions.

With an experimentally determined dilution factor λ for the FA–CoA pool, the FA method provides *in vivo* half-lives of FAs within different brain phospholipids. Short half-lives of arachidonate in PI and PC (5 min in some PC species) are consistent with the role of arachidonic acid as a critical second messenger in signal transduction.[2,3] A 5-fold prolongation of arachidonate half-life in different phospholipids of the rat brain by chronic lithium suggests a heretofore unexpected mechanism of action of lithium in the treatment of bipolar disorder, and furthermore that the FA method can be used to elucidate dynamics of phospholipid metabolism in a variety of other conditions of interest (chronic drug action, development, aging, ischemia). The FA method now can be used with PET to image *in vivo* phospholipid metabolism in humans, where it might help to examine disease states and to assess central toxic effects of drugs and other substances.[8,9]

SUMMARY

An *in vivo* method is presented that allows quantification and imaging of fatty acid incorporation into different brain phospholipids in relation to

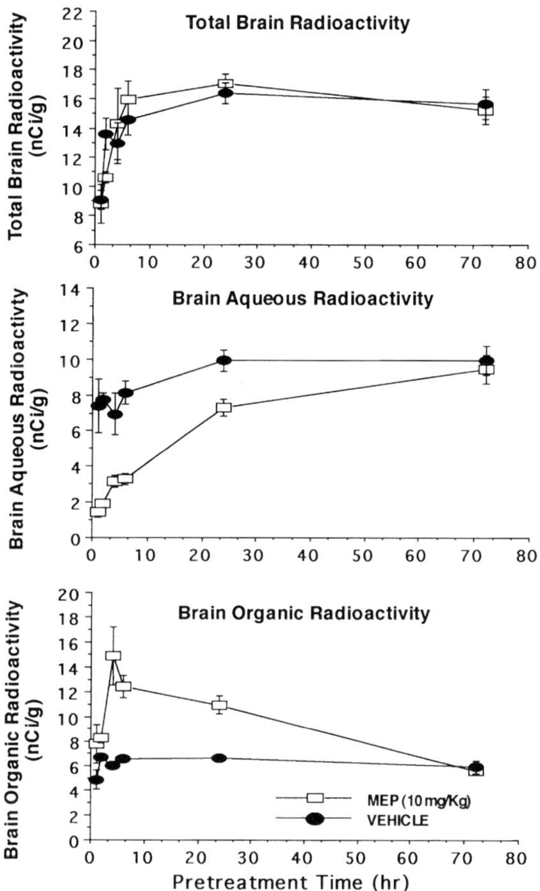

FIGURE 9. [1-^{14}C]palmitate radioactivity in the whole brain and in aqueous and organic (lipid) brain compartments, at various times after p.o. administration of MEP (methyl palmoxirate) to awake rats. Note that MEP does not significantly alter net brain radioactivity (tracer entry), but changes lipid/aqueous radioactivity from 0.6 to 5, thereby reducing the background aqueous radioactivity. (From Chang *et al.*[35] Reproduced by permission.)

membrane synthesis, neuroplasticity, and signal transduction. The method can be used with positron emission tomography, and may help to evaluate brain phospholipid metabolism in humans with brain tumors, neurodegenerative disease, cerebral ischemia or trauma, or neurotoxic effects of drugs or other agents.

REFERENCES

1. PORCELLATI, G., G. GORACCI & G. ARIENTI. 1983. Lipid turnover. *In* Handbook of Neurochemistry, Vol. 5. A. Lajtha, Ed.: 277–294. Plenum. New York, NY.

2. FISHER, S. K. & B. W. AGRANOFF. 1987. Receptor activation and inositol lipid hydrolysis in neural tissues. J. Neurochem. **48:** 999–1017.
3. AXELROD, J., R. M. BURCH & C. L. JELSEMA. 1988. Receptor-mediated activation of phospholipase A_2 via GTP-binding proteins: Arachidonic acid and its metabolites as second messengers. Trends Neurosci. **11:** 117–123.
4. STEPHENSON, D. T., J. V. MANETTA, D. L. WHITE, X. G. CHIOU, L. COX, B. GITTER, P. C. MAY, J. D. SHARP, R. M. KRAMER & J. A. CLEMENS. 1994. Calcium-sensitive cytosolic phospholipase A_2 ($cPLA_2$) is expressed in human brain astrocytes. Brain Res. **637:** 97–105.
5. NARIAI, T., J. J. DEGEORGE, N. H. GREIG & S. I. RAPOPORT. 1991. In vivo incorporation of [9,10-^{3}H]palmitate into a rat metastatic brain-tumor model. J. Neurosurg. **74:** 643–649.
6. FAROOQUI, A. A., L. LISS & L. A. HORROCKS. 1988. Stimulation of lipolytic enzymes in Alzheimer's disease. Ann. Neurol. **23:** 306–308.
7. BAZÁN, N. G. & E. RODRIGUEZ DE TURCO. 1980. Membrane lipids in the pathogenesis of brain edema: Phospholipids and arachidonic acid, the earliest membrane components changed at the onset of ischemia. Adv. Neurol. **28:** 197–205.
8. SINGH, A. K. 1994. Age-dependent neurotoxicity in rats chronically exposed to low level lead ingestion: Phospholipid metabolism in synaptosomes and microvessels. Toxicol. Ind. Health **10:** 89–101.
9. TITHOF, P. K., K. RUEHLE & P. E. GANEY. 1996. Dieldrin and lindane activate neutrophils by a mechanism that involves calcium-independent phospholipase A_2. Toxicologist **30 (No. 1, Part 2):** 54.
10. ROBINSON, P. J., J. NORONHA, J. J. DEGEORGE, L. M. FREED, T. NARIAI & S. I. RAPOPORT. 1992. A quantitative method for measuring regional in vivo fatty-acid incorporation into and turnover within brain phospholipids: Review and critical analysis. Brain Res. Rev. **17:** 187–214.
11. ARAI, T., S. WAKABAYASHI, M. A. CHANNING, B. B. DUNN, M. B. DER, J. M. BELL, P. HERSCOVITCH, W. C. ECKELMAN, S. I. RAPOPORT & M. C. CHANG. 1995. Incorporation of [1-carbon-11]palmitate in monkey brain using PET. J. Nucl. Med. **36:** 2261–2267.
12. YAMAZAKI, S., J. J. DEGEORGE, J. M. BELL & S. I. RAPOPORT. 1994. Effect of pentobarbital on incorporation of plasma palmitate into rat brain. Anesthesiology **80:** 151–158.
13. CHANG, M. C. J., T. ARAI, L. M. FREED, S. WAKABAYASHI, M. A. CHANNING, B. B. DUNN, M. G. DER, J. M. BELL, P. HERSCOVITCH, W. C. ECKELMAN & S. I. RAPOPORT. Brain incorporation of ^{11}C-arachidonate in normocapnic and hypercapnic monkeys: a study using positron emission tomography. Brain Res. In press.
14. GRANGE, E., J. DEUTSCH, Q. R. SMITH, M. CHANG, S. I. RAPOPORT & A. D. PURDON. 1995. Specific activity of brain palmitoyl-CoA pool provides rates of incorporation of palmitate in brain phospholipids in awake rats. J. Neurochem. **65:** 2290–2298.
15. WASHIZAKI, K., Q. R. SMITH, S. I. RAPOPORT & A. D. PURDON. 1994. Brain arachidonic acid incorporation and precursor pool specific activity during intravenous infusion of unesterified [^{3}H]arachidonate in the anesthetized rat. J. Neurochem. **63:** 727–736.
16. PURDON, A. D., T. ARAI & S. I. RAPOPORT. No evidence for direct incorporation of esterified palmitic acid from plasma into brain lipids of awake adult rat. J. Lipid Res. In press.
17. CHANG, M. C. J., E. GRANGE, O. RABIN, J. M. BELL, D. D. ALLEN & S. I. RAPOPORT. 1996. Lithium decreases turnover of arachidonate in several brain phospholipids. Neurochem. Lett. **220:** 171–174.
18. DEGEORGE, J. J., J. G. NORONHA, J. M. BELL, P. ROBINSON & S. I. RAPOPORT. 1989. Intravenous injection of [1-^{14}C]arachidonate to examine regional brain lipid metabolism in unanesthetized rats. J. Neurosci. Res. **24:** 413–423.
19. NORONHA, J. G., J. M. BELL & S. I. RAPOPORT. 1990. Quantitative brain autoradiography of [9,10-^{3}H]palmitic acid incorporation into brain lipids. J. Neurosci. Res. **26:** 196–208.
20. DEGEORGE, J. J., T. NARIAI, S. YAMAZAKI, W. M. WILLIAMS & S. I. RAPOPORT. 1991. Arecoline-stimulated brain incorporation of intravenously administered fatty acids in unanesthetized rats. J. Neurochem. **56:** 352–355.
21. SHETTY, H. U., Q. R. SMITH, K. WASHIZAKI, S. I. RAPOPORT & A. D. PURDON. 1996. Identification of two molecular species of rat brain phosphatidylcholine that rapidly incorporate and turn over arachidonic acid *in vivo.* J. Neurochem. **67:** 1702–1710.

22. HIRASHIMA, Y., A. A. FAROOQUI, J. S. MILLS & L. A. HORROCKS. 1992. Identification and purification of calcium-independent phospholipase A_2 from bovine brain cytosol. J. Neurochem. **59:** 708–714.
23. GRANGE, E., M. C. CHANG, O. RABIN, J. BELL & S. I. RAPOPORT. 1995. Effect of a phospholipase A2 inhibitor, manoalide, on in vivo arachidonic acid incorporation into brain lipids [abstract No. 98]. Symposium on Fatty Acids and Lipids from Cell Biology to Human Disease, 2nd International Conference of the ISSFAL, Bethesda, Maryland, June 7–10, 1995.
24. JONES, C. R., T. ARAI, J. M. BELL & S. I. RAPOPORT. 1996. Preferential in vivo incorporation of [^{3}H]arachidonic acid from blood into rat brain synaptosomal fractions before and after cholinergic stimulation. J. Neurochem. **67:** 822–829.
25. SOKOLOFF, L. 1991. Relationship between functional activity and energy metabolism in the nervous system: Whether, where and why. *In* Brain Work and Mental Activity. Quantitative Studies with Radioactive Tracers. Alfred Benzon Symposium. N. A. Lassen, D. H. Ingvar, M. E. Raichle & L. Friberg, Eds.: 52–67. Munksgaard. Copenhagen.
26. WAKABAYASHI, S., L. M. FREED, J. M. BELL & S. I. RAPOPORT. 1994. In vivo cerebral incorporation of radiolabeled fatty acids after acute unilateral orbital enucleation in adult hooded Long-Evans rats. J. Cereb. Blood Flow Metab. **14:** 312–323.
27. WHITEHOUSE, P. J., D. L. PRICE, R. G. STRUBLE, A. W. CLARK, J. T. COYLE & M. R. DELONG. 1982. Alzheimer's disease and senile dementia: Loss of neurons in the basal forebrain. Science **215:** 1237–1239.
28. NARIAI, T., J. J. DEGEORGE, Y. LAMOUR & S. I. RAPOPORT. 1991. In vivo brain incorporation of [1-^{14}C]arachidonate in awake rats, with or without cholinergic stimulation, following unilateral lesioning of nucleus basalis magnocellularis. Brain Res. **559:** 1–9.
29. ATACK, J. R., H. B. BROUGHTON & S. J. POLLACK. 1995. Inositol monophosphatase—a putative target for Li^+ in the treatment of bipolar disorder. Trends Neurosci. **18:** 343–349.
30. MANJI, H. K., W. Z. POTTER & R. H. LENOX. 1995. Signal transduction pathways. Molecular targets for lithium's actions. Arch. Gen. Psychiatry **52:** 531–543.
31. DE MICHELI, E., M. C. J. CHANG & S. I. RAPOPORT. Evidence for membrane remodeling following unilateral ablation of nucleus basalis magnocellularis: Increased in vivo incorporation of [9,10-^{3}H]palmitic acid into ipsilateral neocortex. Brain Res. In press.
32. DI CHIRO, G., E. OLDFIELD, D. C. WRIGHT, D. DE MICHELE, D. A. KATZ, N. J. PATRONAS, J. L. DOPPMAN, S. M. LARSON, M. ITO & C. V. KUFTA. 1988. Cerebral necrosis after radiotherapy and/or intraarterial chemotherapy for brain tumors: PET and neuropathologic studies. Am. J. Roentgenol. **150:** 189–197.
33. GNAEDINGER, J. M., J. C. MILLER, C. H. LATKER & S. I. RAPOPORT. 1988. Cerebral metabolism of plasma [14-C]palmitate in awake, adult rat: Subcellular localization. Neurochem. Res. **13:** 21–29.
34. TUTWILER, G. F., W. HO & R. J. MOHRBACHER. 1981. 2-Tetradecylglycidic acid. Methods Enzymol. **72:** 533–551.
35. CHANG, M. C. J., S. WAKABAYASHI & J. M. BELL. 1994. The effect of methyl palmoxirate on incorporation of [U-^{14}C]palmitate into rat brain. Neurochem. Res. **19:** 1217–1223.

DISCUSSION

NORA VOLKOW: (*Brookhaven National Laboratory, Upton, N.Y.*): What is the functional significance of transduction that you have decreased your turnover rate of fatty acid?

RAPOPORT: The turnover rate of arachidonic acid in brain phospholipids is decreased by 80 percent at a therapeutic level of lithium. The effect is specific to arachidonic acid, an unsaturated fatty acid esterified at the *sn*-2 position of phospholipids,[17] as turnover of the saturated palmitic acid, which is esterified at the *sn*-1 position, is unaffected. Our findings suggest that lithium inhibits signal transduction involving phospholipase A_2, in addition to its reported effects on adenylate cyclase (A. Mork & A. Geisler, 1989. The effects of lithium *in vitro* and *ex vivo* on adenylate cyclase in brain are exerted by distinct mechanisms. Neuropharmacology **28:** 307–311) and the phosphatidylinositide cycle.[3,7] Phospholipase A_2 is involved in signal transduction mediated by M_1 cholinergic receptors, D_2 dopaminergic receptors, and $5H_2$-serotonergic receptors, among many others. Thus, the high rate of arachidonic turnover in brain represents a high level of neuronal activity mediated by neurotransmitters acting on these receptors. An 80% inhibition of arachidonate turnover by a therapeutic dose of lithium could change cognition and behavior by interfering with this neurotransmission. Furthermore, reported therapeutic efficacy of lithium in manic-depressive disorder may mean that abnormal signal transduction involving phospholipase A_2 contributes to that disorder. This should be explored.

VOLKOW: So has there been work on lithium's effects on adenylate cyclase?

RAPOPORT: Yes. For example, Mork and Geisler (see above) reported that lithium has distinct *in vitro* and *in vivo* effects on adenylate cyclase in rat brain. The *in vitro* effect is demonstrated on forskolin-stimulated enzyme activity in membrane preparations, whereas the *in vivo* effect following chronic lithium treatment is directly on the activated adenylate cyclase. The actual brain concentrations of lithium at therapeutic doses of lithium are too low to produce the *in vitro* effect.

QUESTION: Does the beta oxidation of palmitate give you a useful measure of mitochondrial activity?

RAPOPORT: It might, but it is not what we have focused on. Palmitate is transferred into mitochondria from cytoplasm in the form of palmitoyl-CoA, by means of the enzyme carnitine acyltransferase I. The rate of beta-oxidation of the palmitoyl moieties within mitochondria could be used as a measure of either the transfer rate or of oxidative mechanisms. In human diseases involving mitochondrial mutations, or in animal models of comparable diseases, this rate might be altered and could be measured using labeled palmitate. Secondary effects on the size and turnover of the palmitoyl-CoA pool and on the value of the dilution factor lambda (λ) would be evident, as would secondary effects on transfer and accumulation of palmitate in triglycerides.[23,35] On the other hand, the overall rate of oxidative metabolism in brain is more easily measured by determining rates of glucose utilization and of oxygen consumption with standard methods.

Magnetic Resonance Spectroscopy and Spectroscopic Imaging for the Study of Brain Metabolism[a]

PETER C. M. VAN ZIJL[b,c] AND PETER B. BARKER[d]

[b]*Department of Radiology*
Johns Hopkins University Medical School
217 Traylor Building
720 Rutland Avenue
Baltimore, Maryland 21205-2195

[d]*Department of Neurology*
Henry Ford Hospital
2799 West Grand Boulevard
Detroit, Michigan 48202

INTRODUCTION

Magnetic resonance studies of the brain are generally affiliated with magnetic resonance imaging (MRI), in which the water content and the water relaxation times T_1 and T_2 are used to generate tissue contrast. In addition to this anatomical imaging, there has been a recent surge of interest in so-called functional imaging, in which dynamic properties such as water diffusion, brain blood flow and blood volume, oxygenation, and macromolecule–water proton interactions can be used as image contrast.[1,2] Most of these methods are now standard on many clinical scanners, and, because these methods study water, excellent image resolution in the order of microliters can be attained. It is often forgotten, however, that imaging is only a recent application of nuclear magnetic resonance (NMR) and that its original popularity was due to the study of molecular structure and the possibility of separating out components of chemical mixtures. Obviously, this possibility exists also *in vivo,* and the purpose of this review is to briefly touch upon the most recent advances in MR spectroscopy (MRS) and MR spectroscopic imaging (MRSI) of the brain. It will be shown that, in addition to the measurement of equilibrium levels of brain metabolites and drugs, MRS can also be used to study active brain transport and metabolism. Because of the limited space available, it is impossible to provide an in-depth review of all the literature, and references have been limited to some of the most important original papers and many reviews. Three recent books cover most aspects of localized spectroscopy *in*

[a]This work was supported by the Whitaker Foundation, NIH Grant NS31490. Part of this work was performed during the tenure of an Established Investigatorship from the American Heart Association.

[c]Corresponding author.

vivo and are an excellent methodological guide.[3] Since the present chapter is mainly directed towards brain application scientists, many of whom are not familiar with MRS, the review will focus on some of the basic principles of the methodology and on the available spectral information content of brain spectra of the most important nuclei. This knowledge of the methodological basics is essential to fully appreciate the complexity of MR technology and to avoid overinterpretation of the data. Thus, the purpose is to give an impression of the potential of the technique, rather than to review the abundant literature.

BASIC PRINCIPLES OF MRS

MRS is an extremely versatile method by which any magnetic nucleus can be studied to obtain information about topics ranging from active metabolism to simple concentration studies. However, MR is inherently limited by its low sensitivity, which is illustrated in FIGURE 1. Analogous to other spectroscopic methods, MR measures the result of transitions between energy levels, which are induced by applying radio-frequency (rf) radiation corresponding to the energy difference between the levels. In MR this energy difference is proportional to the magnetic field B_0 and a nuclear constant, the gyromagnetic ratio γ. The MR equipment is characterized by the field strength in Tesla or the resonance frequency at that field $\omega_0 = \gamma B_0$ for the proton nucleus ($\gamma = \gamma_H$). For *in vivo* MRS, fields presently range from 0.5 Tesla (21.4 MHz) to 9.4 Tesla (400 MHz). Most clinical machines that are used for spectroscopy operate at 1.5 Tesla, while a few whole-body machines are available at fields of 3–4 Tesla.

In a pulsed MRS experiment, all nuclei are excited simultaneously, after which the system relaxes back to thermal equilibrium, a process characterized by the so-called longitudinal relaxation time T_1. The MRS signals are measured as a time-dependent response (FIG. 1B), which modulates as a function of the difference in frequency between the excitation frequency and the exact nuclear resonance frequencies. In addition to T_1, the nuclei are relaxed by experiencing the random through-space variation of the magnetic fields of neighboring nuclei, a process called transverse relaxation, described by the constant T_2. *In vivo,* $T_2 \ll T_1$, and the signal decay is described by T_2. The MRS frequency spectrum is calculated from the time-dependent signal using a Fourier transformation (FIG. 1B), and the minimum line width attainable is $1/\pi T_2$. In addition to the random field fluctuations causing irreversible line broadening, the spectral lines can also be broadened by inhomogeneities in the static magnetic field of the spectrometer. This can best be understood from FIGURE 1A, which shows that one field corresponds to one frequency. The true signal decay, including the effect of static field inhomogeneities, is described by T_2^*. Therefore, a standard activity when performing spectroscopy is the removal of static field homogeneities, a process called shimming, to optimize spectral resolution.

Contrary to optical methods, for instance, MR sensitivity is very low. The reason is that sensitivity is proportional to the population difference between the energy levels, which for MR is only about one per million for the field strengths presently in use. Fortunately, MRI can still achieve microliter

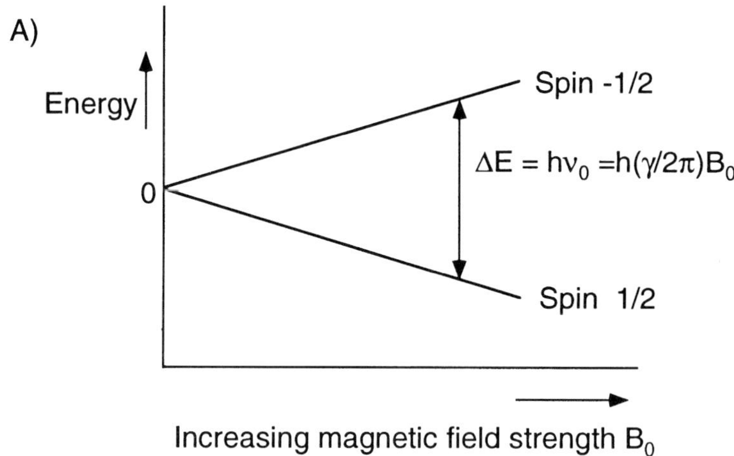

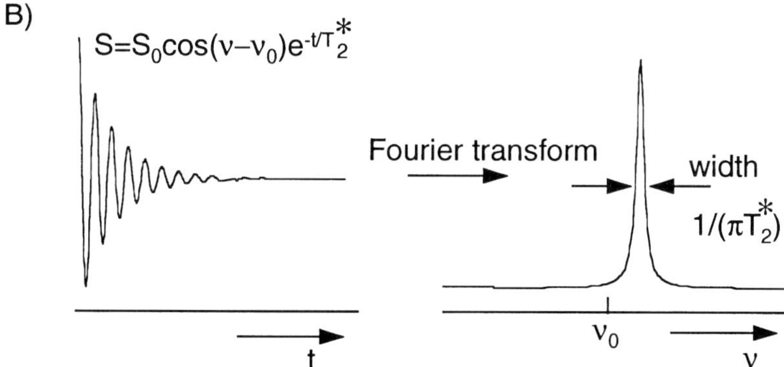

FIGURE 1. **(A)** Diagram showing the energy level separation between the two spin states of a proton as a function of magnetic field. Higher field corresponds to higher frequency ν_0 and to a larger energy separation and resulting higher sensitivity. **(B)** Correspondence between the NMR time domain signal and frequency spectrum. The finite signal decay rate determines the spectral linewidth.

resolution due to the facts that water is highly concentrated *in vivo* (55 M) and that it is the proton nucleus that is measured, which is the most sensitive and fully abundant naturally occurring nucleus. TABLE 1 shows that this situation is clearly less favorable for other nuclei, many of which are used to study

TABLE 1. Gyromagnetic Ratio, Abundance, and Sensitivity of Some Nuclei That Are of Biomedical Interest[a]

Nucleus	$\gamma/2\pi$ (MHz/T)	Natural Abundance	Relative Sensitivity
^{1}H	42.57	100%	1.0
^{19}F	40.05	100%	0.85
^{23}Na	11.26	100%	0.13
^{31}P	17.24	100%	0.083
^{14}N	3.08	99.6%	0.019
^{39}K	1.99	93.1%	0.0010
^{25}Mg	−2.61	10.1%	0.00055
^{13}C	10.71	1.11%	0.00025
^{43}Ca	−2.86	0.145%	0.000018
^{17}O	−5.77	0.037%	0.000019
^{2}H	6.54	0.015%	0.000024
^{15}N	−4.31	0.370%	0.0000068

[a]According to P. G. Morris.[51]

metabolites that are present in millimolar concentrations. In order to improve the situation, one can go to a higher field (increasing the separation of the energy levels in FIG. 1, and thus the population difference) or enrich the metabolites with the magnetic nuclei of interest (e.g., ^{13}C or ^{15}N) to go to higher abundance. The latter is not easy *in vivo,* and going to high field is expensive in a clinical setting. Thus, when spatial resolution is an issue, the best approach is often to just measure the most sensitive nucleus, the proton. However, proton spectroscopy has inherent technical difficulties that have only recently been solved satisfactorily, and the initial pioneering work on *in vivo* spectroscopy therefore used the phosphorus nucleus. To recognize this important history, we will explain the spectral basics using a phosphorus spectrum, before switching to the newer proton methodology. FIGURE 2 shows a brain phosphorus spectrum, which was obtained by spatially selecting a volume of 200 mL in the human brain.[4] This spectrum illustrates both the power and limitation of MRS. The strength of MRS is the ability to separate different molecules (or different nuclei within a molecule) based upon the sensitivity of the magnetic nuclei to their electronic environment. This separation is called the chemical shift and increases when the magnetic field B_0 increases (FIG. 1A). Thus, spectral resolution generally is expected to improve at higher field, although this depends on the inherent line width of the resonances, which may also be field dependent. Because the chemical shift expressed in Hz increases with field, spectra are always normalized by the resonance frequency (in MHz), and the different chemical shifts are expressed in ppm: $\delta(ppm) = 10^6 (\nu - \nu_0)/\nu_0$. Thus, when the chemical shift of one resonance (a reference line) is known, others can be assigned based on their specific chemical shifts, and a true chemical analysis can be attained. Assignments in human brain are generally based on animal data, where MRS spectral analysis of brain extracts can be combined with chemical analysis, such as high-performance liquid chromatography and mass spectroscopy/gas chromatography.

A second important feature in the spectrum in FIGURE 2 is that some of the ATP resonances are not single lines, but have multiple components. These are the so-called scalar couplings, which result from the fact that the nuclei can experience the magnetic fields of their neighboring nuclei through polarization of the electrons in the molecular bonds between them. Although this coupling can provide helpful information about resonance assignments or a means for spectral editing, it often also destroys spectral resolution. When this is the case, the interfering nuclei can be "decoupled" by irradiating them with rf waves. Actually, the ^{31}P spectrum that is given in FIGURE 2 has good resolution because it was acquired with decoupling from the proton nucleus. Thus, only the phosphorus-phosphorus couplings are left in the spectrum.

Finally, the spectrum in FIGURE 2 shows that although a spatial region of

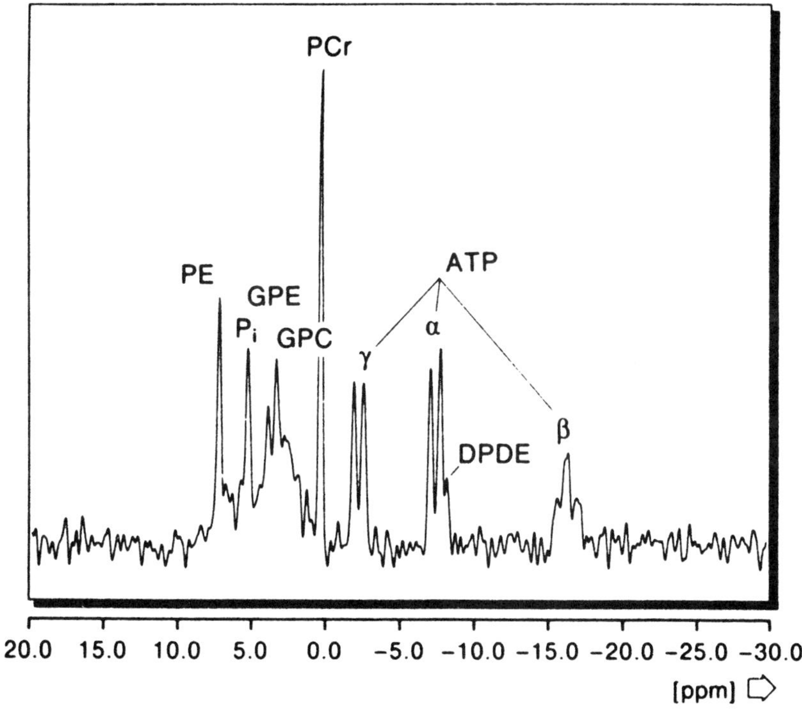

FIGURE 2. ^{1}H-decoupled ^{31}P spectrum of a 200-ml volume localized in the brain of a 6-year-old girl with a history of leukemia. The spectrum was obtained using 256 scans, TR = 3.5 s, and TE = 0 ms (detection directly after excitation, no spin echo sequence). The abbreviations are: PE: phosphoethanolamine; P_i: inorganic phosphate; GPE: glycerophosphoethanolamine; GPC: glycerophosphocholine; PCr: phosphocreatine; ATP: adenosine triphosphate, which has resonances for all three phosphate groups. (Reprinted from P. R. Luyten *et al.*[4] by permission of John Wiley & Sons, Ltd.)

200 mL is studied, the signal-to-noise ratio (S/N) is very low for phosphorus, which is a fully abundant nucleus (TABLE 1). In addition, not all metabolites contain phosphorus, and the MR application of this nucleus has generally been restricted to the study of energy metabolism and lipid metabolism. These applications have been reviewed elsewhere.[5,6] As a consequence of these limitations, work in recent years has concentrated on improving methodology for studying protons, which are more sensitive (TABLE 1) and present in almost all metabolites.

PROTON MRS

There are several problems that have long prohibited the use of proton MRS *in vivo.* The most severe difficulty is the fact that millimolar concentrations of metabolites have to be studied in the presence of the dominating resonances of water and lipids. In addition, the chemical shift range for proton metabolites is very small, and as all metabolites contain protons, the spectrum is very crowded. Finally, the line broadening due to static field nonhomogeneities is proportional to the nuclear gyromagnetic ratio, and the demands for shimming to achieve proper line shapes in a proton spectrum are much more severe than for the other nuclei. Thus, proton MRS methodological development has focused on minimizing unwanted resonances using water and lipid suppression techniques in addition to spectral editing. Fortunately, lipid suppression is straightforward in the brain, since the lipid signals originate from the tissue overlying the brain and are not present inside the brain. The development of spatial localization techniques has especially benefited brain MRS, by allowing any region inside the brain to be studied individually, without lipid contamination. In addition, MRS has the availability of a large arsenal of spectral selection methods, in which the nuclear properties based on chemical shift, scalar coupling, relaxation, and molecular motion can be exploited to select or suppress certain resonances. The applications of most of these methodologies to *in vivo* MRS have recently been reviewed,[7–12] and new techniques are still being developed.

The most common method for spectral selection is the use of selective rf pulses that excite only a certain chemical shift range. Thus, water can be selectively excited and then dephased, or, alternatively, the rest of the spectrum can be selectively excited, without water interference. These selective RF pulses can be combined with gradients in the magnetic field to achieve spatial localization. This is illustrated in FIGURE 3A, which shows that the application of a magnetic field gradient causes a spatial frequency gradient, because each field value corresponds to a characteristic frequency. Thus, through simultaneous application of a gradient and an RF pulse that is selective for a certain frequency range, a certain area in space is selected. This selection is also advantageous with respect to shimming, because the field homogeneity in a small volume (e.g., 1–8 mL) is much better than that over the complete brain. When spatial selection, frequency-selective water suppres-

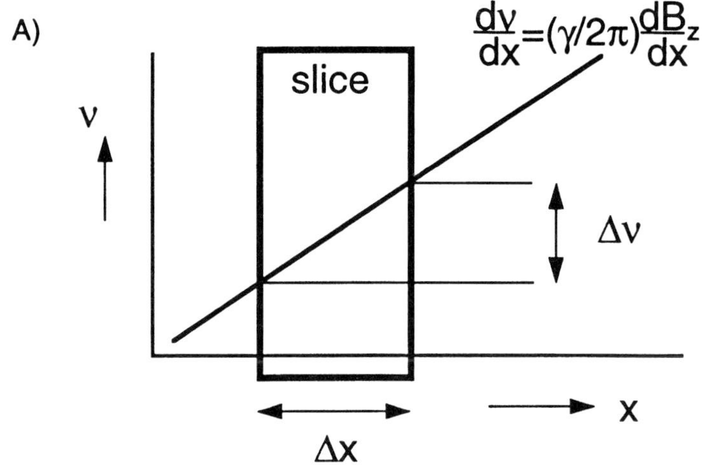

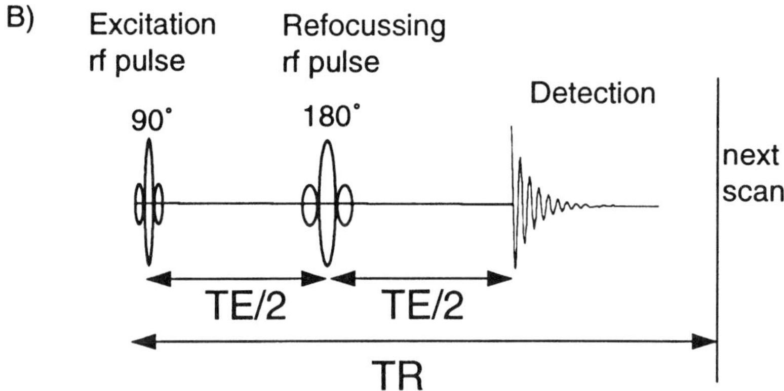

FIGURE 3. (**A**) Diagram showing the principle of slice selection. A magnetic field gradient dB_0/dx causes a frequency gradient over the sample. By applying a frequency-selective rf pulse of width $\Delta\nu$, a spatial region Δx is selected. (**B**) Generalized spin echo experiment. After excitation, the magnetization evolves during the first TE/2 period and refocuses during the second. Detection is initiated on top of the echo, where refocusing is complete. When multiple scans are taken, TR is the total time for excitation, evolution, detection, and waiting until the next scan.

sion, and localized shimming are combined, *in vivo* brain proton spectra of excellent quality can be attained. For example, FIGURE 4 shows a spectrum obtained in a 700-μL volume localized in the cerebral cortex of a cat brain. The overlapping resonances of many metabolites are present in this spectrum; the chemical shifts, concentrations, and structural formulas of the most

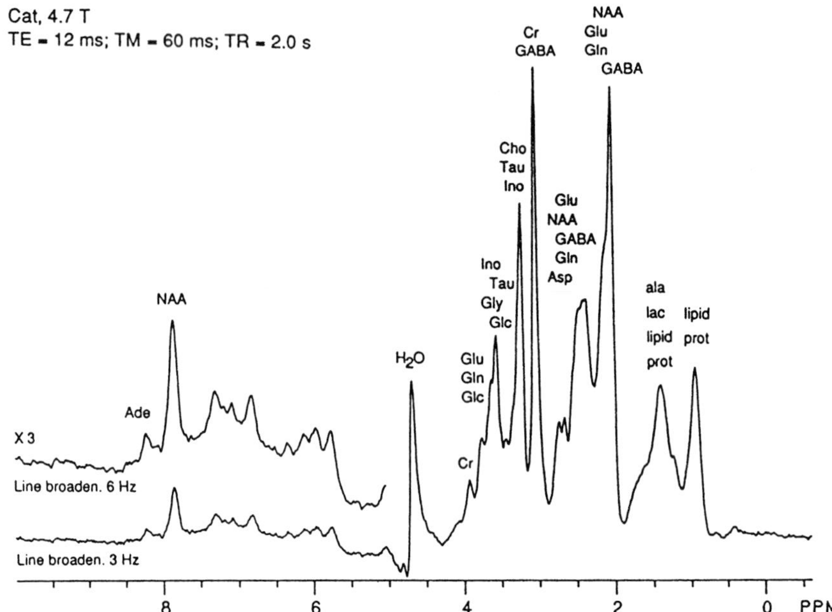

FIGURE 4. Short-TE *in vivo* proton spectrum (2048 scans) of a 700-μL volume localized in the cerebral cortex of a cat. The spectrum was processed with a 2-Hz line broadening. Abbreviations are: NAA: *N*-acetylaspartate; Cho: total choline; Cr: total creatine; Lac: lactate; Ino: inositols; Glu: glutamate; Gln: glutamine; Glc: glucose derivatives; GABA: γ-aminobutyric acid; Asp: aspartate; Gly: glycine; Ala: alanine; Tau: taurine; Ade: adenosines; Prot: protein. Reprinted, with permission, from van Zijl and Moonen.[10]

important compounds are summarized in TABLES 2, 3 and in FIGURE 5.[13–19] The assignments of these resonances are from the pioneering work by Behar *et al.*,[16] who performed brain extract studies and also obtained the first nonlocalized *in vivo* proton spectra. The dominating resonances in the spectrum are from the N(CH3)3 group of total choline (Cho, 3.24 ppm), which consists mainly of phosphoryl choline and glycerophosphoryl choline;[14] the CH3 group of total creatine (Cr, 3.03 ppm), consisting of creatine and phosphocreatine; and the CH3 groups of the combined *N*-acetyl resonances, mainly consisting of *N*-acetyl aspartate (NAA, 2.02 ppm). The reason that Cho is as large as Cr and NAA, despite its low concentration, is the fact that nine protons are measured versus three in Cr and NAA. Other large resonances are inositol and glutamate, which are multiplets due to scalar coupling interactions.

In order to understand the general appearance of the brain spectra, which often varies when obtained by different groups or by the same group at different fields, it is necessary to have some general knowledge about the way these spectra are obtained. The common approach is outlined in FIGURE 3B, which shows a spin echo pulse sequence, consisting of a series of rf pulses.

After excitation by a selective rf pulse (90° pulse), the nuclear spins start evolving with their effective frequencies, which are due to chemical shifts, magnetic field nonhomogeneities, and scalar couplings. The 180° selective pulse inverts the evolution of the chemical shifts and field nonhomogeneities, which are refocussed into a so-called spin echo at the time TE, which is called the echo time. This process is repeated several times, in which the signals of different acquisitions (or scans) are added, and the signal-to-noise ration is improved by the square root of the number of scans. The time of one complete scan is called TR, the repetition time. The signal intensity $S(TE,TR)$ in the spin-echo spectrum is related to the maximum signal intensity $S(0,0)$ and the timing parameters and relaxation times by:

$$S(TE, TR) = S(0, 0)e^{-TE/T_2}(1 - e^{-TR/T_1})f(J) \quad (1)$$

TABLE 2. Chemical Shifts δ[a] of Some Brain Metabolites Measurable by Proton MRS[13–19] [b]

Compound	δ (ppm)	Resonance	Compound	δ (ppm)	Resonance
Ino	3.27	CH(5)	Cho	3.24	$N(CH_3)_3$
	3.53	CH(1,3)		3.56	$CH_2(2)$
	3.59	CH(4,6)		4.07	$CH_2(1)$
	4.05	CH(2)	L-Asp	2.67	$CH_2(3,H\alpha)$
Cr	3.03	CH_3		2.80	$CH_2(3,H\beta)$
	3.93	CH_2		3.90	CH(2)
Glu	2.11	$CH_2(3)$	Tau	3.27	N-CH_2
	2.35	$CH_2(4)$		3.42	S-CH_2
	3.76	CH(2)	GABA	1.91	$CH_2(3)$
NAA	2.02	CH_3		2.30	$CH_2(2)$
	2.50	$CH_2(3,H\alpha)$		3.01	$CH_2(4)$
	2.70	$CH_2(3,H\beta)$	Lac	1.33	$CH_3(3)$
	4.39	CH(2)		4.11	CH(2)
	8.00[c]	NH[c]	Gly	3.56	CH_2
Gln	2.14	$CH_2(3)$	D-Glc[e]	3.20	CH(2β)
	2.46	$CH_2(4)$		3.35	CH(4α,4β) ATP
	3.79	CH(2)		3.40	CH(3β,5β)
	6.13	CH(1′) [d]		3.50	CH(2α)
	8.25	CH(2)		3.66	CH(3α,6β)
	8.54	CH(8)		3.80	CH(5α)
Ade/Inosine	6.10	CH(1′)[d]		3.85	CH(6α)
	8.23	CH(2)		4.60	CH(1β)
	8.33	CH(8)		5.20	CH(1α)
Hypoxanthine	8.18	CH(2)	Ala	1.48	$CH_3(3)$
	8.20	CH(8)		3.79	CH(2)

[a]vs. TSP at 0 ppm.
[b]Abbreviations are in legend to FIGURE 4.
[c]Temperature-dependent chemical shift; *in vivo* δ = 7.85 ppm.
[d]Sugar proton.
[e]In solution (67% β-/33% α-glucopyranose) at 200 MHz, 3 groups of resonances were found with maxima at 3.24, 3.45, and 3.79 ppm.

TABLE 3. Concentrations (μmol/gr Fresh Weight) of Most Abundant Metabolites[13–19]

	Cat	Rat	Rabbit	Average	Human
Ino			10.50	10.5	9.02
Cr			8.34	8.3	9.63
Glu	7.90	8.82	7.43	8.1	9.14
NAA	6.00		5.99	6.0	5.97
Gln	2.80	3.13		3.0	
Cho				1.5	0.49
Asp	1.70	2.13	2.32	2.05	
Tau	2.30		1.66	1.98	1.48
GABA	1.40	1.85	1.62	1.62	1.91
Lac			1.16	1.16	0.40
Gly	0.78	0.82	0.64	0.75	1.02
Ala	0.48	0.47	0.32	0.42	0.93

in which $f(J)$ describes the signal modulation due to the scalar coupling J. The spectrum in FIGURE 4 was obtained at very short TE and therefore contains all resonances. The signal modulation due to T_2 relaxation, and J evolution becomes clear when the echo time is increased (FIG. 6). First of all, water suppression and lipid suppression are improved due to the relatively short T_2 of these compounds. Furthermore, in the cat brain at 4.7 T, signals are reduced by a factor of close to three for the noncoupled CH3 groups of Cho, Cr, and NAA, while the signals for the scalar-coupled resonances have disappeared. Thus, although longer echo times can be used to obtain cleaner spectra, which are more easy to quantify, a heavy toll is paid in terms of signal-to-noise ratio. Finally, it is interesting to compare the short-TE spectra obtained at 4.7 T (FIG. 4) and 2.0 T (FIG. 6). When one studies the Glu/Gln region between 2.0 and 2.5 ppm in the short-TE spectra, it can be seen that the fine structure disappears at higher field. This is due to the fact that the chemical shift differences and line widths are becoming larger than the scalar couplings. Thus, the scalar-coupled resonances can be better resolved at higher field. Judged from the spectra in FIGURES 4 and 6, the resolution of the noncoupled resonances is similar at both field strengths. In principle an improvement in resolution is expected; but the chosen volumes occupy a large part of the brain, and the field nonhomogeneity is worse at higher field. When sufficiently small homogeneous regions can be selected, an improvement in S/N and resolution is expected at high field.

Single-voxel short-TE spectra are now routinely obtained at most clinical instruments for volumes on the order of 4–28 mL. Shimming and data acquisition have been automated and require a total time of about 15–20 min. For smaller volumes the S/N becomes very low, which is due to the method of acquisition. Quantitation of the resonances has also been discussed in detail for these spectra, and many applications to different diseases are being studied. For a recent review of quantitation methods, see Henriksen.[20] While single-voxel methods allow the optimized detection of individual brain regions at short echo times, they also do have a number of disadvantages:

voxel sizes are rather large, and in many conditions choice of voxel location is difficult. For diagnostic purposes, one would in principle like to study the complete brain. Although a contralateral voxel is often also acquired, this directly doubles the study time. To avoid these problems, MRS is nowadays

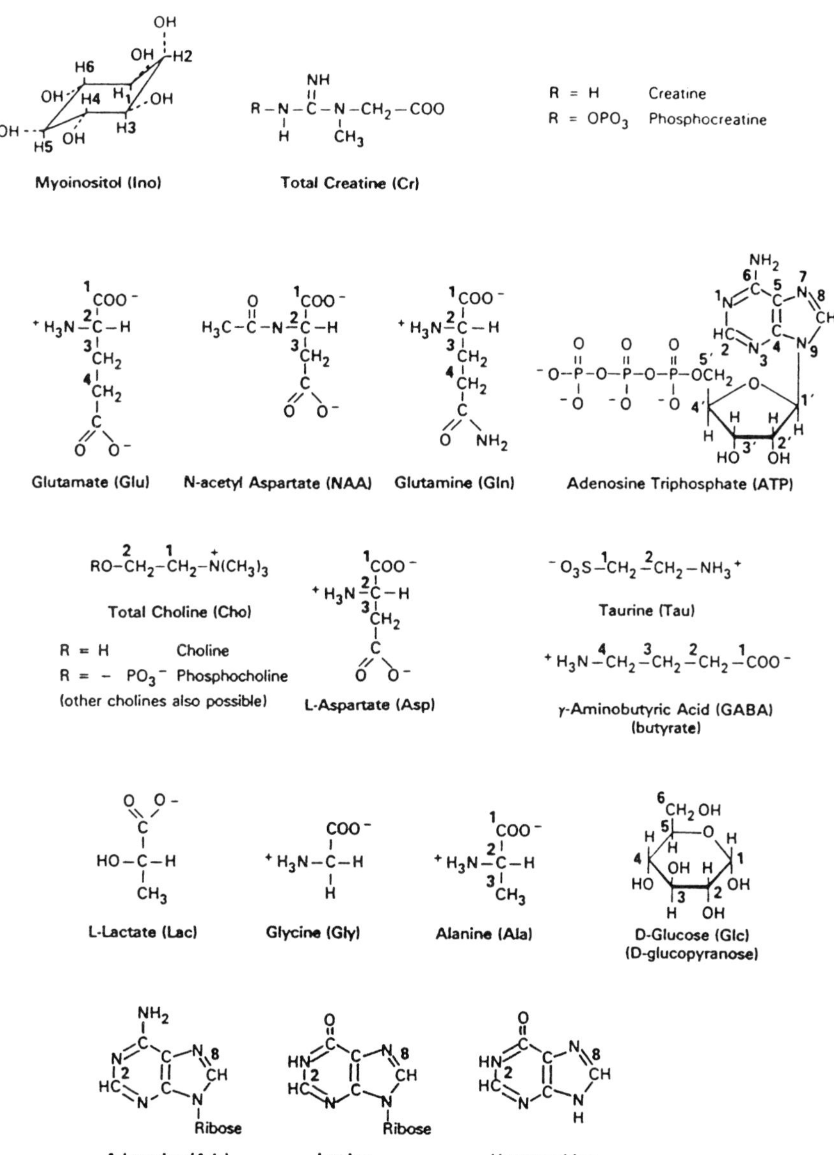

FIGURE 5. Structural formulas for the compounds detected in the short-TE proton MRS spectrum.

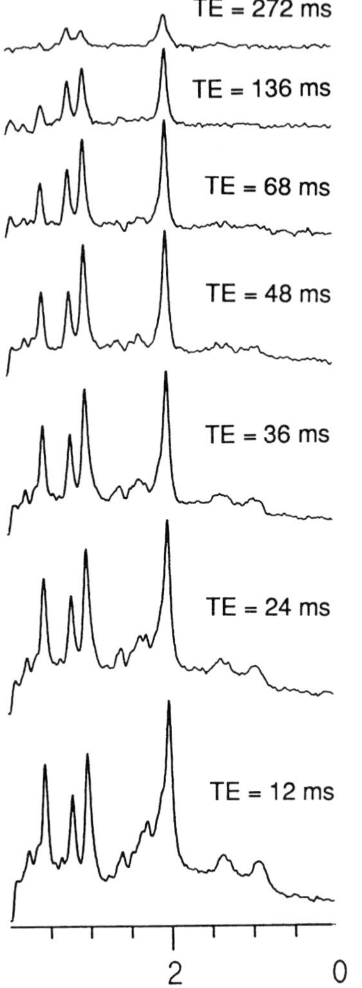

FIGURE 6. *In vivo* proton spectra of a 1-mL volume selected in cat cerebral cortex at 2.0 T as a function of echo time TE. The volume of interest (11 × 8 × 11 mm^3) was in parts of parietal and frontal cortex. Notice the large signal losses at long TE, which are traded for improved spectral resolution.

being combined with imaging[21–24] into so-called MR spectroscopic imaging. In these recent methods, 32 × 32 volumes of about 0.75 mL nominal volume can be obtained in each of four slices in a time of 30 min using single-echo spectroscopy.[23] An example of one application of this method is shown in FIGURE 7, where one of four slices through the brain of a late-stage adrenoleukodystrophy (ALD) patient is shown. This disease, which affects white matter, often progresses from the occipital periventricular regions to the frontal white matter. This progression is clearly seen in FIGURE 7A, where normal spectra are measured in the anterior frontal lobe, while spectra with high Cho, low NAA, and even lactate are found in the most affected region.[25] Both NAA and Cho changes in absolute concentration occur in the initial stages, but the relative Cho changes are much larger: Cho is about doubled in voxel 4, versus a decrease of about 35% in NAA. In the final stage the relative NAA changes are larger. The changes in Cho preceded the changes in the MRI signal, indicating the importance of using MRSI instead of placing a single voxel in a region indicated by MRI. Based on biochemical studies of brains of ALD patients, Cho increases were attributed to an increase in phosphatidyl choline upon demyelination. NAA is a specific neuronal and axonal marker, and its decrease after initial demyelination is presumably due to axonal and neuronal loss in the diseased white matter. Lactate in the most severely affected regions was attributed to inflammation (macrophages present) with possible resulting anaerobic glycolysis or even ischemia. Similar changes in NAA, Cho, and lactate have been found in stroke,[21,26] brain tumors,[27] multiple sclerosis,[28] and many other disorders. Changes in inositol and Glu/Gln have been found in other diseases when using short-TE spectra.[29–31]

The present state of the art in MRSI is the multislice version, which is used in several hospitals. The most advanced method that has been published is a multiecho multislice approach, which can acquire 3 slices of 32 × 32 volumes in 10–12 min and 16 × 16 in 3 min.[32] However, this method is presently not widely available. Improvements in S/N have been reported at higher field,[33,34] but these fields are not generally available in the clinic. Higher resolution using small surface coils has also been reported. Quantitation methods for MRSI are presently also being developed.[35]

MEASUREMENT OF ACTIVE METABOLISM

Although the assessment of changes in equilibrium metabolite levels by MRSI is potentially very powerful and is presently being applied to many diseases, the MRSI spectrum provides only a steady state impression of metabolic changes and does not provide any details about ongoing metabolism. However, in analogy to radiolabel studies, MRS also has the capability to assess active metabolism, namely, by labeling substrates magnetically. This was first demonstrated for ^{13}C-glucose metabolism by Behar *et al.* in the rabbit brain[36] and later by Rothman *et al.* and Beckmann *et al.* in humans.[37,38] Infusion of ^{15}N-labeled ammonia to study glutamine metabolism has been reported by Ross and co-workers.[39] Obviously, these measurements are more complex than MRS of the proton nucleus, since the labeled compound has to be infused in the subject and the clinical scanners are often suitable only for studying protons. Nevertheless, there are presently several laboratories that have this capability. Because there have been several recent reviews of most aspects of the ^{13}C-glucose methodology and of the information content of the ^{13}C metabolic spectra,[40–42] we will restrict ourselves to a brief summary.

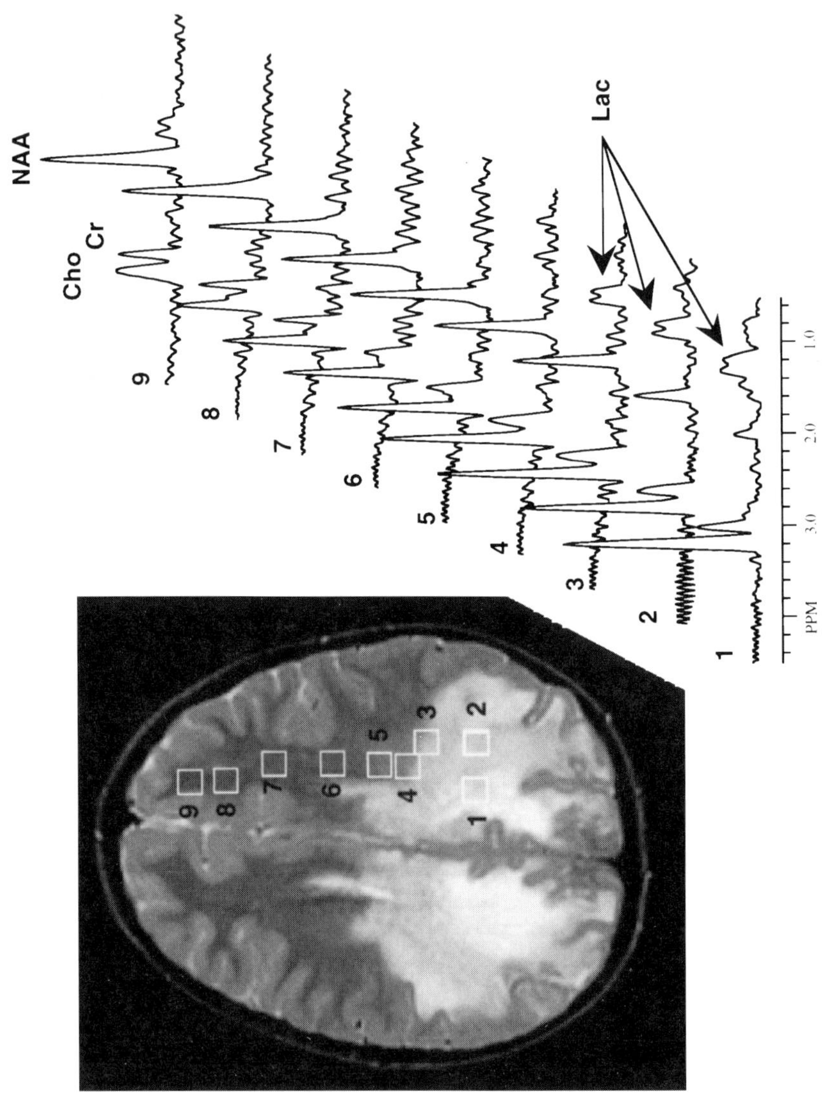
NAA
Cho
Cr
Lac
9
8
7
6
5
4
3
2
1
PPM
3.0
2.0
1.0

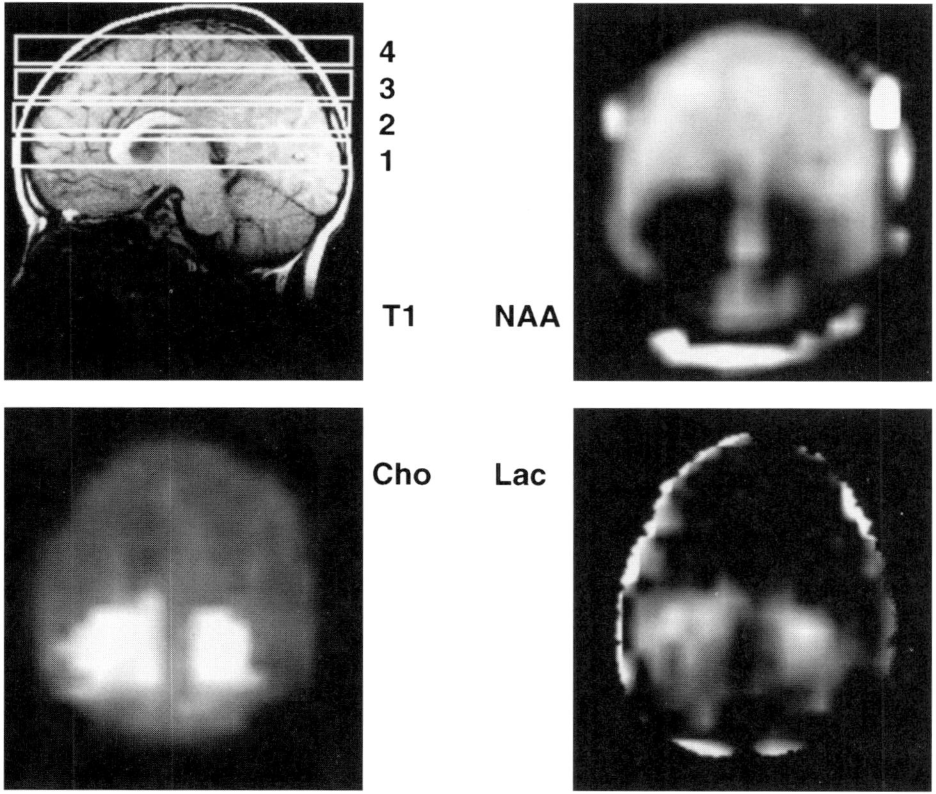

FIGURE 7. (Facing page) T_2-weighted MRI and spectra from 9 voxels selected in a slice containing affected and normal-appearing white matter in a later-stage patient with childhood cerebral-type adrenoleukodystrophy. **(Left)** MRSI slice locations and spectroscopic images of the slice shown above for NAA, Cho, and Lac. The signal hyperintensities in the T_2-weighted MRI indicate demyelination. Clear spectral changes showing increased Cho and slightly decreased NAA are already visible in white matter that appears normal on the MRI. The Cr resonance remains normal, while the most severely affected areas show lactate, which was attributed to inflammation. Reprinted, with permission, from Kruse *et al.*[25]

Although radiolabel methods, such as autoradiography and positron emission tomography (PET), have a much higher sensitivity than MRS, MRS has several advantages that can contribute important additional information about brain metabolism. The main difference between the technologies is the specificity of detection. Radiolabel studies cannot measure the distribution of the label over the different metabolic products and therefore generally use glucose substitutes (e.g., fluorodeoxyglucose), which may have properties that differ from normal glucose. MRS, on the contrary, can measure the metabolic products separately due to their differences in chemical shift of the ^{13}C nucleus; and, as a consequence, the natural compound ^{13}C-glucose can be used for the infusions. The specificity of MRS is demonstrated in FIGURE 8B, which shows *in vivo* two-dimensional proton-detected ^{13}C spectra obtained from a cat brain four hours after the start of a ^{13}C-glucose infusion. FIGURE 8A shows the main pathways for brain glucose transport and metabolism, and thus the origin of the compounds detected in FIGURE 8B. Because MRS can be used to noninvasively perform both steady state concentration measurements

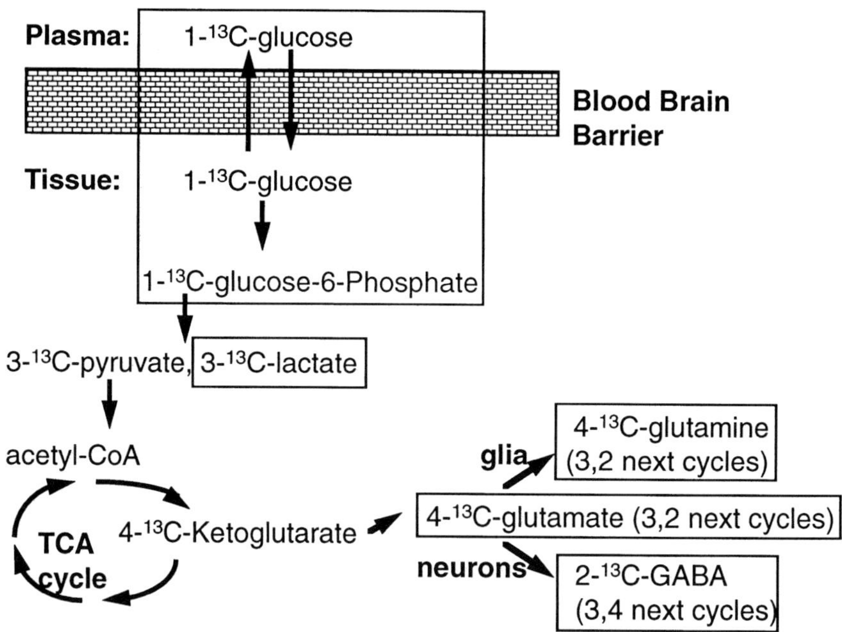

FIGURE 8A. Pathways for uptake and metabolism of 1-^{13}C-glucose in the brain. Numbers denote the position of the label. Metabolites that have been detected *in vivo* or in brain extracts are indicated in a *box*. The resonances for 1-^{13}C-glucose and phosphorylated glucose overlap *in vivo,* but the a- and b-isomers can be separated. Most other compounds can generally be separated using the chemical shifts, but resolution depends on the nucleus observed and the field strength used. Glial and neuronal metabolism can be separated though the production of glutamine versus GABA, respectively.

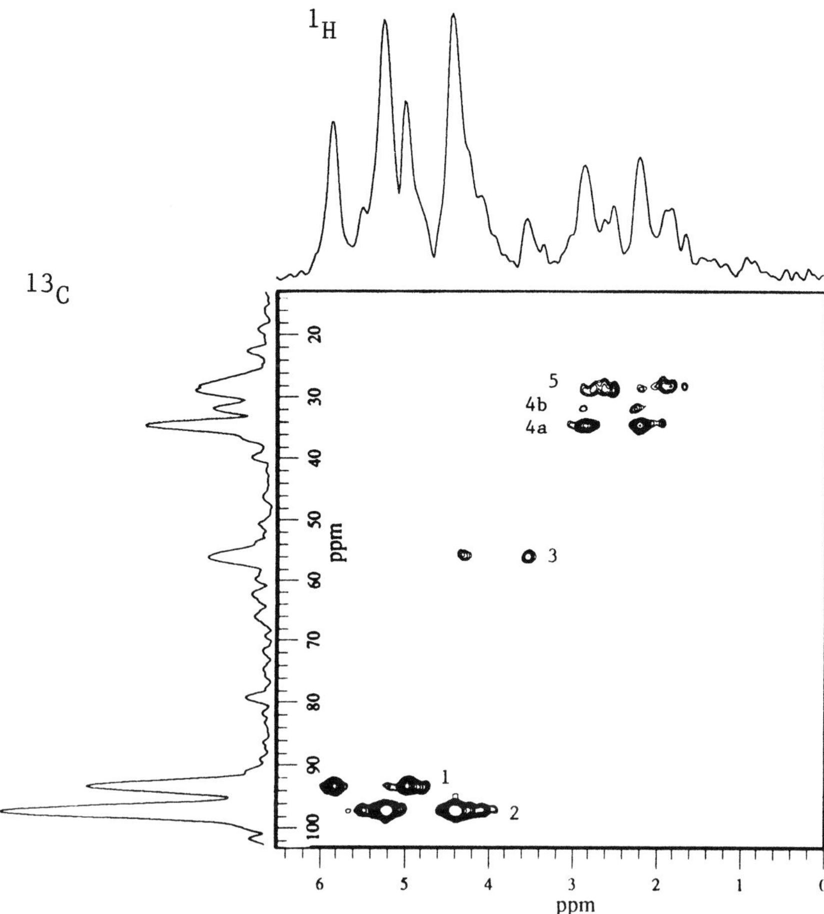

FIGURE 8B. *In vivo* two-dimensional proton-detected ^{13}C-spectrum (4.5-min acquisition time) of an 8-mm slice located in cat brain, acquired 4 h after the start of a ^{13}C-glucose infusion. Assignments are (1) α-1-^{13}C-glucose; (2) β-1-^{13}C-glucose; (3) 2-^{13}C-glutamate/glutamine; (4a) 4-^{13}C-glutamate; (4b) 4-^{13}C-glutamine; (5) 3-^{13}C-glutamate/glutamine. (Reprinted, with permission, from van Zijl *et al.*[50])

and active metabolic rate measurements, both glucose transport[43–45] and metabolism[46–48] can be assessed by MRS. When making specific assumptions about the sources of acetyl-coA, the ^{13}C-glucose data can also be used to assess oxygen metabolism.[48] For details about the different methodological approaches, the reader is referred to the recent reviews.[40–42] From a practical point of view it is important to know that, despite the inherently low sensitivity of MR, the volumes that are expected to be studied are in the same order of magnitude as the volumes in PET, namely, 1–5 mL. The reason is that the subject is made hyperglycemic in the MRS experiment, and that PET is

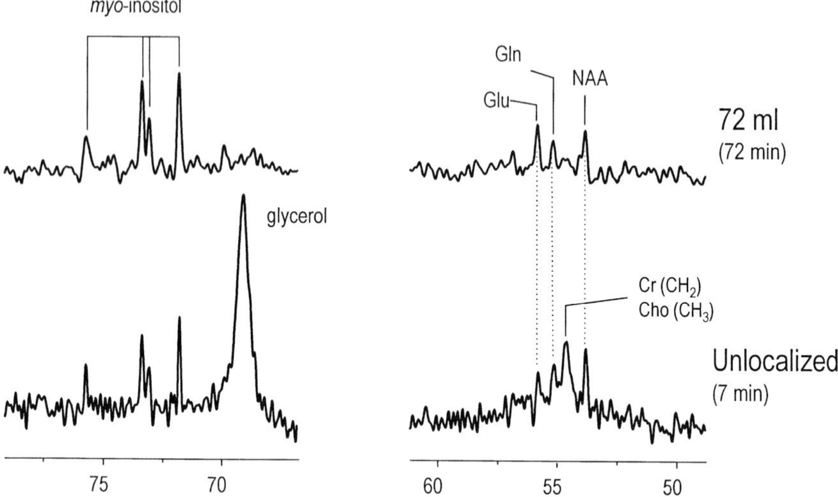

FIGURE 8C. Two sections of a natural abundance NOE-enhanced ^{13}C-spectrum obtained from human brain at 4T, with **(top)** and without **(bottom)** localization. Peaks from myo-inisitol at 72.0, 73.0, 73.3, and 75.1 ppm, as well as the glutamate 2-^{13}C at 55.7 ppm, the glutamine 2-^{13}C at 55.1 ppm and NAA at 54.0 ppm are clearly observed. The peaks of Cr (54.6 ppm) and choline (54.8 ppm) overlap at 54.7 ppm, but were eliminated in the localized spectrum due to the specific pulse sequence used, which selected for ^{13}CH groups only. (Reprinted, with permission, from Gruetter *et al.*[33])

limited in detector resolution. Improved sensitivity is expected at higher fields (4 T), which is demonstrated in FIGURE 8C, where natural abundance ^{13}C spectra of the human brain are shown. The acquisition time for these 72–108-mL volumes is about an hour for natural abundance, indicating that 1-mL volumes should be attainable within a reasonable period of 10–20 min when using ^{13}C-glucose infusion. Depending on the experimental requirements, further improvements are expected using proton-detected ^{13}C spectroscopy,[49,50] where an increase in sensitivity of a factor of 16–32 is expected for protons versus ^{13}C. This latter method is difficult at low field due to poor resolution and increased spectral evolution times for the ^{13}C dimension leading to T_2^* losses. However, proton detection should become more practical at higher fields. Also, the sensitivity is proportional to the number of nuclei; and, for instance, for the $^{13}CH_3$ group of lactate, the sensitivity in proton detection is automatically increased by a factor of three with respect to carbon detection. A second important advantage of MRS over PET is that MRI and MRSI images can be obtained during the same session without moving the subject. PET, on the contrary needs MRI for localization. Finally, MRS scanners are present in most hospitals; if these methods become established, they have the potential to be used on many patients.

SUMMARY

Magnetic resonance imaging is a well-established method for the detailed study of brain anatomy. However, it is less well known that magnetic resonance technology can also be used to study brain metabolite levels and active brain metabolism. In this paper, an overview was given of the state-of-the-art technology for *in vivo* metabolic studies on animals and humans. This includes spectroscopy to study equilibrium levels of metabolites such as creatines, cholines, *N*-acetyl-aspartate, lactate, glutamate, glutamine, γ-aminobutyric acid, alanine, inositols, glycine, glucose, and ATP and its breakdown products. It was shown that metabolite levels in the mM range can be imaged (magnetic resonance spectroscopic imaging) with a spatial resolution of less than 1 mL. An application to human disease was also demonstrated. In addition, magnetic resonance can noninvasively measure the transport and utilization of magnetically labeled (^{13}C) glucose by the brain. Metabolic products that can be detected *in vivo* include several isomers of glutamate as well as glutamine and lactate. The specific advantages and disadvantages of the magnetic resonance magnetic labeling methods were compared with those of radiolabel methods.

CONCLUSIONS

Many methods are presently available to perform magnetic resonance spectroscopy *in vivo,* all of which have been applied successfully to study cells, animals, and humans. Metabolic images of equilibrium levels of metabolites can be obtained on standard clinical equipment, and *in vivo* spectra of active metabolism of ^{13}C glucose have been reported in humans. Metabolic imaging of ^{13}C-labeled glucose and glutamate in animals is already possible, and application to humans is being initiated. Initial work on ^{15}N-enriched metabolites has also been reported. Improved sequences for rapid clinical application will probably be developed in the future.

REFERENCES

1. Le Bihan, D. 1995. Diffusion and Perfusion Magnetic Resonance Imaging. Applications to Functional MRI. Raven Press. New York, NY.
2. Moonen, C. T. W., P. C. M. van Zijl, J. A. Frank, D. Le Bihan & E. D. Becker. 1990. Functional magnetic resonance imaging in medicine and physiology. Science **250:** 53–61.
3. Seelig, J. & M. Rudin. 1992. *In vivo* magnetic resonance spectroscopy, parts I–III. *In* NMR, Basic Principles and Progress, Vols. 26–28. P. Diehl, E. Fluch, H. Günther, R. Kosfeld & J. Seelig, Eds. Springer Verlag. Berlin.
4. Luyten, P. R., G. Bruntink, F. M. Sloff *et al.* 1989. Broadband proton decoupling in human 31P spectroscopy. NMR Biomed. **1:** 177–183.
5. Rudin, M. & A. Sauter. 1992. In vivo phosphorus-31 NMR: Potential and limitations. *In* NMR, Basic Principles and Progress. *In* NMR, Basic Principles and Progress, Vols. 26–28. P. Diehl, E. Fluch, H. Günther, R. Kosfeld & J. Seelig, Eds.: 161–188. Springer Verlag. Berlin.

6. Burt, C. T. 1987. Phosphorus NMR in Biology CRC Press. Boca Raton, FL.
7. Gueron, M., P. Plateau & D. Decorps. 1991. Progr. Nucl. Magn. Reson. Spectr. **23:** 135.
8. Howe, F. A., R. J. Maxwell, D. E. Saunders, M. M. Brown & J. R. Griffiths. 1993. Proton spectroscopy in vivo. Magn. Reson. Quart. **9:** 31–59.
9. Williams, S. R. 1992. In vivo proton spectroscopy: Experimental aspects and potential. *In* NMR, Basic Principles and Progress. P. Diehl, E. Fluch, H. Günther, R. Kosfeld & J. Seelig, Eds.: 55–72. Springer Verlag. Berlin.
10. van Zijl, P. C. M. & C. T. W. Moonen. 1992. Solvent suppression strategies for in vivo magnetic resonance spectroscopy. *In* P. Diehl, E. Fluch, H. Günter, R. Kosfeld & J. Seelig, Eds.: 67–108. NMR, Basic Principles and Progress. Springer-Verlag. Berlin.
11. Ross, B. D. 1991. Biochemical considerations in 1H spectroscopy. Glutamate and glutamine, myoinositol and related metabolites. NMR Biomed. **4:** 59–63.
12. Ross, B., R. Kreis & T. Ernst. 1992. Clinical tools for the 90's: Magnetic resonance spectroscopy and metabolite imaging. Eur. J. Radiol. **14:** 128–140.
13. Arus, C., Y. Chang & M. Barany. 1985. Proton nuclear magnetic resonance spectra of excised rat brain. Assignment of resonances. Physiolog. Chem. Phys. Med. NMR **17:** 23–33.
14. Barker, P. B., S. N. Breiter, B. J. Soher *et al.* 1994. Quantitative proton spectroscopy of canine brain: In vivo and in vitro correlations. Magn. Reson. Med. **32:** 157–163.
15. Fan, T. W-M., R. M. Higashi, A. N. Lane & O. Jardetzky. 1986. Combined use of 1H NMR and GC-MS for metabolite monitoring and in vivo 1H-NMR assignments. Biochim. Biophys. Acta **882:** 154–167.
16. Behar, K. L., J. A. Den Hollander, M. E. Stromski *et al.* 1983. High-resolution ^{1}H NMR study of cerebral hypoxia in vivo. Proc. Natl. Acad. Sci. USA **80:** 4945–4948.
17. McGeer, P. L. & E. G. McGeer. 1989. *In* Basic Neurochemistry. G. J. Siegel, R. W. Albers, B. W. Agranoff & R. Katzman, Eds.: 311. Raven Press. New York, NY.
18. Petroff, O. A. C., T. Ogino & J. R. Alger. 1988. High resolution proton magnetic resonance spectroscopy of rabbit brain: Regional metabolite levels and postmortem changes. J. Neurochem. **51:** 163–171.
19. Petroff, O. A. C., D. D. Spencer, J. R. Alger & J. W. Prichard. 1989. High field proton magnetic resonance spectroscopy of human cerebrum obtained during surgery for epilepsy. Neurology **39:** 1197–1202.
20. Henriksen, O. 1995. In vivo quantitation of metabolite concentrations in the brain by means of proton MRS. NMR Biomed. **8:** 139–148.
21. Berkelbach van der Sprenkel, J. W., N. M. Knufman, P. C. van Rijen, P. R. Luyten, J. A. den Hollander & C. A. Tulleken. 1992. Proton spectroscopic imaging in cerebral ischaemia. Where we stand and what can be expected. Adv. Tech. Stand. Neurosurg. **19:** 3–17.
22. Moonen, C. T. W., G. Sobering, P. C. M. van Zijl, J. Gillen, M. von Kienlin & A. Bizzi. 1992. Proton spectroscopic imaging of human brain. J. Magn. Reson. **98:** 556–575.
23. Duyn, J. H., J. Gillen, G. Sobering, P. C. M. van Zijl & C. T. W. Moonen. 1993. Multislice proton MR spectroscopic imaging of the brain. Radiology **188:** 277–282.
24. Spielman, D., J. Pauly, A. Macovski & D. Enzmann. 1991. Spectroscopic imaging with multidimensional pulses for excitation: SIMPLE. Magn. Reson. Med. **19:** 67–84.
25. Kruse, B., P. B. Barker, P. C. M. van Zijl, J. H. Duyn, C. T. W. Moonen & H. W. Moser. 1994. Multislice proton magnetic resonance spectroscopic imaging in X-linked adrenoleukodystrophy. Ann. Neurol. **36:** 595–608.
26. Barker, P. B., J. H. Gillard, P. C. M. van Zijl *et al.* 1994. Serial magnetic resonance proton spectroscopic imaging of acute stroke. Radiology **192:** 723–732.
27. Alger, J. R., J. A. Frank, A. Bizzi *et al.* 1990. Metabolism of human gliomas: Assessment with H-1 MR spectroscopy and F-18 fluorodeoxyglucose PET [see comments]. Radiology **177:** 633–41.
28. Davie, C. A., C. P. Hawkins, G. J. Barker *et al.* 1993. Detection of myelin breakdown products by proton magnetic resonance spectroscopy. Lancet **341:** 630–631.
29. Frahm, J., H. Bruhn, M. L. Gyngell, K. D. Merboldt, W. Hänicke & R. Sauter. 1989. Localized proton NMR spectroscopy in different regions of the human brain in vivo; relaxation times and concentrations of cerebral metabolites. Magn. Reson. Med. **11:** 47–63.

30. KREIS, R., B. D. ROSS, N. A. FARROW & Z. ACKERMAN. 1992. Metabolic disorders of the brain in chronic hepatic encephalopathy detected with H-1 MR spectroscopy. Radiology **182:** 19–27.

31. KREIS, R. & B. D. ROSS. 1992. Cerebral metabolic disturbances in patients with subacute and chronic diabetes mellitus: Detection with proton MR spectroscopy. Radiology **184:** 123–130.

32. DUYN, J. H. & C. T. W. MOONEN. 1993. Fast proton spectroscopic imaging of human brain using multiple spin echoes. Magn. Reson. Med. **30:** 409–414.

33. GRUETTER, R., M. GARWOOD, K. UGURBIL & E. R. SEAQUIST. 1996. Observation of resolved glucose signals in 1H NMR spectra of the human brain at 4 Tesla. Magn. Reson. Med. **36:** 1–6.

34. HETHERINGTON, H. P., G. F. MASON, J. W. PAN *et al.* 1994. Evaluation of cerebral gray and white matter metabolite differences by spectroscopic imaging at 4.1 T. Magn. Reson. Med. **32:** 565–571.

35. SOHER, B. J., P. C. M. VAN ZIJL, J. H. DUYN & P. B. BARKER. 1996. Quantitative proton spectroscopic imaging of the human brain. Magn. Reson. Med. **35:** 356–363.

36. BEHAR, K. L., O. A. C. PETROFF, J. W. PRICHARD, J. R. ALGER & R. G. SHULMAN. 1986. Detection of metabolites in rabbit brain by 13C NMR spectroscopy following administration of 1-13C-glucose. Magn. Reson. Med. **3:** 911–920.

37. BECKMANN, N., J. TURKALJ, J. SEELIG & U. KELLER. 1991. 13C NMR for the assessment of human brain glucose metabolism in vivo. Biochemistry **30:** 6362–6366.

38. ROTHMAN, D. L., E. J. NOVOTNY, G. I. SHULMAN, *et al.* 1992. ^{1}H-{^{13}C} NMR measurements of {4-^{13}C}-glutamate turnover in human brain. Proc. Natl. Acad. Sci. USA **89:** 9603–9606.

39. KANAMORE, K. & B. D. ROSS. 1995. Selective in vivo observation of [5-15N] glutamine amide protons in rat brain by 1H-15N multiple-quantum coherence transfer NMR. J. Magn. Reson. B **107:** 107–115.

40. BECKMANN, N. 1992. In vivo 13C spectroscopy in humans. *In* NMR, Basic Principles and Progress. M. Rudin & J. Seelig, Eds.: 73–100. Springer-Verlag. Berlin.

41. BECKMANN, N. 1995. 13C Magnetic resonance spectroscopy as a noninvasive tool for metabolic studies on humans. *In* Carbon-13 NMR Spectroscopy of Biological Systems. N. Beckmann, Ed.: 269–322. Academic Press. New York, NY.

42. VAN ZIJL, P. C. M. & D. ROTHMAN. 1995. NMR studies of brain 13C-glucose uptake and metabolism: Present status. Magn. Reson. Imag. **13:** 1213–1221.

43. GRUETTER, R., E. J. NOVOTNY, S. D. BOULWARE *et al.* 1992. Direct measurement of brain glucose concentrations in humans by 13C NMR spectroscopy. Proc. Natl. Acad. Sci. USA **89:** 1109–1112 (erratum 89: 12208).

44. GRUETTER, R., E. J. NOVOTNY, S. D. BOULWARE, D. L. ROTHMAN & R. G. SHULMAN. 1996. 1H NMR studies of glucose transport in the human brain. J. Cereb. Blood Flow Metab. **16:** 427–438.

45. VAN ZIJL, P. C. M., C. T. W. MOONEN, D. DAVIS, D. DESPRES, L. ANDERSON & R. PARKER. 1992. Direct monitoring of Glucose Transport in the Brain. Society of Magnetic Resonance in Medicine. Works in Progress: 550. Berlin.

46. GRUETTER, R., E. J. NOVOTNY, S. D. BOULWARE *et al.* 1994. Localized 13C NMR spectroscopy in the human brain of amino acid labeling from 13C glucose. J. Neurochem. **63:** 1377–1385.

47. MASON, G. F., K. L. BEHAR, D. L. ROTHMAN & R. G. SHULMAN. 1992. NMR determination of intracerebral glucose concentration and transport kinetics in rat brain. J. Cereb. Blood Flow Metab. **12:** 448–455.

48. MASON, G. F., R. GRUETTER, D. L. ROTHMAN, K. L. BEHAR, R. G. SHULMAN, & E. J. NOVOTNY. 1995. Simultaneous determination of the rates of the TCA cycle, glucose utilization, α-ketoglutarate/glutamate exchange, and glutamine synthesis in human brain by NMR. J. Cereb. Blood Flow Metab. **15:** 12–25.

49. ROTHMAN, D. L., K. L. BEHAR, H. P. HETHERINGTON *et al.* 1985. 1H-observe 13C-decouple spectroscopic measurements of lactate and glutamate in the rat brain in vivo. Proc. Natl Acad. Sci. USA **82:** 1633–1637.

50. VAN ZIJL, P. C. M., A. S. CHESNICK, D. DESPRES, C. T. W. MOONEN, J. RUIZ-CABELLO & P. VAN GELDEREN. 1993. In vivo proton spectroscopy and spectroscopic imaging of {1-13C}-glucose and its metabolic products. Magn. Reson. Med. **30:** 544–551.
51. MORRIS, P. G. 1986. Nuclear Magnetic Resonance Imaging in Medicine and Biology. Oxford University Press. New York, NY.

DISCUSSION

QUESTION: Given the sensitivity that you talked about is, there an ability to use the glucose measurement in activation studies? Have you been able to witness changes?

VAN ZIJL: At Yale, Dr. Rothman *et al.* have done a study where they looked at visual activation; they say they saw the oxidative glucose metabolism, doubled by a factor of two. They did that in a volume localized in the back of the brain. I have seen it shown at a conference. I don't think it has been published yet. So researchers *are* trying to do these studies.

Multiecho Approaches to Spectroscopic Imaging of the Brain[a]

R. V. MULKERN,[b,c] H. CHAO,[d] J. L. BOWERS,[e] AND D. HOLTZMAN[f]

[b]*Department of Radiology*
[f]*Department of Neurology*
Children's Hospital and Harvard Medical School
Boston, Massachusetts 02115

[d]*Harvard/MIT Division of Health Science Technology*
Cambridge, Massachusetts 02138

[e]*Department of Radiological Sciences*
Deaconess Hospital
Boston, Massachusetts 02215

CONVENTIONAL, RARE, AND CPMG MODE SPECTROSCOPIC IMAGING

Conventional spectroscopic imaging as originally presented by Brown *et al.*[1] involves exciting the spin system, phase encoding the resulting transverse magnetization with brief field gradient pulses, and reading out each signal in the absence of applied field gradients. The volume initially excited may be restricted with the use of section-selective radio frequency (rf) pulses, examples being the point resolved echo spectroscopy (PRESS) or stimulated echo acquisition mode (STEAM) selective rf trains[2,3] for exciting cube-like volumes. With the signal readout in the absence of field gradients, direct Fourier transform yields the spectral information. The longer the signal readout duration, the higher the spectral resolution. Typical readouts in conventional SI methods are on the order of 1 s, providing a 1-Hz spectral resolution.

From a total acquisition time perspective, the slow part of conventional SI lies in the phase encoding process used to provide the spatial mapping of the spectral peaks within the excited volume. The phase encoding process requires that the entire sequence be repeated at some repetition time (TR) interval until the desired number of phase encoding steps along each dimension, a quantity proportional to the spatial resolution along that dimension, is

[a]This work was supported in part by grants from the Whitaker Foundation (R.V.M.), The Radiological Society of North America (J.B.), and National Institute of Health Grant 1-RO1 NS 26371 (D.H.).

[c]Address for correspondence: R. V. Mulkern, Ph.D., Department of Radiology, Children's Hospital, 300 Longwood Avenue, Boston, Massachusetts 02115. Phone: (617) 730-0737; fax: (617) 730-0645; e-mail: mulkern@bwh.harvard.edu

obtained. As an example, consider a three-dimensional (3D) acquisition in which all three spatial dimensions are to be phase encoded with 32 phase encoding steps. In this case, the sequence must be repeated 32 × 32 × 32 or 32,768 times. Even using a relatively short TR period of 1 s, a scan time of approximately 9 h results.

More practical SI scans of the brain utilize one-dimensional (1D) or two-dimensional (2D) phase encoding formats with a tailored excitation volume of either a column (1D) or a slice (2D). For instance, if a selected slice is to be spatially phase encoded using an in-plane 32 × 32 spatial matrix, a total of 1,024 signals must be acquired. Thus, even with a reasonably long TR of 2 s, which allows for substantial relaxation between spin excitations, a scan time of 34 minutes results. This is more practical than the 3D SI example considered above. Nevertheless, the 2D example serves to demonstrate how conventional SI studies, which acquire a single phase encoded spectroscopic signal each TR period, tend to have much longer scan times than the few minutes generally associated with modern MRI scans of the brain.[4] As Brown *et al.* noted,[1] more reasonable resolutions and imaging times for SI might be achieved if there were "some way to sample different k values while simultaneously refocussing the spins. . .". The term *k-values* refers to the different phase encoding steps associated with the spatial mapping process. The multiecho approach described herein utilizes Carr-Purcell-Meiboom-Gill (CPMG) echo trains[5,6] to refocus the spins, sampling a different k-value for every echo generated and so realizing the suggestion of Brown *et al.*

The first article describing the multiecho approach for reducing SI scan times refered to the method as spectroscopic imaging with rf echo plaNar (SIRFEN) technique.[7] This acronym employs terminology most consistent with the technique as an rf echo planar variant. Namely, different echoes are used for distinct phase encoding steps, accelerating the data collection process as envisioned by Mansfield and Maudsley[8] in early discussions of echo planar imaging (EPI). In this work we shall refer to this rapid multiecho SI technique as the RARE mode due to its similarity to the more commonly known rapid acquisition with relaxation enhancement (RARE) fast imaging technique.[9–12]

Another multiecho SI mode that does not decrease scan time but is useful for optimizing scan time reduction strategies and SI quality is to encode each echo of a CPMG train with the same set of phase encoding gradients.[13–16] The gradients are then incremented from TR interval to TR interval, as in conventional SI, until the desired spatial matrix is full. Unlike the conventional method, however, spectroscopic images are obtained at several echo times (TE's). The resulting data sets are useful for determining minimum echo readout durations for resolving spectral lines as well as for determining the spectral transverse relaxation times T_2, which determine how much signal different peaks contribute at different echo times. These features are important since tranverse relaxation and J-coupling effects modulate the amplitudes of the echo signals, the former causing diminished signal in later echoes and the latter causing sinusoidal echo time oscillations. We shall refer to multiecho spectroscopic imaging performed in this manner as the CPMG mode.

All three methods, conventional, RARE, and CPMG multiecho mode SI schemes are shown in FIGURE 1 for a one-dimensional spectroscopic imaging format. In working towards reduced scan times with the multiecho methods, it has proved useful to initially employ the slower CPMG mode in order to determine the optimal set of sequence timing parameters for RARE mode acquisitions. We demonstrate below how both modes are used to explore the potential of multiecho scan time reduction strategies for ^{1}H and ^{31}P SI studies of the brain. First, however, we discuss several key technical aspects of multiecho methods.

T_2 DECAY, SPECTRAL RESOLUTION, AND NUMBER OF ECHOES: CPMG MODE CONSIDERATIONS

As echoes are generated following a spin excitation, there is a gradual loss of signal due to T_2 decay processes. The T_2 decay time is typically defined in terms of a monoexponential decay of signal strength S with echo time TE:

$$S = S_o \exp(-TE/T_2), \tag{1}$$

where S_o is the signal immediately after excitation. T_2 depends on many factors and differs among spectral peaks. In practical terms, T_2 decay limits the amount of signal available from a given peak in successive echoes. The generation of spin-echoes beyond a given peak's T_2 decay envelope leads to diminishing returns in signal-to-noise. This feature highlights an important practical consideration in performing multiecho SI studies—how to determine the number of useable echoes that can be acquired within the limitations imposed by the T_2 decay time. This number depends not only upon the T_2 decay time but also on how long a time period is used for acquiring each individual echo. This echo "readout" duration is in turn inversely related to the spectral resolution—the longer the readout, the higher the spectral resolution. The essential problem thus becomes one of deciding on the minimum spectral resolution required for a given SI problem. This determines the minimum echo readout duration, which, combined with a knowledge of the spectral T_2 decay times, determines the number of echoes that can be gainfully collected.

The CPMG mode is best suited for studying the fundamental trade-offs between T_2 decay, spectral resolution, and the total number of useable echoes for any given task. As an example, it has been found from CPMG SI studies of vertebral bone marrow that a 32-ms echo readout is sufficient for spectral quantitation of the fat (combined methylene plus methyl triglyceride resonances) and water at 1.5 T.[15] In addition, spectral T_2 values of approximately 80 and 120 ms were measured from the CPMG data sets for the water and fat marrow resonances, respectively. The conclusion is that 3 to 6 useable echoes can be acquired for RARE mode SI studies of vertebral marrow when the goal

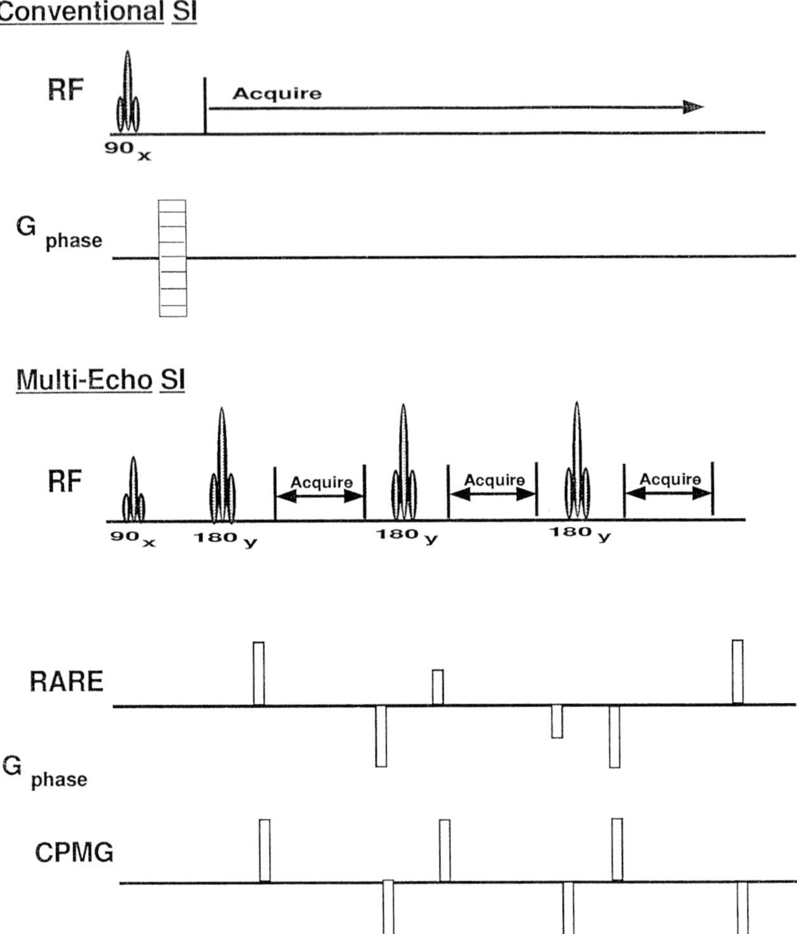

FIGURE 1. Pulse sequence diagrams for 1D spectroscopic image (SI) data acquisitions using a conventional SI method (**top**) and the two multiecho SI methods discussed in the text, RARE and CPMG. The data acquisition periods of the conventional SI methods are longer then the acquisition periods of the CPMG and RARE methods, which subsequently suffer from reduced spectral resolution. However, the breakup of the conventional SI readout period into multiple smaller readouts in the form of spin echos generated with 180° refocusing pulses allows for the collection of several different spatial phase encode steps in RARE mode, reducing scan times compared to conventional SI. In CPMG mode, the scan time is equivalent to conventional SI, but data sets are collected at the various echo times, allowing for detailed studies of the spectral resolution vs. T_2-decay tradeoffs necessary to optimize RARE mode scan time reduction strategies. In both multiecho sequences, the phase encode gradient applied immediately prior to echo readout is "unwound" following readout with an oppositely polarized phase encode gradient to return the spin system to the central k-space line prior to the next refocusing pulse.[7,9–12]

is to provide information on relative fat/water concentrations in minimal scan times.

k-SPACE, PHASE ENCODE ORDERING, AND EFFECTIVE ECHO TIMES: RARE MODE CONSIDERATIONS

Once CPMG mode SI studies have been applied to determine optimal echo readout durations and the number of useable echoes for a given problem, the transition to RARE mode SI for reducing scan times can be made. The k-space formalism for describing MR imaging[17] serves to describe the spatial phase encoding process in RARE SI mode as well. The term *k-space* refers to the raw data matrices whose rows are the time signals acquired following the different spin excitations. Fourier transformation of these raw data matrices yields the final MR images or MR spectroscopic images.

Let us consider the k-space data of a RARE mode SI collected with just one-dimensional phase encoding (FIGURE 1). Ultimately, the SI generated will be a 2D image in which one dimension is spatial and the other dimension is spectral. The k-space matrix for such an acquisition is defined by a k_y (vertical) axis and a k_x (horizontal) axis. Each horizontal line of the matrix is an echo that has been read out symetrically about its center and in the absence of any field gradients to retain the spectroscopic information. Fourier transformation along the k_x axis provides the spectral information. The vertical k_y location of each line in the k-space matrix is determined by the specific amplitude of the phase encode gradient that preceded that particular echo readout. Fourier transformation along the k_y axis leads to the spatial mapping along one spatial dimension. In RARE mode, the k-space lines are filled with successive echoes, and several lines are filled each TR interval.[7]

FIGURE 2 illustrates the filling of such a k-space matrix with a four-echo RARE sequence. As shown, four lines of the k-space matrix are filled each TR period. Using conventional SI, only one line of the k-space matrix is filled each TR period. Similarly, in CPMG mode, four separate k-space matrices are generated for each echo time but are filled, as in conventional SI, at a rate four times slower than the single k-space matrix obtained from a four-echo RARE mode sequence. What is significant about the RARE mode acquisition is that the k-space matrix is a "mixed bag" of lines formed from different echoes collected at different echo times following the initial excitation. The question then arises as to which echo time should be used in Eq (**1**) to adequately describe the T_2-weighting of a RARE spectroscopic image. In addition, how does this k-space "T_2-filter" affect SI quality?

Fortunately, these kinds of questions have been extensively considered for the closely associated RARE imaging technique where an effective echo time (ETE) that best characterizes the T_2-weighting factor has been identified as that echo which has been encoded with the smallest phase encoding gradients.[10–12] These echoes contain low-frequency component spatial information but most of the tissue contrast information in the form of the T_2-weighting

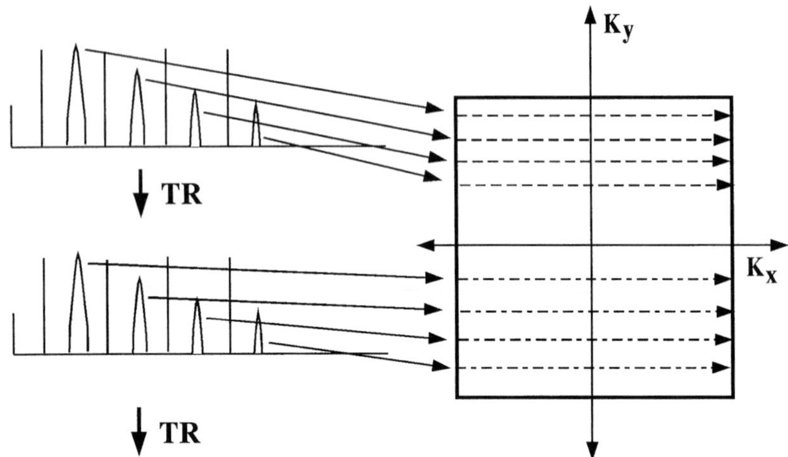

FIGURE 2. Schematic of a RARE mode filling of k-space for a 1D SI data matrix. Each line in the k-space matrix is an echo generated as one of several during a CPMG echo train. Thus the k_x-axis is essentially individual time points during a single echo collection. The echoes are read out without applied field gradients so that Fourier transformation over the k_x-axis yields the spectral information. With a four-echo RARE mode acquisition, four echoes fill four different lines, or four different k_y positions, of the k-space matrix. The vertical position of each line, or echo, is determined by the amplitude of the phase encode gradient preceding the readout. Fourier transformation along the k_y-axis results in the spatial mapping along the direction of the phase encode gradient. In conventional SI, one line of k-space is filled each TR interval, making it four times slower than the RARE mode filling shown in the figure.

factor given by Eq (**1**) with TE replaced by ETE. The echoes encoded with the larger phase encoding gradients in turn contain the higher frequency component spatial information and determine such properties as the quality of edge definition between different tissues and overall blurriness of the images along the spatial dimension encoded with multiple echoes.

The relationship between the phase encode amplitude and the type of information encoded into a given echo allows for a considerable flexibility in choosing the ETE and subsequent T_2-weighting of RARE mode SI's. FIGURE 3a and b illustrate how two different ETE settings may be made with a 4-echo, 8-shot sequence collecting a total of 32 phase encode steps in 8 TR intervals (the number of "shots" of the sequence). In these diagrams, the signal attenuation with echo time due to T_2-decay is plotted along the y-axis as a function of phase encode step from the least negative to the most positive (x-axis). The amplitudes associated with each k_y line of the k-space matrix are plotted in this manner. With conventional SI methods, such a plot would be a straight horizontal line since phase encode steps are not collected at different echo times but rather at the same time following each excitation. The scheme shown in FIGURE 3a uses the first echo of each shot for encoding the smallest phase encode gradients near the center of k-space. Thus, the phase encode steps around the central zero phase encode step show the least signal attenuation, insuring the shortest possible ETE, which will be equal to the minimum echo spacing. This scheme leads to the most signal while sacrificing some edge definition (blurring) along the spatial dimension encoded with multiple echoes. FIGURE 3b shows an alternative phase encode reordering strategy in which the second and third echoes of the four-echo CPMG train are used for the smaller phase encode gradients, the so-called straight phase encode order.[18] The ETE in this case is approximately equal to the time between the second and third echo times. The resultant SI will be more T_2-weighted than one acquired with the scheme of FIGURE 3a. For those spectral peaks with long enough T_2 values to be present in all four echoes, however, a higher quality spatial mapping will result from this phase encode ordering due to the greater signal available for some of the high-frequency spatial components.

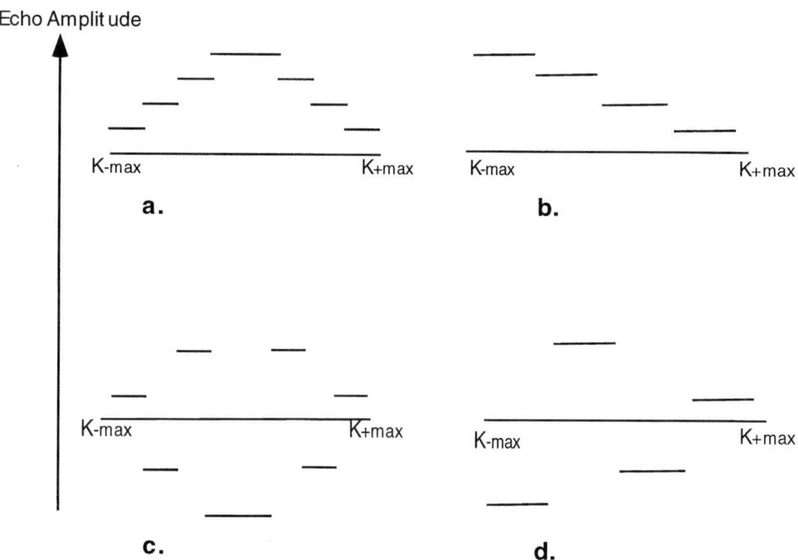

FIGURE 3. Diagrams illustrating echo amplitude vs. phase encode gradient amplitude along the k_y-axis for four echo RARE mode SI acquisitions. The top two diagrams (**a and b**) represent two different manipulations of the effective echo time (ETE) for different T_2-weightings. In **a**, the earliest echoes are used for phase encode gradient amplitudes around 0, resulting in minimal T_2 weighting with an ETE equal to the echo spacing. In **b**, a "straight" phase encode order is shown in which the ETE is pushed to the middle echoes for increased T_2-weighting (longer ETE) and more signal for some of the larger k_y values, improving edge definition. References 10–12 discuss these effects from a RARE imaging perspective but are completely relevant to the SI case. The lower figures (**c and d**) depict how J-coupling modulations among lactate protons or ATP ^{31}P nuclei affect the diagrams in **a** and **b**, which show only the T_2-decay effects. The sinusoidal variations with echo time can result in negative weighting factors, complicating the spatial mapping process.

Diagrams like FIGURE 3a and b illustrate different phase encoding schemes for manipulating effective echo times of RARE acquisitions and show how the different k-space lines are weighted by the "T_2-filter" of k-space. In some cases echoes are further modulated by J-coupling interactions between the nuclei under observation. In this case the k-space lines attain sinusoidal-type weighting factors in addition to the exponential T_2 decay attenuation. The effect on the k-space lines is illustrated in FIGURE 3c and d, where the possibility of some k-space lines acquiring negative weighting factors is observed. J-coupling interactions turn out to be quite important for multiecho studies of some metabolites like lactate and ATP, and so we discuss them in more detail.

J-COUPLING EFFECTS ON RARE MODE k-SPACE DATA; SPATIAL MISREGISTRATION

The J-coupling phenomenon is well known in high field NMR spectroscopy, where it is manifested as a splitting of individual resonances into multiplets.[19] Not all nuclei are affected by J-coupling, including some very important signals like the proton resonance from water and the most prominent brain metabolite signals in ^{1}H brain spectra. Most observable J-coupling interactions occur between groups of nuclei with different chemical shifts that are at adjacent sites along a molecule. The bonding electrons holding these groups together also have magnetic moments that serve to mediate the J-coupling interactions between the chemically distinct, adjacent groups. For example, the lactate molecule has a methyl group (CH_3) adjacent to a methine proton (CH). Furthermore, the methyl protons (one group) and methine proton (the other "group") have different chemical shifts. This sets the stage for a J-coupling interaction between the two groups. A high field spectrum of lactate thus reveals a doublet for the methyl resonance, a splitting due to the "up" or "down" state of the methine proton. Similarly a quartet of lines is observed for the methine resonance, which is split into four levels by the effective spin $3/2 = \frac{1}{2} + \frac{1}{2} + \frac{1}{2}$ of the three adjacent methyl protons.

The effects of J-coupling in CPMG and RARE mode SI acquisitions appear as echo time–dependent amplitude modulations. These modulations can be calculated from a knowledge of the spin Hamiltonian and some basic quantum mechanics.[19,20] For instance, the lactate proton signal arises from a so-called weakly coupled AX_3 system whose Hamiltonian reads:

$$H = w_1 I_z + w_2(S_z + S'_z + S''_z) + J(I_z S_z + I_z S'_z + I_z S''_z), \qquad (2)$$

where I_z and the S_z, S'_z , S''_z are the z-component spin angular momentum operators for the A and three X spins of the lactate system, w_1 and w_2 are the chemical shifts of the A and X spins, respectively, and J is the coupling constant between the A and X spins. The term "weakly coupled" refers to the fact that the coupling constant J is much smaller than the chemical shift difference $|w_1 - w_2|$. This allows one to neglect the nonsecular terms $I_x S_x$,

I_yS_y, etc., which would otherwise be in the Hamiltonian of Eq **(2)**. Using standard quantum mechanical principles,[19,20] the lactate signal modulations with echo time are readily calculated with Eq **(2)**. For an echo spacing of 2t in a CPMG train, the amplitudes for the A and X spins at the center of the nth echo at TE = n2t are given by

$$S_A = \cos(3JTE/2) + 3\cos(JTE/2) \quad \textbf{(3a)}$$

and

$$S_X = 12\cos(JTE/2), \quad \textbf{(3b)}$$

where J is in radians/s. For lactate J is approximately $2\pi \times 7$ Hz, and Eq **(3b)** indicates that spin echo amplitudes of the X spins will swing from maximally negative to maximally positive values at intervals of approximately 143 ms. Equation **(3)** predicts a somewhat more complex behavior for the A spins with TE. Both signal behaviors are readily verified. FIGURE 4 shows signal intensities of the A spins and X spins of lactate measured experimentally from a series of single spin-echo (so-called Hahn spin-echo) spectra acquired at 7 T

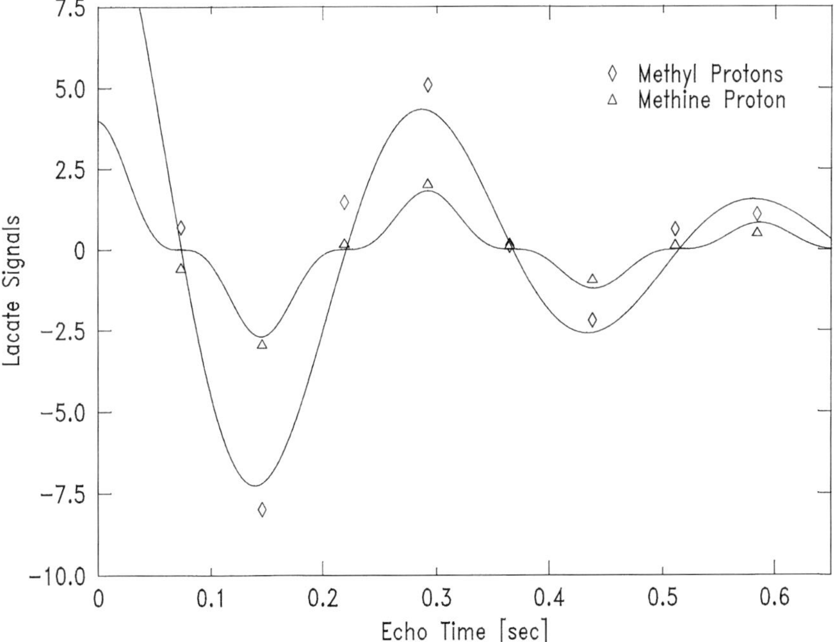

FIGURE 4. Experimentally observed J-coupling modulations with echo time of the methyl protons (X spins) and the methine proton (A spins) of the AX_3 system of the lactate molecule. The data, measured from lactate solution spectra at 7 T, shows the predicted modulations (*solid lines*) calculated from basic quantum mechanical principles. These effects must be accounted for to make proper spatial maps of coupled spin systems with multiecho SI methods.

from a 100-mM lactate solution in 99% D_2O. Shown with the experimentally measured points are theoretical fits using Eq **(3)** multiplied by a monoexponential T_2 decay factor **(1).** The spin-echo modulations of both proton groups of the lactate molecule are seen to conform to the theory.

Lactate is an important metabolite detectable in proton brain spectroscopy in a number of pathologic states. The echo time oscillations due to J-coupling shown in FIGURE 4 complicate lactate mapping with multiecho SI methods. Duyn *et al.* have considered implementations of RARE mode SI methods that specifically address the lactate detection problem.[21] In particular, they selected echo spacings that are multiples of $2\pi/J$ (about 143 ms), so that the lines in k-space from odd and even echoes have opposite signs for the methyl spins of lactate. This results in phase encode–echo amplitude correlations like those shown in FIGURE 3c and d. These in turn lead to severe spatial misregistration upon Fourier transformation. Simply reversing the sign of the odd echoes restores the k-space data to a standard data set for lactate methyl protons, which can then be mapped with only the usual T_2-decay–associated problems discussed above.

For *in vivo* ^{31}P multiecho spectroscopic imaging studies, J-coupling effects among the three phosphorus nuclei of the ATP molecule also play a prominent role. The ^{31}P nuclei are chemically distinct and in a linear array along the molecule. As such they form a weakly coupled AMX system. The Hamiltonian is given by

$$H = w_\gamma I_{z\gamma} + w_\alpha I_{z\alpha} + w_\beta I_{z\beta} + J_{\gamma\alpha} I_{z\gamma} I_{z\alpha} + J_{\gamma\beta} I_{z\gamma} I_{z\beta} + J_{\alpha\beta} I_{z\alpha} I_{z\beta}, \quad \textbf{(4)}$$

where $J_{\alpha\beta}$, $J_{\beta\gamma}$, and $J_{\alpha\gamma}$ are the coupling constants and the chemical shifts w and I_z components of the nuclei are labeled with the α, β, and γ subscripts.

Using basic quantum mechanics again leads to expressions for the nth echo amplitudes of the α, β and γ resonances which read

$$S_\alpha = \cos((J_{\alpha\beta} - J_{\alpha\gamma})TE/2) + \cos((J_{\alpha\beta} + J_{\alpha\gamma})TE/2) \quad \textbf{(5a)}$$

$$S_\beta = \cos((J_{\alpha\beta} - J_{\beta\gamma})TE/2) + \cos((J_{\alpha\beta} + J_{\beta\gamma})TE/2) \quad \textbf{(5b)}$$

$$S_\gamma = \cos((J_{\alpha\gamma} - J_{\beta\gamma})TE/2) + \cos((J_{\alpha\gamma} + J_{\beta\gamma})TE/2). \quad \textbf{(5c)}$$

It should be noted that $J_{\alpha\beta}$ and $J_{\beta\gamma}$ are the coupling constants between adjacent nuclei, while $J_{\alpha\gamma}$ is the coupling constant between the α and γ ATP nuclei, which are two chemical bonds apart. As we shall see below, this constant is largely negligible. Furthermore, the two adjacent bond coupling constants are nearly equal. This considerably simplifies the complex echo time oscillations given by Eq **(5a–c)** (vide infra).

MULTIECHO ^1H SPECTROSCOPIC IMAGING STUDIES OF BRAIN

The spectral peaks that have attracted the most attention in ^1H spectroscopic studies of the brain arise from methyl groups (CH_3) of *N*-acetylaspartate (NAA), choline (Cho)–containing compounds, and total creatine (Cr) compounds including phosphocreatine.[22–24] These three resonances appear at approximately 2.0 ppm (NAA), 3.2 ppm (Cho), and 3.0 ppm (Cr). They are the most prominent peaks in normal, water suppressed brain spectra. The methyl group of lactate at a spectral location around 1.3 ppm often appears in pathological brain tissue.[25–27] The preeminent role that NAA, Cho, and Cr signals have played in the literature of proton spectroscopic brain studies is largely a consequence of their relatively long T_2 values compared to other metabolites, a feature that would tend to favor multiecho acquisitions.

Duyn and Moonen first performed ^1H RARE mode SI studies of brain at 1.5 T.[28] They utilized 32 × 32 2D in-plane matrices with one phase encoding dimension acquired with multiple echoes. The 3D k-space matrices were completely filled in approximately 10 minutes using a 2.7-s TR. With conventional SI, these same acquisition parameters would lead to scan times exceeding 30 minutes. Though the scan time reduction is impressive, a major price is paid with loss in spectral resolution compared to conventional SI. Namely, despite the use of 128-ms echo readouts with an absolute spectral resolution of 8 Hz, there was a poor separation of the Cho and Cr resonances, which at 1.5 T are approximately 13 Hz apart. Longer echo readouts to increase the spectral resolution and solve the Cho/Cr resolution problem would, unfortunately, introduce greater T_2 decay loss, leading to increased spatial blurring and a reduction in the number of usable echoes and increased scan times.

The Cho/Cr resolution problem in the brain at 1.5 T is not confined to RARE mode acquisitions. Mulkern *et al.*[13] generated CPMG mode multiecho SI's of the brain using five echoes with echo readouts and spacings similar to those employed by Duyn and Moonen.[28] The long scan times associated with the CPMG as opposed to RARE mode acquisitions for 2D SI acquisitions (30 minutes vs. 10 minutes) were avoided by employing a 1D phase encoding format in combination with a "line scan" mode.[13,15,16,18] The latter employs slice selective 180° pulses that refocus spins in a plane perpendicular to the plane excited by the initial 90° pulse. The resulting echoes arise from spins nominally confined to the intersection of the two planes. With this method, only 1D spatial encoding is required to localize signal along the column. With 30 phase encode steps, a 2.2-s TR and 8 signal averages per phase encoding step, 5-echo CPMG data sets of the selected columns were obtained in approximately 9 minutes.[13]

FIGURE 5 shows some representative 1.5-T line scan CPMG mode SI's of a 15 × 15–mm² column oriented anteriorly to posteriorly through the brain of a healthy 22-year-old male. The column targeted for spectroscopic interrogation is outlined as a black band in FIGURE 5a using a presaturation technique coupled with a rapidly acquired scout image.[18] FIGURE 5b,c, and d are the first, second, and third echo SI's with TE's of 114, 228, and 342 ms, respectively. The vertical axis is spatial and the horizontal axis is spectroscopic. The echo spacing of 114 ms accommodated echo readouts of 96 ms with a 10-Hz

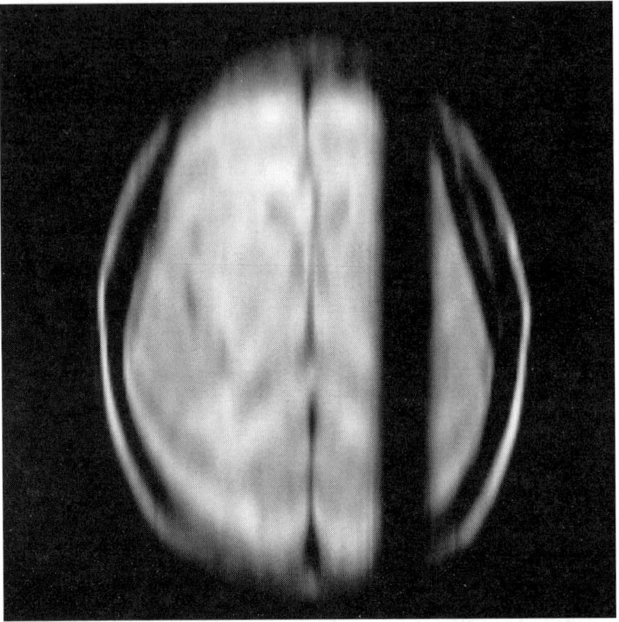

a.

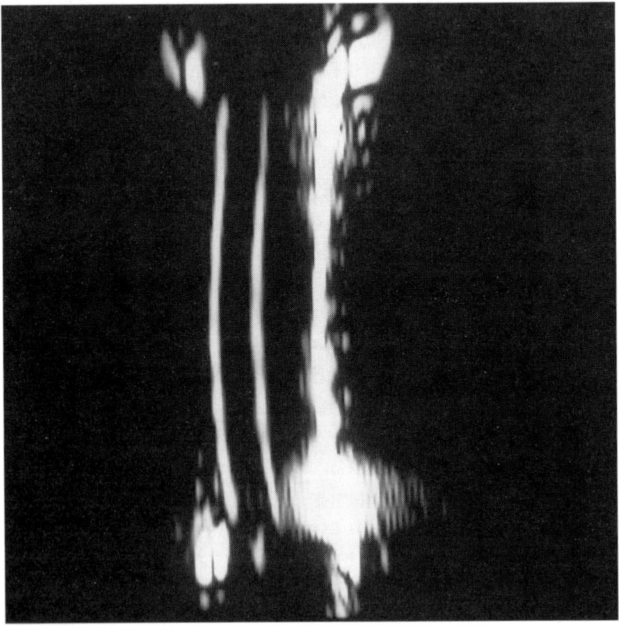

b

FIGURE 5

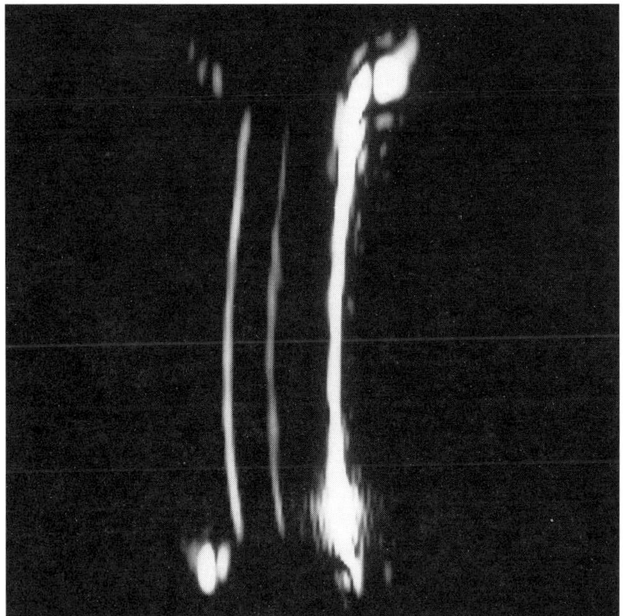

c

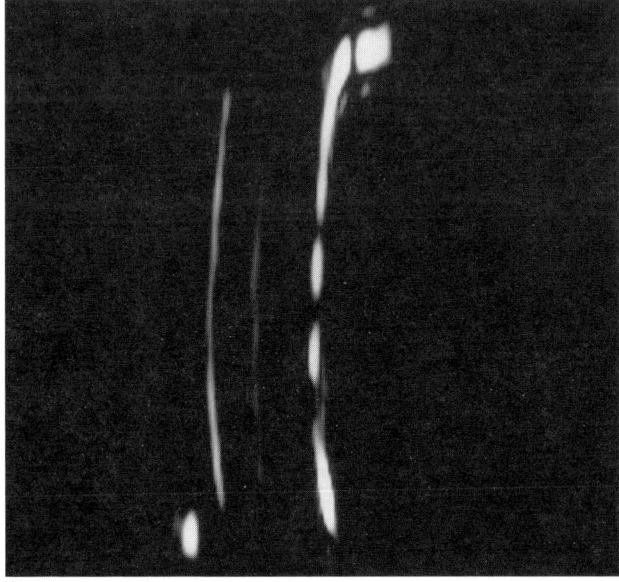

d

FIGURE 5

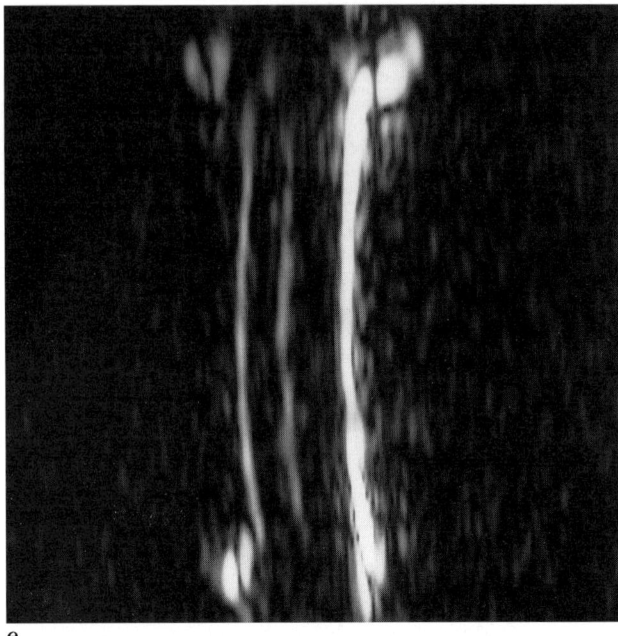

e

FIGURE 5 (*Above and preceding pages*). (**a**) Axial scout image of the column targeted for spectroscopic interrogation. The 15 × 15–mm² column is outlined with a saturation band oriented anteriorly to posteriorly through the brain. CPMG mode SI's of the column at echo times of 114 ms, 228 ms, and 342 ms collected in approximately 9 minutes are shown in **b–c**. The spectroscopic axis is horizontal with lipid peaks visible at scalp locations (left side of SI) and the residual water band furthest to the right. The NAA band and the combined Cho + Cr band both traverse the length of the column (peak assignment in text). Note the presence of these metabolite bands in all three echoes. (**e**) RARE mode SI of the same column acquired in only three minutes using a three-echo RARE acquisition with all other parameters the same as CPMG acquisition (see text for acquisition parameters).

absolute spectral resolution. Two lipid resonances from CH_3 and CH_2 groups appear at scalp locations towards the top and bottom of the column at spectral locations furthest to the left. These resonances have been greatly reduced by the use of an inversion pulse placed 150 ms prior to the CPMG train[13] but still provide signals as strong or stronger than the brain metabolite signals. Proceding from left to right along the spectral axis, the first vertical band that traverses the entire length of the brain is the NAA resonance. The next full-length band consists of both Cho + Cr protons since these two peaks are generally unresolvable at the spectral resolution afforded by 96-ms echo readouts at 1.5 T. The residual water band furthest to the right provides the strongest signal in all these images despite the use of three frequency-selective water suppression pulses.[13]

FIGURE 5b,c, and d demonstrate the T_2-decays of the individual metabolite peaks as they fade with echo time. They also demonstrate, however, that signal from these primary brain resonances, NAA and Cho + Cr, are present at all three echo times. Indeed, spectral T_2 values measured from such data sets were all 175 ms or longer,[13] indicating that three echoes can be gainfully used in RARE mode acquisitions, reducing nine-minute acquisitions to three minutes while retaining essentially the same spectral information. FIGURE 5e is the three-echo RARE mode SI of the column acquired in only three minutes using parameters identical to the CPMG mode acquisitions. Note that the same resonances are mapped but with some degradation in signal-to-noise and increased spatial blurring traded for the decreased scan time.

FIGURE 6 presents results from another CPMG and RARE mode SI study designed to push the limits of data speed acquisition with the multiecho approach at 1.5 T. The horizontally oriented column depicted in FIGURE 6a was initially interrogated with a line scan CPMG sequence consisting of 5 echoes with a 78-ms echo spacing and 64-ms echo readouts. The reduced readout period compared to the previous study made the spectral resolution even smaller (16 vs. 10 Hz). The advantage is that all five echoes of the CPMG acquisition contained signal from both the NAA band and the combined Cho + Cr band. FIGURE 6b demonstrates the strong signals remaining in the third echo CPMG SI with a TE of 234 ms. The implication for the RARE mode acquisitions is that five echoes may be used to decrease k-space filling by a factor of five with the 78-ms echo spacing. FIGURE 6c is a RARE mode SI of the brain column acquired in approximately 15 s using only one signal average per phase encode, a 2.2 s TR and all five echoes to fill the 30 phase encodes in just six "shots." The effective TE for this image is 234 ms since the third echo was used for the smallest phase encoding gradients. The NAA band and the combined Cho + Cr band are mapped quite nicely across the brain. Blurring along the spatial dimension from the residual water and lipid peaks in the scalp is more evident than in the CPMG image due to the T_2 filter effects discussed above. FIGURE 7 is a brain spectrum ($15 \times 15 \times 15$–mm^3 voxel) extracted from the rapid scan SI of FIGURE 6c. The spectral quality is quite reasonable given the 15-s acquisition time, with the major limitation being the lack of Cho + Cr separation.

Despite the shortening of brain SI scan times demonstrated with ^{1}H RARE mode SI studies of the brain at 1.5 T performed to date, the overall results are somewhat disappointing in that the reduced echo readouts required to capture several useful echoes do not provide sufficient spectral resolution for separating Cho and Cr resonances. In some applications a measure of the NAA/(Cho + Cr) ratios may be of utility. In these cases, RARE mode SI studies can be useful in facilitating the clinical examinations. However, the primary advantages of multiecho ^{1}H SI studies in the brain will probably be more fully realized at field strengths greater than 1.5 T. This is due not only to improved signal-to-noise ratio but, more fundamentally, because of a greater chemical shift dispersion. Shungu and Hilal have utilized echo readouts of 55 ms at 4.7 T and demonstrated separation of Cho and Cr resonances in the rat brain.[29]

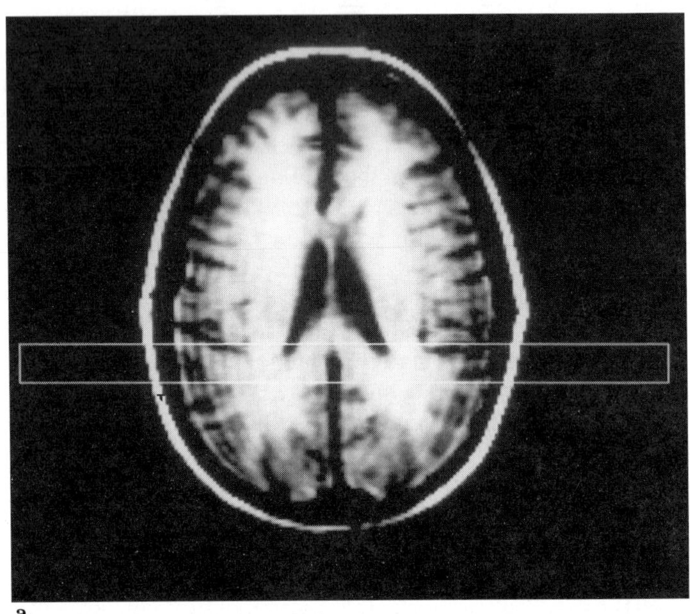

a

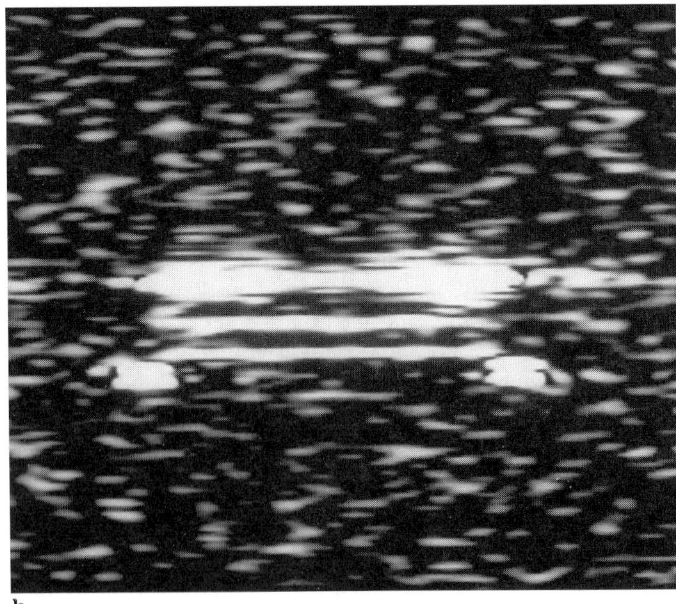

b

FIGURE 6

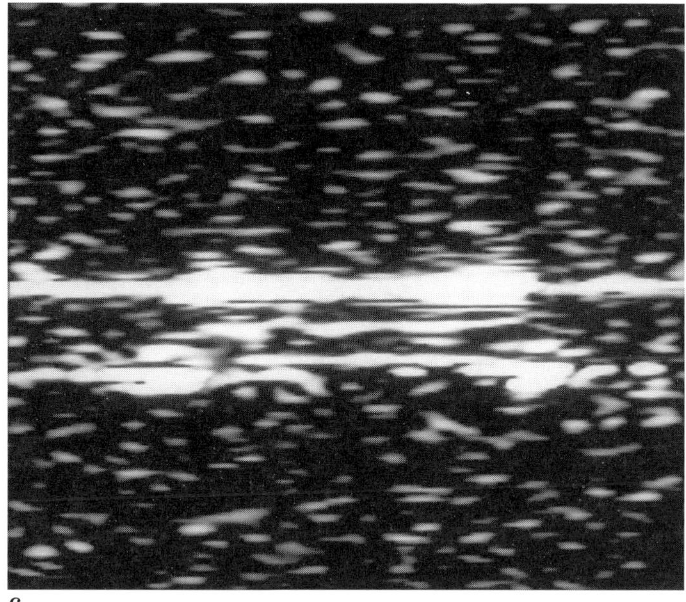

c

FIGURE 6 (*Above and facing page*). (**a**) Tissue column (15 × 15 mm^2) for spectroscopic study oriented left-to-right through the axial brain image. A reduced echo spacing of 78 ms and 64 ms readout was used to generate five-echo CPMG mode SI's in approximately two minutes. The third echo SI with TE = 234 ms is shown in **b** , with the Cho + Cr and NAA bands between the residual brain water (*top*) and lipid peaks in the scalp. Spectroscopic axis is vertical in these SI's, and signal from the NAA and Cho + Cr bands were present in all five echoes. This allows for acquisition of five-echo RARE mode SI's with 30 phase encode steps in approximately 15-s scan times using a 2.2-S TR. The 15-s RARE mode SI of the column is given in **c**, demonstrating the extremely rapid mapping of brain metabolites along the column.

Dreher and Leibfritz have demonstrated that 128-ms echo readouts are more than sufficient for separating Cho from Cr in animal brains at 3 T.[14] These studies demonstrate that the primary problem associated with CPMG and RARE mode SI studies of the brain at the most widely used clinical field strength of 1.5 T should not be an impediment at 3 T and above. The ongoing development of high field systems for both functional and spectroscopic studies suggests that the multiecho approach will play an important future role in ^{1}H brain SI studies. The high field systems should also make possible ^{31}P multi-echo SI studies of the brain, a topic we now discuss.

MULTI ECHO ^{31}P SPECTROSCOPIC IMAGING STUDIES AT 4.7 T

^{31}P NMR *in vivo* contains unique information about the energy state of tissue.[30–34] Resonances from ATP, phosphocreatine (PCr), and inorganic phosphorus (Pi) all contribute to *in vivo* ^{31}P spectra. Because of the low sensitivity and concentration of ^{31}P nuclei, even conventional SI methods applied in 1D spatial encoding formats have characteristically required scan times of 20 minutes or more.[32] The multiecho approach to ^{31}P spectroscopic imaging *in vivo* may thus prove very useful in reducing scan times. We have now performed some initial testing that demonstrates the feasibility of CPMG/RARE mode techniques for ^{31}P studies;[33,34] it is an area that had been neglected for reasons discussed below.

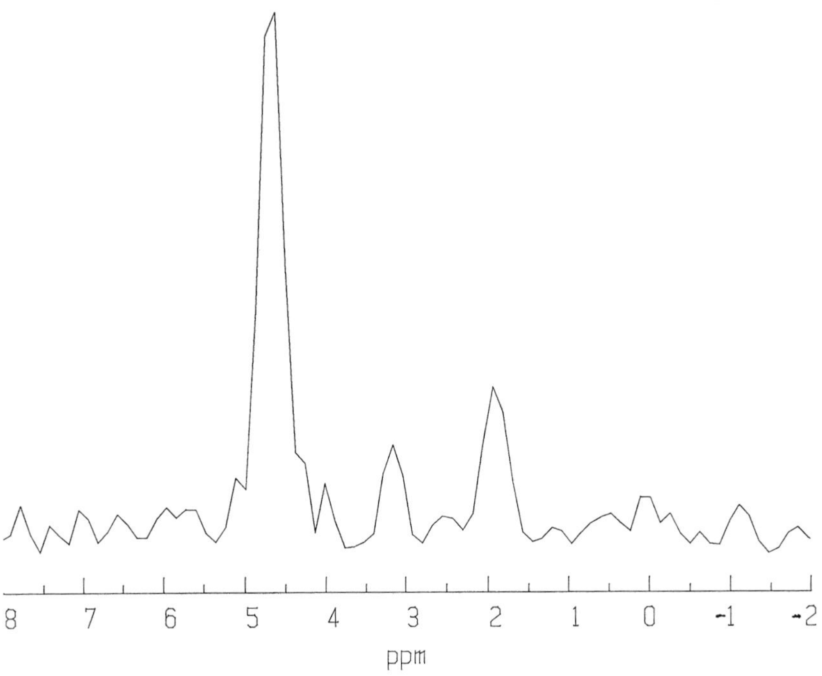

FIGURE 7. Brain spectrum extracted from a 15 × 15 × 15–mm^3 voxel of the 15-s RARE mode SI data of FIGURE 6c. Residual water at 4.7 ppm, Cho + Cr combined peak at 3.1 ppm, and NAA peak at 2.0 ppm all clearly visualized in the magnitude spectrum with an effective TE (ETE) of 234 ms. Reduced spectral resolution due to 64-ms echo readouts prohibits separation of Cho and Cr peaks but allows for a decrease in scan time by a factor of five.

The lack of attention paid to multiecho methods for ^{31}P SI to date may be due to a long-standing misconception that T_2 values of ATP resonances are short, in the 8- to 40-ms range.[35–38] If this were the case, multiecho SI methods would be of little value for mapping some of the most informative ^{31}P resonances. Several recent reports provide more accurate assessments of *in vivo* ATP T_2 values by properly taking into account the J-coupling effects among the ATP nuclei.[39–42] These reports find ATP T_2 values *in vivo* to be longer than previously thought and in the 65- to 100-ms range. This important finding has led us to consider multiecho approaches for ^{31}P studies, particularly at high field, where short echo readouts suffice to resolve the individual peaks of *in vivo* ^{31}P spectra.

The first consideration for ^{31}P multiecho studies of ATP is to determine precisely how J-coupling interactions modulate echo signal intensities and how these modulations affect spatial mapping. From 7 T spectroscopic studies of ATP solutions we determined that the $J_{\alpha\beta}$ and $J_{\beta\gamma}$ coupling constants were approximately equal, with a value of $J/2\pi = 19.3$ Hz.[33,34] The long range coupling constant was too small to accurately measure and so was taken to be 0. Eqs 5a–c then simplify, so that the spin-echo modulations of the ATP peaks obey the relations

$$S_\alpha = 2\cos(JTE/2) \quad \textbf{(6a)}$$

$$S_\beta = 1 + \cos(JTE) \quad \textbf{(6b)}$$

$$S_\gamma = 2\cos(JTE/2). \quad \textbf{(6c)}$$

These equations predict that for TE values that are integer multiples of $2\pi/J$, the β peak will be consistently maximized while the α and γ peaks will oscillate from negative to positive maximal values. This is precisely what is shown in FIGURE 8, which presents high field (7 T) Hahn spin-echo spectra of a 50-mM ATP solution. The echo times of 52, 104, 156, and 208 ms are all multiples of $2\pi/J$. The α and γ doublets oscillate from negative to positive values from odd to even echoes, as expected from Eq **(6a)** and **(6c).** The β peak is a triplet that is consistently positive as, expected from Eq **(6b)** for these echo times.

As discussed above, these modulations result in additional weighting factors for RARE mode k-space lines as illustrated in FIGURE 3c and d. The usual T_2-weighting with echo time (FIGURE 3a and b) is further modulated so that some k-space lines become negative, a situation never occurring for uncoupled spins. This has profound effects on spatial registration following Fourier transformation along the phase encode dimension. FIGURE 9a and b are RARE mode 1D SI's of a 50-mM ATP phantom acquired at 4.7 T with a 4-echo, 8-shot sequence and an 8-echo, 4-shot sequence, respectively. The phantom also contained 50 mM Pi, which appears as the top spectral band in the images. The RARE SI's mapped the spatial dimension (horizontal axis) with 32 phase encode steps and were acquired in only 36 and 18 s, respectively, using a 2.2-s TR and 2 signal averages per phase encode. The corresponding CPMG images required 140-s scan times (4 and 8 times longer than the RARE SI's of FIGURE 9) but demonstrated that signal from all three ATP resonances and the Pi peak were present in most of the echoes due to their long T_2 values in solution. The echo spacing employed in these CPMG/RARE studies was 52 ms or nearly $2\pi/J$ so that the α and γ resonances oscillated from negative to positive values from echo to echo. This is why these resonances, appearing as the two central bands in FIGURE 9a and b, appear severely ghosted along the phase encode (horizontal) dimension. The J-coupling oscillations have lead to spatial misregistration for these bands but

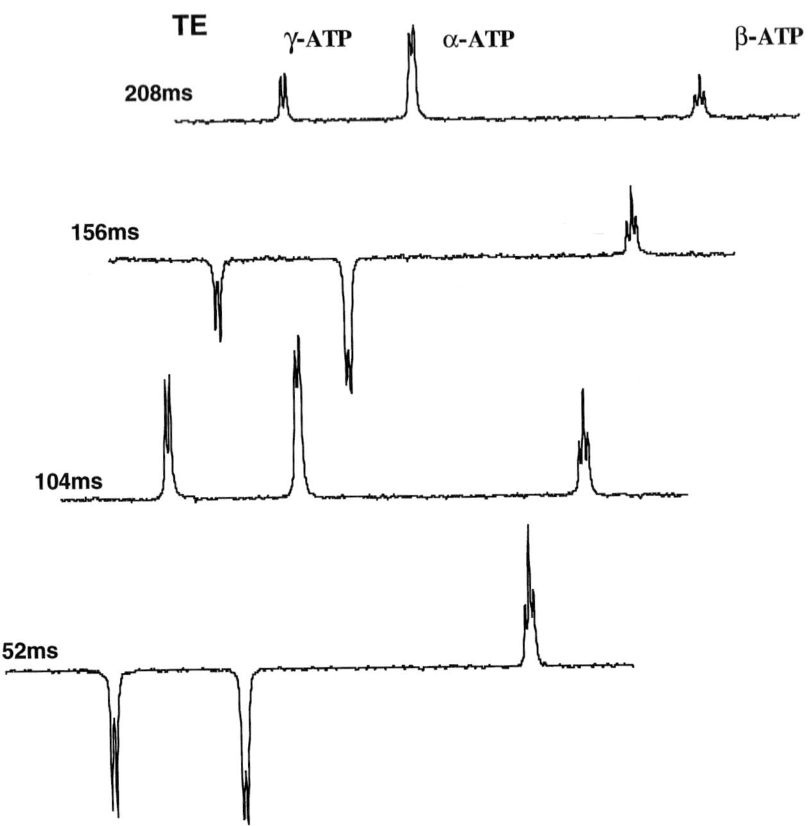

FIGURE 8. Hahn spin-echo spectra (90_x − TE/2 − 180_y − TE/2 − acquire) of the ^{31}P nuclei in a 50-mM ATP solution. TE values that are the first four integer multiples of $2\pi/J$ with J = 19.3 Hz are shown with the oscillations of the ATP peaks with echo time consistent with those predicted by theory. Spectra were acquired with a 7-T spectrometer.

not for the uncoupled Pi resonance or for the β resonance since this peak is consistently positive for echo times that are multiples of $2\pi/J$ (FIGURE 8).

Fortunately, the J-coupling effects on spatial registration can be completely corrected. FIGURE 9c and d are the RARE mode SI's of the phantom in which odd echo lines of the k-space matrices used to construct the SI's in FIGURES 9a and c have been multiplied by −1 prior to Fourier transformation. Note how the α and γ ATP bands are now nicely mapped, while the Pi and β bands have become misregistered due to the additional k-space processing. Thus it appears that the only deleterious effect of J-coupling in mapping ATP peaks in solution with RARE mode SI methods is the need to perform separate reconstructions—not acquisitions—for the different spectral peaks.

An *in vivo* demonstration of the ^{31}P multiecho approach in the rat brain is shown in FIGURE 10. A surface coil was placed on the top of the skull, and a volume coil was used to transmit the hard 90° and 180° pulses. An echo spacing of 20 ms corresponding to approximately $2\pi/3J$ (with $J/2\pi = 16$ Hz *in vivo*) was used. In this case, all peaks show some J-coupling oscillations, and the more general equations **(6a– c)** must be used for k-space corrections of RARE mode data sets. FIGURES 10a–c are the CPMG SI's at echo times of 20, 40, and 60 ms, respectively. They were acquired in 17 minutes using a 1.0-s TR, 16 phase encodes, and 64 signal averages. The spectral axis is vertical, with the strongest band arising from PCr. The β-ATP peak is seen as

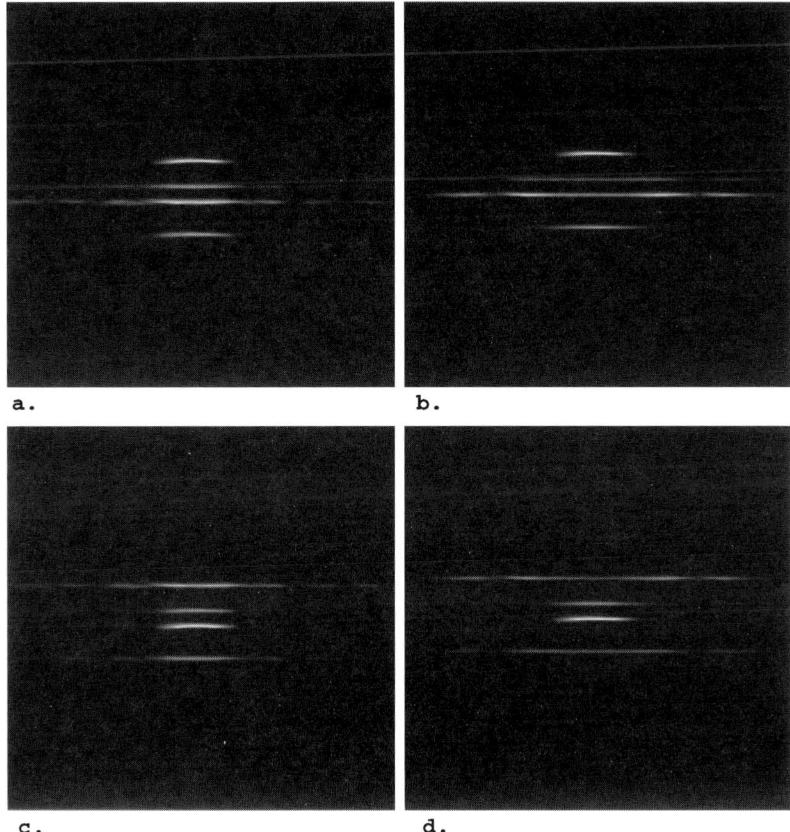

FIGURE 9. Phosphorus RARE mode SI data sets at 4.7 T (Bruker Biospec, Bruker Instruments, Billerica, MA) are shown, with **a** and **b** being four- and eight-echo RARE mode 1D SI's of a 50-mM ATP, 50-mM Pi phantom acquired in 36 and 18 s, respectively. The horizontal axis is spatial, and the vertical axis is spectroscopic, with bands, from top to bottom, of Pi, γ, α, and β ATP peaks. The echo spacing was $2\pi/J = 52$ ms, and the α and γ peaks are considerably ghosted due to the negative amplitudes for the odd echoes (FIGURE 3c and d and FIGURE 8). Correction of the raw data matrices to account for these modulations can be made prior to Fourier transformation resulting in the improved spatial maps for these resonances shown in **c** and **d**.

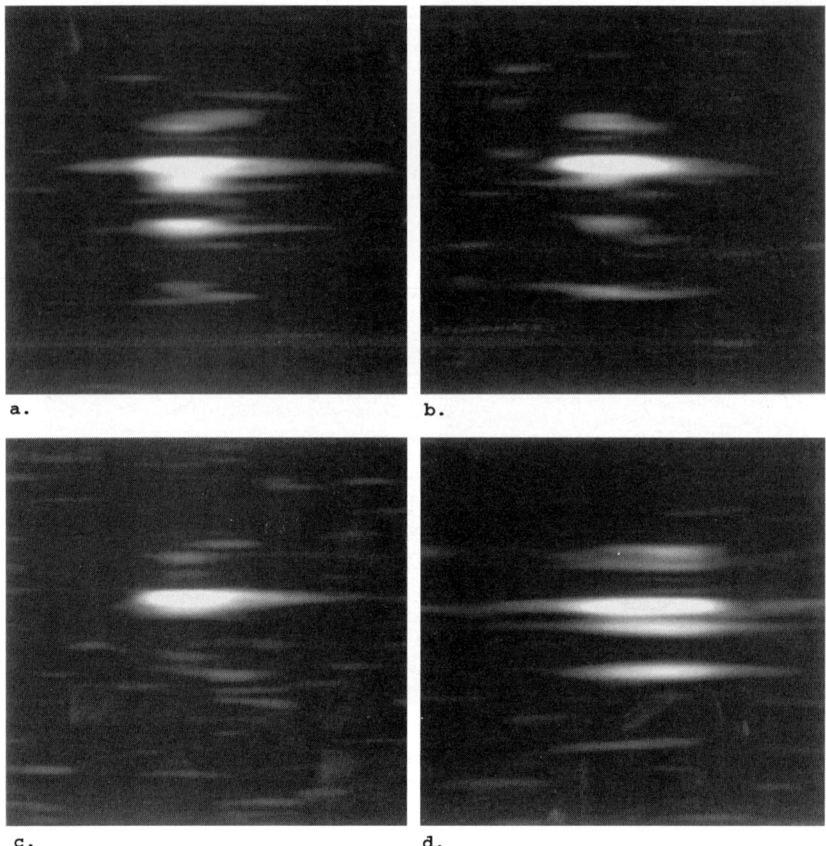

FIGURE 10. *In vivo* ^{31}P CPMG mode and RARE mode 1D SI data sets of a rat brain at 4.7 T, with **a–c** showing the CPMG SI's at echo times of 20, 40, and 60 ms. Signal from PCr is the strongest, though some signal is observed from the ATP peaks in the first two echoes and to a lesser degree in the third echo (same spectral/spatial configuration as FIGURE 9). The RARE mode SI data set shown in **d** was acquired in under six minutes and demonstrates reasonable spatial mapping of all three ATP resonances and PCr with a three-fold reduction in scan time compared to conventional SI methods with the same acquisition parameters.

the lowest spectral band and is clearly present in the first two echoes. The third echo (FIGURE 10c) has very diminished ATP peaks due to both shorter T_2 values *in vivo* as well as J-coupling effects. Using all three echoes in a RARE mode acquisition resulted in the SI of FIGURE 10d, which was acquired in only 5 minutes and 40 seconds. All three ATP resonances are mapped through the brain along with the strong PCr peak. The quality of the spatial map is quite reasonable but shows some blurring and ghosting due to both T_2-decay and, for the ATP peaks, J-coupling ghosts in this uncorrected image. FIGURE 11 is a spectrum extracted from this data set and demonstrates reasonable spectral separation of the ^{31}P peaks despite the low spectral resolution afforded by the 18-ms echo readouts.

In conclusion, *in vivo* ^{31}P multiecho studies are feasible at field strengths of 4.7 T. There are particular problems beyond simple T_2-decay for the ATP peaks in that J-coupling modulations result in spatial misregistration. These problems appear amenable to correction by k-space postprocessing. The ability to perform 1D SI studies of the brain in approximately 5 minutes or less should facilitate studies of hypoxia, stroke, and other disorders affecting brain energy metabolism.

SUMMARY

Spectroscopic imaging (SI) with nuclear magnetic resonance (NMR) is one of the most powerful tools available for studying brain chemistry *in vivo.* Both proton (^{1}H) and phosphorus (^{31}P) NMR offer valuable biochemical information that can in principle be mapped throughout the entire brain, thereby enhancing our understanding of brain function. With the exception of protons from tissue water and the triglycerides of adipose tissue, however, nuclei contributing to the NMR signals of living tissue are in relatively small (millimolar) concentrations. The low concentration of metabolite nuclei reduces the overall sensitivity of conventional SI techniques, making high-

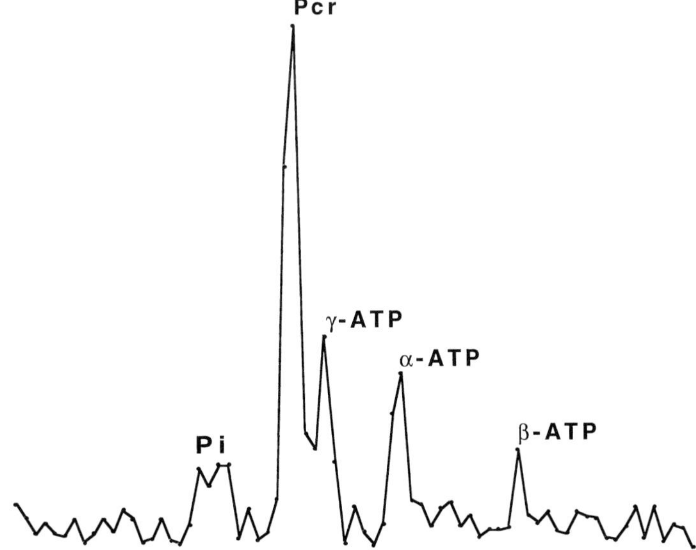

FIGURE 11. *In vivo* ^{31}P spectrum extracted from the data set of FIGURE 10d, showing spectral quality of RARE mode ^{31}P SI in the rat brain. Note that even with spectral readouts of approximately 18 ms, the major ^{31}P resonances are well resolved at 4.7 T.

quality metabolite mapping a lengthy procedure. This problem has led to the development and testing of nonconventional methods for reducing SI scan times, including techniques based on the collection of multiple spin-echoes. The extent to which multiecho methods can be used to decrease SI scan times and maintain high-quality metabolite mapping depends on several factors. These include the spectral transverse relaxation times, the spectral resolution required, and J-coupling interactions. We have discussed these various technical aspects of multiecho SI methods as applied to ^{1}H and ^{31}P spectroscopic imaging of the living brain.

ACKNOWLEDGMENTS

We thank Jiqun Meng, Ph.D. and Koichi Oshio, M.D., Ph.D. for invaluable assistance with pulse sequence design and programming.

REFERENCES

1. Brown, T. R., B. M. Kincaid & K. Ugurbil. 1982. NMR chemical shift imaging in three dimensions. Proc. Natl. Acad. Sci. (USA) **79:** 3523–3526.
2. Frahm, J., K. D. Merboldt & W. Hanicke. 1987. Localized proton spectroscopy using stimulated echoes. J. Magn. Reson. **72:** 502–508.
3. Bottomley, P. A. 1987. Spatial localization in NMR spectroscopy in vivo. Ann. N.Y. Acad. Sci. **508:** 333–348.
4. Ahn, S. S., M. T. Mantello, K. M. Jones, R. V. Mulkern, P. S. Melki, N. Higuchi & P. D. Barnes. 1992. Rapid MR imaging of the pediatric brain using the fast spin-echo technique. AJNR **13:** 1169–1177.
5. Carr, H. Y. & E. M. Purcell. 1954. Effects of diffusion on free precession in nuclear magnetic resonance experiments. Phys. Rev. **94:** 630–638.
6. Meiboom, S. & D. Gill. 1958. Modified spin-echo method for measuring nuclear relaxation times. Rev. Sci. Instrum. **29:** 688–691.
7. Mulkern, R. V., P. S. Melki, H. S. Lilly & F. A. Hoffer. 1991. 1D spectroscopic imaging with RF echo planar (SIRFEN) methods. Magn. Reson. Imaging **9:** 909–916.
8. Mansfield, P. & A. A. Maudsley. 1977. Planar spin imaging by NMR. J. Magn. Reson. **27:** 101–119.
9. Hennig, J., A. Naureth & H. Friedburg. 1986. RARE imaging: A fast imaging method for clinical MR. Magn. Reson. Med. **3:** 823–833.
10. Mulkern, R. V., S. T. S. Wong, C. Winalski & F. A. Jolesz. 1990. Contrast manipulation and artifact assessment of 2D and 3D RARE sequences. Magn. Reson. Imaging **8:** 557–566.
11. Mulkern, R. V., P. S. Melki, P. Jakab, N. Higuchi & F. A. Jolesz. 1991. Phase encode order and its effect on contrast and artifact in single-shot RARE sequences. Med. Phys. **18:** 1032–1037.
12. Melki, P. S., F. A. Jolesz & R. V. Mulkern. 1992. Partial RF echo planar imaging with the FAISE method: I. Experimental and theoretical assessment of artifact. Magn. Reson. Med. **26:** 328–341.
13. Mulkern, R. V., J. Meng, K. Oshio & A. A. Tzika. 1996. Line scan imaging of brain metabolites with CPMG sequences at 1.5 T. J. Magn. Reson. Imaging **6:** 399–405.
14. Dreher, W. & D. Leibfritz. 1995. Parametric multiecho proton spectroscopic imaging: Application to the rat brain in vivo. Magn. Reson. Imaging **13:** 753–761.
15. Mulkern, R. V., J. Meng, K. Oshio, C. R. G. Guttmann & D. Jaramillo. 1994. Bone marrow characterization in the lumbar spine with inner volume spectroscopic CPMG imaging studies. J. Magn. Reson. Imaging **4:** 585–589.

16. MULKERN, R. V., J. MENG, K. OSHIO, D. S. WILLIAMSON, H. S. LILLY, C. R. G. GUTTMANN & D. JARAMILLO. 1995. Spectroscopic imaging of the knee with line scan CPMG sequences. J. Comput. Assisted Tomogr. **19:** 247–255.
17. TWIEG, D. B. 1983. The k-space trajectory formulation of the NMR imaging process with applications in analysis and synthesis of imaging methods. Med. Phys. **10:** 610–621.
18. OSHIO, K. & R. V. MULKERN. 1992. Rapid fat/water assessment in knee cavity bone marrow by inner volume spectroscopic imaging with RARE. J. Magn. Reson. Imaging **2:** 601–604.
19. CORIO, P. L. 1960. The analysis of nuclear magnetic resonance spectra. Chem. Rev. **60:** 363–429.
20. MULKERN, R. V. & J. L. BOWERS. 1994. Density matrix calculations of AB spectral modulations: Quantum mechanics meets in vivo spectroscopy. Conc. Magn. Reson. **6:** 1–23.
21. DUYN, J. H., A. FRANK & C. T. W. MOONEN. 1995. Incorporation of lactate measurement in multi-spin-echo proton spectroscopic imaging. Magn. Reson. Med. **33:** 101–107.
22. FRAHM, J., H. BRUHN, M. L. GYNGELL, K. D. MERBOLDT, W. HANICKE & R. SAUTER. 1989. Localized proton NMR spectroscopy in different regions of the human brain in vivo. Relaxation times and concentrations of cerebral metabolites. Magn. Reson. Med. **11:** 47–63.
23. KREIS, R., T. ERNST & B. D. ROSS. 1993. Development of the human brain: In vivo quantification of metabolite and water content with proton magnetic resonance spectroscopy. Magn. Reson. Med. **30:** 424–437.
24. WEBB, P. G., N. SAILASUTA, S. J. KOHLER, T. RAIDY, R. A. MOATS & R. E. HURD. 1994. Automated single-voxel proton MRS: Technical development and multisite variation. Magn. Reson. Med. **31:** 365–373.
25. ALGER, J. R., J. A. FRANK, A. BIZZI, M. J. FULHAM, B. X. DESOUZA, M. O. DUHANEY, S. W. INSCOE, J. L. BLACK, P. C. M. VAN ZIJL, C. T. W. MOONEN & G. DI CHIRO. 1990. Metabolism of human gliomas: Assessment with H-1 MR spectroscopy and F-18 fluorodeoxyglucose PET. Radiology **177:** 633–641.
26. SEGERBARTH, C. M., D. F. BALERIAUX, P. R. LUYTEN & J. A. DEN HOLLANDER. 1990. Detection of metabolic heterogeneity of human intracranial tumors in vivo by ^{1}H NMR spectroscopic imaging. Magn. Reson. Med. **13:** 62–76.
27. BARKER, P. B., J. D. GLICKSON & R. N. BRYAN. 1993. In vivo magnetic resonance spectroscopy of human brain tumors. Top. Magn. Reson. Imaging **5:** 32–45.
28. DUYN, J. H. & C. T. W. MOONEN. 1993. Fast proton spectroscopic imaging of human brain using multiple spin echoes. Magn. Reson. Med. **30:** 409–414.
29. SHUNGU, D. C. & S. K. HILAL. 1995. Multislice proton spectroscopic imaging of the brain with retention of spectral selectivity. Proceedings of the Society of Magnetic Resonance, Third Scientific Meeting, Nice, France: 329.
30. BOTTOMLEY, P. A., H. C. CHARLES, P. B. ROEMER, D. FLAMIG, H. ENGESETH, W. A. EDELSTEIN & O. M. MUELLER. 1988. Human in vivo phosphate metabolite imaging with ^{31}P NMR. Magn. Reson. Med. **7:** 319–336.
31. BUCHLI, R., O. DUC, E. MARTIN & P. BOESIGER. 1994. Assessment of absolute metabolite concentrations in human tissue by ^{31}P MRS in vivo. Part 1: Cerebrum, cerebellum, cerebral gray and white matter. Magn. Reson. Med. **32:** 447–452.
32. TSUJI, M. K., R. V. MULKERN, C. U. COOK, R. L. MEYERS & D. HOLTZMAN. 1996. Relative phosphocreatine and nucleoside triphosphate concentrations in cerebral gray and white matter measured in vivo by ^{31}P nuclear magnetic resonance. Brain Res. **707:** 146–154.
33. MULKERN, R. V., H. CHAO, C. U. COOK, D. HOLTZMAN & J. L. BOWERS. 1996. Multi-echo spectroscopic imaging considerations for ^{31}P NMR studies of ATP. Proceedings of the International Society of Magnetic Resonance in Medicine, Fourth Meeting: 1216.
34. CHAO, H., J. L. BOWERS, D. HOLTZMAN & R. V. MULKERN. Multi-echo ^{31}P spectroscopic imaging of ATP: A scan time reduction strategy. J. Magn. Reson. Imaging. In press.
35. TURNER, J. C. & P. B. GARLICK. 1984. One- and two-dimensional ^{31}P spin-echo studies of myocardial ATP and phosphocreatine. J. Magn. Reson. **57:** 221–227.
36. THOMSEN, C., K. E. JENSEN & O. HENRIKSEN. 1989. ^{31}P NMR measurements of T_2 relaxation times of metabolites in human skeletal muscle in vivo. Magn. Reson. Imaging **7:** 557–559.

37. ALBRAND, J. P., M. F. FORAY, M. DECORPS & C. REMY. 1986. ^{31}P NMR measurements of T_2 relaxation times of ATP with surface coils: Suppression of J modulation. Magn. Reson. Med. **3:** 941–945.
38. MERBOLDT, K. D., D. CHIEN, W. HANICKE, M. G. GYNGELL, H. BRUHN & J. FRAHM. 1990. Localized ^{31}P spectroscopy of the adult brain in vivo using stimulated-echo (STEAM) sequences. J. Magn. Reson. **89:** 343–361.
39. STRAUBINGER, K., W-I. JUNG, M. BUNSE, O. LUTZ, K. KUPER & G. DIETZE. 1994. Spin-echo methods for the determination of ^{31}P transverse relaxation times of the ATP signals of human skeletal muscle in vivo. Magn. Reson. Imag. **12:** 121–129.
40. JUNG, W-I., K. STRAUBINGER, M. BUNSE, F. SCHICK, K. KUPER, G. DIETZE & O. LUTZ. 1992. ^{31}P transverse relaxation times of the ATP signal NMR signals of human skeletal muscle in vivo. Magn. Reson. Med. **28:** 305–310.
41. JUNG, W-I., K. STRAUBINGER, M. BUNSE, S. WIDMAIER, F. SCHICK, K. KUPER, G. DIETZE & O. LUTZ. 1993. A pitfall associated with determination of transverse relaxation times of the ^{31}P NMR signals of ATP using the Hahn spin-echo. Magn. Reson. Med. **30:** 138–141.
42. JUNG, W-I., S. WIDMAIER, M. BUNSE, U. SEEGER, K. STRAUBINGER, F. SCHICK, K. KUPER, G. DIETZE & O. LUTZ. 1993. ^{31}P transverse relaxation times of ATP in human brain in vivo. Magn. Reson. Med. **30:** 741–743.

DISCUSSION

QUESTION: What are some of the downsides of super high field strengths, other issues that may impact the measurements?

MULKERN: The downside of going from 4 teslas or 4.7 teslas for proton is that your resonance frequency starts to get pretty high, like 200 megahertz, so you have rf penetration problems. At 65 megahertz you have no trouble getting the radio frequency that you need deep inside the brain through the whole body. When you go to those higher field strengths, you start to run into this problem. In a 1978 paper in *Physics in Medicine and Biology* (**23:** 630–643) Bottomley and Andrew suggested that at NMR operating frequencies above 30 megahertz "magnetic field amplitude and phase variations . . . may cause serious distortions in an image of a human torso." Imaging is now performed routinely at GS megahertz without any such distortions. At very much higher field strengths (427 megahertz for protons at 10 tesla, for instance), the image distortions predicted by Bottomley and Andrew for whole body torso imaging may be anticipated.

For phosphorous it is not that big a deal because at 4.7 teslas the frequency you are using for phosphorous is only around 80 megahertz. When people start talking about 10-tesla machines, now the technology will be here, you really are going to start talking about microwave-type electronics, and I think that is a downside. I think the rf penetration problem is also coupled with the rf power deposition problem, and heating people up might become a real source of degradation.

New Histological and Physiological Stains Derived from Diffusion-Tensor MR Images

PETER J. BASSER[a]

Biomedical Engineering and Instrumentation Program
National Center for Research Resources
National Institutes of Health
Bethesda, Maryland 20892

INTRODUCTION

The measurement of the self-diffusivity of water (and other solvents) using the phenomenon of nuclear magnetic resonance was first reported more than four decades ago.[1] Methodological improvements in these diffusion measurements[2] and the subsequent development of magnetic resonance imaging,[3] together created the possibility to measure diffusion properties of water in tissues on a voxel by voxel basis. Diffusion imaging (DI), which was first realized in 1985,[4–6] consists of measuring an apparent diffusion constant (ADC)[7] in each voxel. Both its theoretical underpinnings and its applications are well-known and are described in a number of excellent books and review articles.[7,8]

While in tissues such as brain gray matter the ADC measured by diffusion imaging is largely independent of the orientation of the tissue, in brain white matter the ADC depends strongly upon the orientation of the tissue.[9–16] Since the ADC characterizes molecular displacements in only one direction, it inherently does not provide enough information to describe the three-dimensional translational displacements of protons (or other labeled nuclei) necessary to characterize diffusion in brain white matter and other anisotropic media. This additional information, however, is provided by the effective or apparent diffusion *tensor* of water, $\underline{D}$, in each voxel. The measurement of $\underline{D}$ in each voxel and the analysis and display of the information derived from it is called diffusion tensor imaging (DTI).[17] Of particular interest are new scalar parameters that possess properties of a quantitative histological or physiological stain and can be displayed as images that elucidate intrinsic features or characteristics of diffusion in tissues. Examples include images or maps of the mean diffusivity and the degree of diffusion anisotropy.

[a]Address for correspondence: Peter J. Basser, Ph.D., NIH/NCRR/BEIP, Building 13, Room 3N-17, 13 South Drive, Bethesda, Maryland 20892–5766.

BACKGROUND

In diffusion imaging (DI), one measures a single scalar apparent diffusion constant (ADC) in each voxel from a series of diffusion-weighted images (DWIs). These are just conventional MRIs whose contrast is sensitized or weighted by the local diffusivity in each voxel. Specifically, from these DWIs, one uses linear regression of Eq. **(1)** below to estimate an ADC in each voxel:

$$\ln\left(\frac{A(b)}{A(0)}\right) = -\,b\,D = -\,b\,\mathrm{ADC}, \tag{1}$$

where A(b) is the measured echo magnitude in each voxel; b is a constant called the b-value or b-factor, which is calculated for each gradient pulse sequence[18]; and A(0) is the echo magnitude without any applied diffusion gradients. Whether one is acquiring DWIs or maps of the ADC, DI is inherently a *one-dimensional* technique, that is, it can only meaningfully measure molecular displacements along one direction.

Diffusion tensor imaging (DTI)[17] is a new MRI modality that was developed to describe diffusion in anisotropic medium for which Eq. **(1)** is no longer valid. With DTI, one estimates an effective diffusion tensor, $\underline{D}$, from DWIs using a more general relationship between the measured echo magnitude in each voxel and the applied magnetic field gradient sequence[19–21]:

$$\begin{aligned}\ln\left(\frac{A(\underline{b})}{A(\underline{0})}\right) &= -\sum_{i=1}^{3}\sum_{j=1}^{3} b_{ij}D_{ij} = -\,\mathrm{Trace}\,(\underline{b}\,\underline{D}) \\ &= -\,(b_{xx}D_{xx} + 2b_{xy}D_{xy} + 2b_{xz}D_{xz} + b_{yy}D_{yy} + 2b_{yx}D_{yx} + b_{zz}D_{zz})\end{aligned} \tag{2}$$

Above, b_{ij} is a component of the symmetric b-matrix, $\underline{b}$, and $A(\underline{b})$ the echo magnitude for a gradient sequence whose b-matrix is $\underline{b}$. Whereas in DI a b-factor is usually calculated for a gradient sequence applied in one direction, in DTI the b-matrix is always calculated from all applied gradient sequences (including all imaging and diffusion gradient sequences).[19–21]

To understand the role of the b-matrix in DTI, it is useful to view the diffusion process in the principal frame of the anisotropic medium, by diagonalizing $\underline{D}$ as follows:

$$\underline{D} = \underline{E}\,\underline{\Lambda}\,\underline{E}^{T} \tag{3}$$

Above, $\underline{E}$ is the matrix whose columns are the eigenvectors or principal directions of $\underline{D}$: ϵ_1, ϵ_2, and ϵ_3; and $\underline{\Lambda}$ is the diagonal matrix whose diagonal elements are the corresponding eigenvalues or principal diffusivities of $\underline{D}$: λ_1, λ_2, and λ_3. Using Eq. **(3),** and the fact that $\mathrm{Trace}(\underline{M}\,\underline{N}) = \mathrm{Trace}\,(\underline{N}\,\underline{M})$ for two matrices $\underline{M}$ and $\underline{N}$, Eq. **(2)** can be rewritten as:

$$\ln\left(\frac{A(\underline{b})}{A(\underline{b}=\underline{0})}\right) = -\ \mathrm{Trace}(\underline{b}\ \underline{E}\ \underline{\Lambda}\ \underline{E}^{T}) = -\ \mathrm{Trace}(\underline{E}^{T}\ \underline{b}\ \underline{E}\ \underline{\Lambda})$$

$$= -\ \mathrm{Trace}\ (\underline{b}'\ \underline{\Lambda}). \qquad \textbf{(4)}$$

The matrix $\underline{b}' = \underline{E}^{T}\ \underline{b}\ \underline{E}$ is just the b-matrix in the principal frame of $\underline{D}$. The diagonal elements of $\underline{b}'$: b_{11}', b_{22}', and b_{33}' represent the projections of the original b-matrix (measured in the laboratory frame) along the principal directions of $\underline{D}$. Now, expanding Eq. **(4),** we obtain the following simple formula:

$$\ln\left(\frac{A(\underline{b}')}{A(\underline{b}'=\underline{0})}\right) = -\ b_{11}'\lambda_1 - b_{22}'\lambda_2 - b_{33}'\lambda_3 \qquad \textbf{(5)}$$

In the principal frame of the anisotropic medium, the contribution of each principal diffusivity on the echo attenuation is seen to be weighted by its corresponding b′-matrix element. Whereas in isotropic diffusion there is a single b-factor premultiplying the diffusion coefficient, in anisotropic diffusion there are three coefficients premultiplying each of the three principal diffusivities.

Once a b-matrix element has been calculated for each DWI, we estimate $\underline{D}$ from all the DWIs using multivariate linear regression[b] of Eq. **(2).** One requirement of DTI is that we apply diffusion gradients in a multiplicity (at least six) noncollinear direction.[21]

Diffusion tensor imaging subsumes diffusion imaging; the former reduces to the latter when the sample is isotropic. In such cases, it can be shown that Eq. **(2)** reduces to Eq. **(1).**

Diffusion of a Water in an Isotropic, Homogeneous Medium

Diffusion isotropy describes the case in which the translational mobility of the diffusing molecule is independent of the medium's orientation. Homogeneous diffusion refers to the case in which the translational mobility of the diffusing molecule is independent of the position within the medium. If a medium is both isotropic and homogeneous, then the translational displacement profile is given by[22]:

$$\rho(\mathbf{r}|\tau_d) = \frac{1}{\sqrt{(4\pi D\tau_d)^3}}\exp\left(-\frac{\mathbf{r}^{T}\mathbf{r}}{4D\tau_d}\right) = \frac{1}{\sqrt{(4\pi D\tau_d)^3}}\exp\left(-\frac{x^2+y^2+z^2}{4D\tau_d}\right). \qquad \textbf{(6)}$$

[b]Multivariate linear regression is just one of a number of statistical techniques that could be used to estimate $\underline{D}$ from the echo data.

Above, $\rho(\mathbf{r}|\tau_d)$ is the probability that a particle located initially at position $\mathbf{r} = \mathbf{0}$ is located at position $\mathbf{r}$ at a later time τ_d. Surfaces of constant $\rho(\mathbf{r}|\tau_d)$ are concentric spheres ("diffusion spheres"), as we see by setting the exponent of Eq. **(6)** equal to a constant. When we choose the constant to be ½,

$$x^2 + y^2 + z^2 = (\sqrt{2D\tau_d})^2 = 2D\tau_d. \qquad \mathbf{(7)}$$

Then, the radius of the diffusion sphere, $\sqrt{2D\tau_d}$, is also the standard deviation of $\rho(\mathbf{r}|\tau_d)$, σ, defined by the well-known Einstein formula[22]:

$$\sigma = \sqrt{2D\tau_d} \qquad \mathbf{(8)}$$

Thus, the radius of this particular diffusion sphere has the physical interpretation of being the mean-squared displacement of a particle released at the center of the sphere at time τ_d. The translational displacement profile of water is spherically symmetric in this case, and is completely specified by a single scalar constant, D, the diffusion coefficient; and the diffusion time, τ_d.

Diffusion of a Water in an Anisotropic, Homogeneous Medium

Recall that diffusion anisotropy is a property of certain media in which the translational mobility of the diffusing molecule depends upon the medium's orientation. In biological tissues such as brain white matter, we can ascribe anisotropic diffusion (observed in MR spectroscopy or imaging studies) to spatial variations of molecular mobility (heterogeneity) at micron and submicron length scales. This phenomenon appears to be caused primarily by the spatial arrangement of macromolecular, membranous, and fibrous constituents and their interfaces. In such tissues, diffusion anisotropy can be characterized within a macroscopic voxel by an effective diffusion tensor, $\underline{D}$. The voxel-averaged displacement distribution is now slightly more complicated:

$$\rho(\mathbf{r}|\tau_d) = \frac{1}{\sqrt{|\underline{D}|(4\pi\tau_d)^3}} \exp\left(\frac{-\mathbf{r}^T\underline{D}^{-1}\mathbf{r}}{4\tau_d}\right). \qquad \mathbf{(9)}$$

Whereas in an isotropic medium D appears in the variance of the distribution [Eq. **(6)**], in an anisotropic medium $\underline{D}$ appears in the "matrix of variances and covariances"[23] [Eq. **(9)**]. Whereas D^3 appeared in the normalization factor of $\rho(\mathbf{r}|\tau_d)$ in Eq. **(6)**, $|\underline{D}|$ (the determinant of $\underline{D}$) appears in its place in Eq. **(9).** When we construct surfaces of constant probability (again by setting the exponent of $\rho(\mathbf{r}|\tau_d)$ to a constant), we now obtain instead:

$$\begin{aligned}(D_{yy}D_{zz} - D_{yz}^2)x^2 + 2(D_{xz}D_{yz} - D_{xy}D_{zz})xy + (D_{xx}D_{zz} - D_{xz}^2)\,y^2 \\ 2(D_{xy}D_{yz} - D_{xz}D_{yy})xz + 2(D_{xy}D_{xz} - D_{xx}D_{yz})yz \\ + (D_{xx}D_{yy} - D_{xy}^2)z^2 = |\underline{D}|\tau_d,\end{aligned} \qquad \mathbf{(10a)}$$

which, rewritten in a more familiar form,

$$a\,x^2 + 2b\,xy + dy^2 + 2c\,xz + 2e\,yz + f\,z^2 = 1, \qquad \mathbf{(10b)}$$

is easily recognized as the equation of a three-dimensional ellipsoid,[c] called the "diffusion ellipsoid."[17,24]

Clearly, in an anisotropic medium, six independent parameters (a—f in Eq. **(10b)** or equivalently the six independent coefficients of $\underline{D}$: D_{xx}, D_{yy}, D_{zz}, D_{xy}, D_{xz}, and D_{yz}) are required to describe the three-dimensional displacements of particles, whereas in an isotropic medium, only one parameter, D, is sufficient. These additional parameters are required because in anisotropic media, displacements generally appear to be *correlated* in both parallel and perpendicular directions, whereas in isotropic media they do not. In fact, the elements of the diffusion tensor represent the magnitude of the correlations between the translational displacements in parallel and perpendicular directions. Specifically, the diagonal elements of $\underline{D}$, D_{xx}, D_{yy}, and D_{zz} represent the strength of correlations between molecular displacements along the same directions (i.e., along x, y, and z, respectively), while its off-diagonal elements, D_{xy}, D_{xz}, D_{yz}, represent strength of correlations in molecular displacements along perpendicular directions (i.e., between x and y, x and z, and y and z, respectively). In anisotropic media the diagonal elements of the diffusion tensor are generally unequal, whereas in isotropic media they are all equal. Moreover, in anisotropic media the off-diagonal elements are generally non-zero and may be large (i.e., comparable in magnitude to the diagonal elements), whereas in isotropic media they all equal zero.

For an anisotropic medium, we can always find a preferred frame of reference, generally other than the laboratory frame, in which translational displacements in orthogonal directions appear to be uncorrelated. This is called the "principal frame." Thus, in this frame all off-diagonal elements of the diffusion tensor vanish. The new coordinate axes are now coincident with the principal axes of the diffusion ellipsoid, and the equation describing the diffusion ellipsoid, Eq. **(10),** assumes a simpler, familiar form:

$$\left(\frac{x'}{\sqrt{2\lambda'_{xx}\tau_d}}\right)^2 + \left(\frac{y'}{\sqrt{2\lambda'_{yy}\tau_d}}\right)^2 + \left(\frac{z'}{\sqrt{2\lambda'_{zz}\tau_d}}\right)^2 = 1. \qquad \mathbf{(11)}$$

Above λ_{xx}', λ_{yy}', and λ_{zz}' are the principal diffusivities along the three respective principal directions; and $\sqrt{2\lambda'_{xx}\tau_d}$, $\sqrt{2\lambda'_{yy}\tau_d}$, $\sqrt{2\lambda'_{zz}\tau_d}$, are the mean-squared displacements of a molecule along the (three principal) x′, y′, and z′ directions at time τ_d, respectively. The mean-squared displacements are represented as the lengths of the major and minor axes of the diffusion ellipsoid. It is important to note that in most MRI applications, the principal

[c]Both $\underline{D}$ and the coefficient matrix are positive definite.

axes of the diffusion ellipsoid are not known *a priori,* and generally do not coincide with the x-y-z laboratory axes.[20]

In summary, the diagonal and off-diagonal elements of $\underline{D}$ are essential in specifying the probability distribution in Eq. **(9),** and characterizing the *size, shape,* and *orientation* of the diffusion ellipsoid in the (x-y-z) laboratory coordinate frame. Below we will see that they are also required to calculate new MRI stains.

QUANTITATIVE DIFFUSION TENSOR IMAGING—DEVELOPING AND USING MRI "STAINS"

Characterizing Diffusion Isotropy

Moseley and colleagues discovered in animals[25–27] and Warach *et al.* later showed in humans[28,29] that a reduction in the ADC is a sensitive indicator of the onset and severity of a cerebral ischemic event. However, Moseley also showed that while in gray matter (where diffusion is approximately isotropic) the ADC is independent of the direction of the diffusion sensitizing gradients, in white matter this is not the case.[13] In white matter, the contrast of the DWI (or of the ADC) in a voxel also depends on the direction in which the diffusion sensitizing gradient is applied with respect to the direction of the white matter fiber tracts in that voxel. This introduces an additional source of image contrast which complicates the interpretation of diffusion images in anisotropic white matter. Why? In white matter, one cannot ascertain whether the measured image contrast results from a structural/physiologic change (brought on by the ischemic event itself), or arises from diffusion anisotropy in the tissue (i.e., the dependence of the ADC to the relative orientation of the applied diffusion gradient and the local fiber orientation). Clearly, in ischemia monitoring, diffusion anisotropy in white matter produces an unwanted artifact that complicates the interpretation of diffusion images.

Diffusion tensor spectroscopy[20,30] and diffusion tensor imaging[17,31] provided new imaging parameters that solved this and other vexing MR imaging problems. Associated with each diffusion tensor are scalar quantities known as *invariants* that are *intrinsic* to the medium. Specifically, these parameters (and functions of them) are independent of the orientation of the tissue structures, their relative orientation to the patient's body within the MR magnet, the direction of the applied imaging and diffusion sensitizing gradients, and the choice of the laboratory coordinate system (in which the components of the diffusion tensor and magnet field gradients are measured).[20,21] In 1992, the scalar invariants of $\underline{D}$ were first proposed as novel MR parameters and were shown experimentally to be independent of fiber tract direction in anisotropic skeletal muscle.[30]

The three fundamental scalar invariants of $\underline{D}$, I_1, I_2, and I_3, are the coefficients of the characteristic equation of $\underline{D}$:

$$\lambda^3 - I_1\lambda^2 + I_2\lambda - I_3 = 0, \quad (12)$$

which is used to calculate the three principal diffusivities (λ_1, λ_2 and λ_3) of $\underline{D}$. I_1, I_2, and I_3 can be calculated directly from the diffusion tensor, or expressed in terms of λ_1, λ_2 and λ_3:

$$I_1 = \lambda_1 + \lambda_2 + \lambda_3; \quad I_2 = \lambda_1\lambda_2 + \lambda_2\lambda_3 + \lambda_1\lambda_3; \quad I_3 = \lambda_1\lambda_2\lambda_3. \quad (13)$$

Another desirable property of the scalar invariants is that each is independent of the assignment or order of the principal diffusivities or eigenvalues. Therefore, if we permute the subscripts of the eigenvalues, the value of a scalar invariant is unchanged. The same property holds for functions of the scalar invariants. Moreover, each scalar invariant has a distinct geometrical (and physical) interpretation. I_1 is proportional to the sum of the squares of the major and minor axes of the diffusion ellipsoid, I_2 is proportional to the sum of the squares of the areas of the three principal ellipses of the diffusion ellipsoid, and I_3 is proportional to the square of the volume of the diffusion ellipsoid.

The First Invariant—The Trace of the Diffusion Tensor

The first scalar invariants, I_1 can be written in several ways:

$$I_1 = \mathrm{Trace}(\underline{D}) = D_{xx} + D_{yy} + D_{zz} = 3\langle D\rangle = \lambda_1 + \lambda_2 + \lambda_3 = 3\langle\lambda\rangle. \quad (14)$$

It is proportional to the orientationally averaged apparent diffusivity.[32] To see this, note that according to the Einstein equation, the mean-squared displacement in the ith principal direction, $\langle r_i^2\rangle$, is given by:

$$\langle r_i^2\rangle = 2\lambda_i\tau \quad (15)$$

in a diffusion time τ, so the mean-squared displacement averaged along the three principal directions, $\langle\langle r^2\rangle\rangle$ is

$$\langle\langle r^2\rangle\rangle = \frac{\langle r_x^2\rangle + \langle r_y^2\rangle + \langle r_z^2\rangle}{3} = 2\frac{\lambda_1 + \lambda_2 + \lambda_3}{3}\tau = 2\langle\lambda\rangle\tau. \quad (16)$$

This is the same result one obtains by averaging the mean-squared displacement uniformly over all directions.[32]

Characterizing Diffusion Anisotropy

Although $\mathrm{Trace}(\underline{D}) = I_1$ characterizes the mean diffusion properties in a voxel, it provides no information about diffusion anisotropy within a voxel. However, the second and third invariants of $\underline{D}$ do. One potentially useful measure of diffusion anisotropy is their ratio, I_2/I_3, which can be interpreted as the square of the surface-to-volume ratio of the diffusion ellipsoid. We would expect this quantity be a minimum in an isotropic medium in which the diffusion ellipsoid is a sphere, and to increase monotonically as the diffusion ellipsoid becomes more eccentric. However, the surface-to-volume ratio has units of inverse length. Since we prefer to have a non-dimensional measure of anisotropy, we can normalize it accordingly:

$$\text{"S-to-V"} = \frac{(2\mathrm{I}_2)^{3/2}}{\mathrm{I}_3} = \frac{(2(\lambda_1\lambda_2 + \lambda_2\lambda_3 + \lambda_1\lambda_3))^{3/2}}{\lambda_1\lambda_2\lambda_3}. \tag{17}$$

Rotational invariance of "S-to-V" is assured because it depends solely on the ratio of two scalar invariants.

Another approach to characterizing diffusion anisotropy is to determine the magnitude of the anisotropic part of the diffusion tensor in each voxel. This can be done by decomposing $\underline{\mathrm{D}}$ into its isotropic and anisotropic parts[33]:

$$\underline{\mathrm{D}} = \underbrace{\langle \mathrm{D} \rangle \underline{\mathrm{I}}}_{\substack{\text{isotropic} \\ \text{tensor}}} + \underbrace{(\underline{\mathrm{D}} - \langle \mathrm{D} \rangle \underline{\mathrm{I}})}_{\substack{\text{anisotropic} \\ \text{tensor}}}. \tag{18}$$

The isotropic part of the diffusion tensor is the familiar mean diffusivity, $\langle \mathrm{D} \rangle$, multiplied by the identity tensor, $\underline{\mathrm{I}}$, while the anisotropic part of $\underline{\mathrm{D}}$ is what we call the "diffusion deviatoric" or "diffusion deviation tensor," $\underline{D}$[33]:

$$\underline{D} = \underline{\mathrm{D}} - \langle \mathrm{D} \rangle \underline{\mathrm{I}} \tag{19}$$

The first invariant of $\underline{D}$, $\mathrm{I}_1' = \mathrm{Trace}\,(\underline{D})$ can be shown to be zero,[33] while the other scalar invariants of $\underline{D}$, I_2' and I_3', are simply related to I_1, I_2 and I_3 (e.g., see Ref. 34):

$$\mathrm{I}_2' = \mathrm{I}_2 - \frac{1}{3}\mathrm{I}_1^2 \quad \text{and} \quad \mathrm{I}_3' = \mathrm{I}_3 - \frac{1}{3}\mathrm{I}_1\mathrm{I}_2 + \frac{2}{27}\mathrm{I}_1^3 \tag{20}$$

While in their present form I_2' and I_3' are not too informative, they can be rewritten[d] to reveal interesting features about tissue microstructure. In particular, I_2' can be shown to be proportional to the mean-squared deviation of the eigenvalues or principal diffusivities with respect to their mean value:

$$\mathrm{I}_2' = \frac{(\lambda_1 - \langle\lambda\rangle)^2 + (\lambda_2 - \langle\lambda\rangle)^2 + (\lambda_3 - \langle\lambda\rangle)^2}{2} = \frac{3}{2}\,\mathrm{Variance}(\lambda). \tag{21}$$

[d] I_2' and I_3' are easily expressed as functions of the form Trace ($\underline{D}^n$) (where $\underline{D}^n$ signifies multiplication of $\underline{D}$ by itself n times).

$$\mathrm{I}_2' = \frac{1}{2}\mathrm{Trace}(\underline{D}^2) \quad \text{and} \quad \mathrm{I}_3' = \frac{1}{3}\mathrm{Trace}(\underline{D}^3)$$

This method to generate scalar invariants is well-known in the continuum mechanics literature.[34]

It was recently proposed as a measure of diffusion anisotropy[35] as it (i) is a scalar invariant quantity and it (ii) measures the magnitude of the anisotropic part of the diffusion tensor, $\underline{D}$ in Eq. **(18)**.[33] In the context of the DTI experiment, I_2' can also be interpreted as being proportional to the sample variance of the *estimated* eigenvalues in each voxel.

While I_2' measures the amount by which the measured eigenvalues of $\underline{D}$ deviate from their sample mean, it does not reflect how they are distributed about it. Conturo *et al.*[36] recently intimated that higher moments could. When might this information be useful? Suppose diffusivity were large along one principal direction, and were much smaller in the two transverse directions, that is, $\lambda_1 \gg \lambda_2 \approx \lambda_3$. Then, the corresponding diffusion ellipsoid would be "cigar"-shaped. This shape has recently been observed in white matter fibers in the corpus callosum and in the pyramidal tract in monkeys[37] and in humans.[38] Now, suppose that $\lambda_1 \approx \lambda_2 \gg \lambda_3$. This corresponds to a diffusion ellipsoid that is "pancake"-shaped. While in general, I_2' cannot distinguish between these two cases, the third moment or skewness should be able to.

$$I_3' = \frac{(\lambda_1 - \langle\lambda\rangle)^3 + (\lambda_2 - \langle\lambda\rangle)^3 + (\lambda_3 - \langle\lambda\rangle)^3}{3} = \text{Skewness}(\lambda), \qquad \textbf{(22)}$$

For the cigar-shaped diffusion ellipsoid, the skewness of the estimated eigenvalues would be negative, while for the pancake-shaped ellipsoid, it would be positive (depending on whether $\langle\lambda\rangle$ is significantly greater than or less than λ_2). Higher moments of the eigenvalues of $\underline{D}$ may furnish additional information about their distribution, although they may be increasingly susceptible to noise (e.g., see Ref. 37).

Other potentially informative anisotropy indices are the ratios of the principal diffusivities.[17] These dimensionless ratios measure the relative effective diffusivities in the three principal directions. Effectively, they measure the prolateness or eccentricity of the diffusion ellipsoid, independent of its size and orientation. If we number the principal diffusivities in decreasing order, the dimensionless anisotropy ratio, λ_2/λ_3, then measures the degree of cylindrical symmetry (with $\lambda_2/\lambda_3 = 1$ indicating perfect cylindrical symmetry). To measure the relative magnitude of the diffusivities along the fiber-tract direction and the two transverse directions, we can calculate λ_1/λ_2 and λ_1/λ_3, or, as above, measure the eccentricities of the two remaining great ellipses obtained from the diffusion ellipsoid that also contain its major axis (i.e., the axis along the fiber tract direction).[e] Pierpaoli and Basser[37] recently showed that while in principle these quantities are physically meaningful, in practice they are highly susceptible to noise in the MRIs, which introduces a bias when the eigenvalues are sorted according to size.[37,39]

[e]While the ratios of the eigenvalues of $\underline{D}$ represent the ratios of its principal diffusivities, it may be preferable to measure the ratios of the mean squared diffusion distances. This can be done simply by taking the square roots of the ratios presented above, i.e. $\sqrt{\lambda_i/\lambda_j}$

In summary, diffusion anisotropy is an intrinsic feature of the tissue, so its measures should be independent of the sample's placement or orientation with respect to the (laboratory) x-y-z reference frame.[35] Characterizing the degree of diffusion anisotropy is tantamount to characterizing features of the shape of a three-dimensional diffusion ellipsoid, independent of its orientation, and size. Thus, it is easy to see that knowing only the diagonal elements of the diffusion tensor is not adequate to characterize diffusion anisotropy. One should know at least the three eigenvalues of the diffusion tensor, and preferably higher moments of their distribution. In most MRI applications we typically do not know the eigenvalues *a priori.* We generally calculate them from the estimated diagonal *and* off-diagonal elements of $\underline{D}$.

COMBINING STAINS OF ISOTROPIC AND ANISOTROPIC DIFFUSION

One way to display information simultaneously about isotropic and anisotropic diffusion using a single image is by representing the three (sorted) principal diffusivities, λ_1, λ_2, and λ_3, using red, green, and blue (R-G-B) intensities, respectively.[40] Ideally, isotropic regions should appear as a shade of gray, whereas anisotropic tissues should appear colored. However, this display method still requires sorting the eigenvalues in each voxel, (for example, in decreasing order), making it susceptible to the same bias that afflicts images of the ratios of the principal diffusivities.[37] Still, this color imaging scheme is superior to one proposed in which R-G-B colors are assigned to the DWIs measured in the x-, y-, and z- directions, respectively.[41,42] Latour's method[40] does not introduce an orientational artifact, i.e., a change in hue or intensity if the laboratory frame or the sample is rotated, whereas Nakada's method[41] does.

OTHER STAINS DERIVED FROM THE DIFFUSION TENSOR

One might think of a stain as a scalar quantity, but it does not have to be. The diffusion ellipsoid that we construct in each voxel is also an invariant quantity whose size, shape, and orientation do not vary with respect to translation or rotation of the laboratory coordinate system. The same holds for the eigenvectors of the diffusion tensor.

One of the most intriguing applications of diffusion tensor imaging is in developing MRI stains that reveal new *architectural* features of anisotropic structures such as fiber tract directions in brain and other tissues. So far, we have concentrated our efforts on developing MRI stains based upon diffusion tensors measured within each voxel. However, useful information also is found in the *pattern* of diffusion tensors or quantities derived from them, which could provide additional insights about tissue organization, structure, and function. For example, if we take the local nerve fiber tract direction in each voxel (given by the eigenvector associated with the largest eigenvalue), we can surmise that the fiber-tract *pattern* or direction field contains useful biological and clinical information. Its temporal evolution from the embryonic to adult stages may be of interest in understanding dynamical processes in normal and abnormal brain development. Moreover, subsequent alterations may indicate degeneration, aging, or disease. The geometry of various cortical regions, in particular, the curving and twisting of fiber tracts may be useful in elucidating organizing principles of information processing within the brain.

While we have previously used tensor algebraic approaches to obtain information about the *pattern* of diffusion tensors in an image,[33] we can also apply concepts from differential geometry to identify new and useful features of the *diffusion tensor field.* One way to exploit constructs of differential geometry is to treat each diffusion tensor estimated in each voxel as a discrete, volume-averaged sample of a diffusion tensor field. In some cases, we can establish a correspondence between the three normalized orthogonal eigenvectors of the diffusion tensor: ϵ_1, ϵ_2, and ϵ_3, and the three orthogonal vectors that describe a space curve, $\mathbf{r}(\mathrm{s})$, in three dimensions: $\mathbf{t}(\mathrm{s})$, $\mathbf{n}(\mathrm{s})$, and $\mathbf{b}(\mathrm{s})$ (where s is the arc length). Above, $\mathbf{t}(\mathrm{s})$ is the unit tangent vector to the curve, $\mathbf{n}(\mathrm{s})$ is the principal normal vector, and $\mathbf{b}(\mathrm{s})$ is the binormal vector. Together, they constitute a "moving trihedron" that follows the space curve.[43] These vectors also define three mutually orthogonal planes, the normal plane, the rectifying plane, and the osculating plane which are normal to $\mathbf{t}(\mathrm{s})$, $\mathbf{n}(\mathrm{s})$, and $\mathbf{b}(\mathrm{s})$, respectively. If we assume that the fiber tracts are continuous from voxel to voxel, we can use the spatial variation of these vectors to characterize *intrinsic* local features of these curves, namely, their *torsion* and *curvature.* The curvature vector, $\mathbf{k}(\mathrm{s})$, is defined below as follows:

$$\mathbf{k}(\mathrm{s}) = \frac{\mathrm{d}\mathbf{t}}{\mathrm{ds}} \tag{23}$$

and its magnitude is the curvature, $\kappa(\mathrm{s})$. The torsion, $\tau(\mathrm{s})$, is defined as

$$\tau(\mathrm{s}) = -\frac{\mathrm{d}\mathbf{b}}{\mathrm{ds}} \cdot \mathbf{n}. \tag{24}$$

Once $\mathbf{t}(\mathrm{s})$, $\mathbf{n}(\mathrm{s})$, and $\mathbf{b}(\mathrm{s})$ are determined in each voxel, we can plot scalar functions of them, $\kappa(\mathbf{r})$ and $\tau(\mathbf{r})$ in each voxel so that now the curvature and torsion are displayed in each voxel. These intrinsic, rotationally and translationally invariant parameters specify new characteristics of the fiber-tract pattern within each voxel. (N.B.: In tissues like skeletal muscle and white matter, we can safely assign the tangent vector to be parallel to the eigenvector associated with the largest eigenvalue in a voxel. However, the eigenvectors are known to within a factor of -1. Therefore, a convention for determining a positive and negative fiber direction must be established. To this author's knowledge, developmental or histological reasoning do not suggest such a convention at the present time. A right-handed coordinate system can then be constructed coincident with all three eigenvectors. The assignment of the **n** and **b** vectors could be performed on the basis of the relative magnitudes of the remaining eigenvalues.)

VECTOR CALCULUS OPERATIONS APPLIED TO THE FIBER DIRECTION FIELDS

Other vector operations applied to the diffusion tensor field should provide new information. The divergence of a vector field produces a scalar field that is rotationally and translationally invariant, like the other stains we have discussed so far. Such is the case if we compute the divergence of the tangent vector field given as a function of **r**, **t** (**r**), as well as for **n**(**r**), and **b**(**r**):

$$\nabla \cdot \mathbf{t}(\mathbf{r}); \quad \nabla \cdot \mathbf{n}(\mathbf{r}); \quad \nabla \cdot \mathbf{b}(\mathbf{r}); \tag{25a}$$

where

$$\nabla \cdot \mathbf{t}(\mathbf{r}) = \frac{\partial t_x(\mathbf{r})}{\partial x} + \frac{\partial t_y(\mathbf{r})}{\partial y} + \frac{\partial t_z(\mathbf{r})}{\partial z}. \tag{25b}$$

The divergence of a vector field is often used to identify whether and where there are sources or sinks of a flowing quantity, such as charge or heat. In our application, it would be used to identify regions of convergence or divergence of the fiber tracts. In voxels where fiber tracts radiate or terminate, we expect $\phi(\mathbf{r}) = \nabla \cdot \mathbf{t}(\mathbf{r})$ to be non-zero. Peskin proposed that the direction field vector, **t**(**r**), describing the muscle fiber directions in the heart are divergence-free, i.e., $\nabla \cdot \mathbf{t}(\mathbf{r}) = 0$.[44] One would not expect this to apply in the brain, where nerve fiber tracts cross and terminate in certain regions. Using diffusion tensor imaging, one can, in principle, test these hypotheses directly.

Since we estimate a diffusion tensor in each voxel, we only obtain a discrete sample of the tensor field. Thus, we must calculate the gradients of the direction vectors **t**(**r**), **n**(**r**), and **b**(**r**) numerically. A reasonable approach is to use centered differences to obtain a discrete approximation to $\nabla \cdot \mathbf{t}(\mathbf{r})$:

$$\nabla \cdot \mathbf{t}(\mathbf{r}) = \frac{t_x(\mathbf{r} + \Delta x\mathbf{i}) - t_x(\mathbf{r} - \Delta x\mathbf{i})}{2\Delta x} + \frac{t_y(\mathbf{r} + \Delta y\mathbf{j}) - t_y(\mathbf{r} - \Delta y\mathbf{j})}{2\Delta y} + \frac{t_z(\mathbf{r} + \Delta z\mathbf{k}) - t_z(\mathbf{r} - \Delta z\mathbf{k})}{2\Delta z} \tag{26}$$

Another potentially revealing vector operation that produces a scalar invariant of a vector field is the magnitude of the curl or circulation of the direction vector field:

$$\left|\nabla \times \mathbf{t}(\mathbf{r})\right| \tag{27a}$$

where

$$\nabla \times \mathbf{t}(\mathbf{r}) = \mathbf{i}\left(\frac{\partial t_z(\mathbf{r})}{\partial y} - \frac{\partial t_y(\mathbf{r})}{\partial z}\right) + \mathbf{j}\left(\frac{\partial t_x(\mathbf{r})}{\partial z} - \frac{\partial t_z(\mathbf{r})}{\partial x}\right) + \mathbf{k}\left(\frac{\partial t_y(\mathbf{r})}{\partial x} - \frac{\partial t_x(\mathbf{r})}{\partial y}\right). \tag{27b}$$

If all the fibers in a local area were straight, $|\nabla \times \mathbf{t}(\mathbf{r})|$ would vanish; where they curl, $|\nabla \times \mathbf{t}(\mathbf{r})|$ is positive. Owing to previously acquired fiber maps in human and animal brains, it is reasonable to expect that this quantity will not be zero everywhere. We would expect it to be large in the cortical area of the brain, where there are many convolutions and U-fibers that have recently been made visible using diffusion tensor MRI methods.[38]

A discrete approximation to this expression is obtained by using the formula:

$$\begin{aligned}\nabla \times \mathbf{t}(\mathbf{r}) \approx\ & \mathbf{i}\left(\frac{t_z(\mathbf{r} + \Delta y\mathbf{j}) - t_z(\mathbf{r} - \Delta y\mathbf{j})}{2\Delta y} - \frac{t_y(\mathbf{r} + \Delta z\mathbf{k}) - t_y(\mathbf{r} - \Delta z\mathbf{k})}{2\Delta z}\right) \\ & + \mathbf{j}\left(\frac{t_x(\mathbf{r} + \Delta z\mathbf{k}) - t_x(\mathbf{r} - \Delta z\mathbf{k})}{2\Delta z} - \frac{t_z(\mathbf{r} + \Delta x\mathbf{i}) - t_z(\mathbf{r} - \Delta x\mathbf{i})}{2\Delta x}\right) \\ & + \mathbf{k}\left(\frac{t_y(\mathbf{r} + \Delta x\mathbf{i}) - t_y(\mathbf{r} - \Delta x\mathbf{i})}{2\Delta x} - \frac{t_x(\mathbf{r} + \Delta y\mathbf{j}) - t_x(\mathbf{r} - \Delta y\mathbf{j})}{2\Delta y}\right).\end{aligned} \tag{28}$$

One obvious problem with implementing differential geometric measures with real data is that they are inherently noisy. These measures require taking spatial derivatives of vectors, like local direction vectors, which are themselves random variables. Differentiation just amplifies the uncertainty. Filtering methods will undoubtedly have to be developed to obtain smoothed maps of these quantities. However, as the signal-to-noise ratio, quality, and acquisition rate in DWI increase, differential geometry–based measures should play an increasingly important role as MRI stains.

In summary, new invariant MR stains can also be derived from the diffusion tensor field *per se,* not just from the individual diffusion tensors measured in each voxel. In regions (e.g., along some white matter tracts and in the cortex) where this tensor field is expected to be continuous, invariant measures of fiber tract or sheet architecture (torsion, twisting, etc.) should be informative. Moreover, at interfaces between tissue types where we expect the diffusion tensor fields to be discontinous (e.g., at the boundary of white matter fiber tracts and CSF-filled ventricles), differential geometric approaches should aid in identifying these boundaries, both in normal and pathological tissues.

CONCLUDING REMARKS

Diffusion tensor MRI provides a new paradigm for probing tissue structure at different levels of hierarchical organization. While experimental diffusion times are consistent with measurements of molecular displacements on the order of microns, these molecular motions are ensemble-averaged within a voxel, and then subsequently assembled into multislice or 3-D images of tissues or organs. Thus, this single imaging method permits us to study and elucidate complex structural features spanning length scales from the macromolecular to the macroscopic!

If one is interested in using a scalar quantity to characterize an intrinsic feature of an anisotropic medium, such as its degree diffusion anisotropy, that parameter should be invariant to translation and rotation of the laboratory coordinate system. If, in addition, that parameter is physically meaningful, it should possess characteristics of a quantitative physiological or histological stain. Scalar invariants of the diffusion tensor and functions of them possess these desirable properties.

The development of fast, high-quality, high-resolution DWI sequences[38,45] and user-friendly software with which to estimate diffusion tensors and produce images of quantitative "stains" derived from them have greatly facilitated the clinical implementation of DT-MRI.

REFERENCES

1. CARR, H. Y. & E. M. PURCELL. 1954. Effects of diffusion on free precession in nuclear magnetic resonance experiments. Phys. Rev. **94:** 630–638.
2. STEJSKAL, E. O., J. E. TANNER. 1965. Spin diffusion measurements: Spin echoes in the presence of time-dependent field gradient. J. Chem. Phys. **42:** 288–292.
3. LAUTERBUR, P. C. 1972. Image formation by induced local interactions: examples employing nuclear magnetic resonance. Nature **242:** 191–192.
4. TAYLOR, D. G. & M. C. BUSHELL. 1985. The spatial mapping of translational diffusion coefficients by the NMR imaging technique. Phys. Med. Biol. **30:** 345–349.
5. MERBOLDT, K. D., W. HANICKE & J. FRAHM. 1985. Self-diffusion NMR imaging using stimulated echoes. J. Magn. Reson. **64:** 479–486.
6. LE BIHAN, D. & E. BRETON. 1985. Imagerie de diffusion in-vivo par resonance magnetique nucleaire. C. R. Acad. Sci. (Paris) **301:** 1109–1112.
7. LE BIHAN, D. 1991. Diffusion NMR imaging. Magn. Reson. Quarterly **7:** 1–30.
8. LE BIHAN, D. 1995. Diffusion and Perfusion Magnetic Resonance Imaging. Raven Press. New York.
9. TURNER, R., D. LE BIHAN, J. MAIER, R. VAVREK, L. K. HEDGES & J. PEKAR. 1990. Echo-planar imaging of intravoxel incoherent motion. Radiology **177:** 407–414.
10. GARRIDO, L., V. J. WEDEEN, K. K. KWONG, U. M. SPENCER & H. L. KANTOR. 1994. Anisotropy of water diffusion in the myocardium of the rat. Circ. Res. **74:** 789–793.
11. CLEVELAND, G. G., D. C. CHANG, C. F. HAZLEWOOD & H. E. RORSCHACH. 1976. Nuclear magnetic resonance measurement of skeletal muscle: anisotropy of the diffusion coefficient of the intracellular water. Biophys. J. **16:** 1043–1053.
12. HENKELMAN, R. M., G. J. STANISZ, J. K. KIM & M. J. BRONSKILL. 1994. Magn. Reson. Med. **32**(5): 592.

13. MOSELEY, M. E., Y. COHEN, J. KUCHARCZYK, J. MINTOROVITCH, H. S. ASGARI, M. F. WENDLAND, J. TSURUDA & D. NORMAN. 1990. Diffusion-weighted MR imaging of anisotropic water diffusion in cat central nervous system. Radiology **176:** 439–445.
14. TANNER, J. E. 1979. Self diffusion of water in frog muscle. Biophys. J. **28:** 107–116.
15. DORAN, M., J. V. HAJNAL, N. VAN BRUGGEN, M. D. KING, I. R. YOUNG & G. M. BYDDER. 1990. Normal and abnormal white matter tracts shown by MR imaging using directional diffusion weighted sequences. J. Comput. Assist. Tomogr. **14:** 865–873.
16. CHENEVERT, T. L., J. A. BRUNBERG & J. G. PIPE. 1990. Anisotropic diffusion in human white matter: Demonstration with MR techniques in vivo. Radiology **177:** 401–405.
17. BASSER, P. J., J. MATTIELLO & D. LE BIHAN. 1994. MR diffusion tensor spectroscopy and imaging. Biophys. J. **66:** 259–267.
18. LE BIHAN, D. 1991. Molecular diffusion nuclear magnetic resonance imaging. Magn. Reson. Q. **7:** 1–30.
19. MATTIELLO, J., P. J. BASSER & D. LE BIHAN. 1994. Analytical expression for the b matrix in NMR diffusion imaging and spectroscopy. J. Magn. Reson. **A 108:** 131–141.
20. BASSER, P. J., J. MATTIELLO & D. LE BIHAN. 1992. Diagonal and off-diagonal components of the self-diffusion tensor: Their relation to and estimation from the NMR spin-echo signal. *In:* 11th Annual Meeting of the SMRM, Berlin, 1992, p. 1222.
21. BASSER, P. J., J. MATTIELLO & D. LE BIHAN. 1994. Estimation of the effective self-diffusion tensor from the NMR spin echo. J. Magn. Reson. B **103:** 247–254.
22. EINSTEIN, A. 1926. Investigations on the Theory of the Brownian Movement. Dover Publications. New York, NY.
23. RAO, C. R. 1965. Linear Statistical Inference and Its Applications. John Wiley. New York, NY.
24. CRANK, J. 1975. The Mathematics of Diffusion. Oxford University Press. Oxford, England.
25. MOSELEY, M. E., J. KUCHARCZYK, J. MINTOROVITCH, Y. COHEN, J. KURHANEWICZ, N. DERUGIN, H. ASGARI & D. NORMAN. 1990. Diffusion-weighted MR imaging of acute stroke: Correlation with T2-weighted and magnetic susceptibility-enhanced MR imaging in cats. Am. J. Neuroradiol. **11:** 423–429.
26. MOSELEY, M. E., Y. COHEN, J. MINTOROVITCH, L. CHILEUITT, H. SHIMIZU, J. KUCHARCZYK, M. F., WENDLAND & P. R. WEINSTEIN. 1990. Early detection of regional cerebral ischemia in cats: Comparison of diffusion- and T2-weighted MRI and spectroscopy. Magn. Reson. Med. **14:** 330–346.
27. MINTOROVITCH, J., M. E. MOSELEY, L. CHILEUITT, H. SHIMIZU, Y. COHEN & P. R. WEINSTEIN. 1996. Comparison of diffusion- and T2-weighted MRI for the early detection of cerebral ischemia and reperfusion in rats. Magn. Reson. Med. **18:** 39–50.
28. CHIEN, D., K. K. KWONG, D. R. GRESS, F. S. BUONANNO, R. B. BUXTON & B. R. ROSEN. 1992. MR diffusion imaging of cerebral infarction in humans. Am. J. Neuroradiol. **13:** 1097–1102; discussion, 1103–1105.
29. WARACH, S., D. CHIEN, W. LI, M. RONTHAL & R. R. EDELMAN. 1992. Fast magnetic resonance diffusion-weighted imaging of acute human stroke [published erratum appears in Neurology 1992 **42(11):** 2192]. Neurology **42:** 1717–1723.
30. BASSER, P. J. & D. L. BIHAN. 1992. Fiber orientation mapping in an anisotropic medium with NMR diffusion spectroscopy. 1221, 11th Annual Meeting of the SMRM, Berlin.
31. BASSER, P. J., J. MATTIELLO, R. TURNER & D. L. BIHAN. 1993. Diffusion tensor echo-planar imaging of human brain. 1404, 12th Annual Meeting of the SMRM, New York, NY.
32. KÄRGER, J., H. PFEIFER & W. HEINK. 1988. Principles and applications of self-diffusion measurements by nuclear magnetic resonance. *In* Advances in Magnetic Resonance. J. Waugh. Eds. Vol. 12: 1. Academic Press, New York, NY.
33. BASSER, P. J. & C. PIERPAOLI. 1996. Microstructural and physiological features of tissues elucidated by quantitative-diffusion-tensor MRI. J. Magn. Reson. **B(111):** 209–219.
34. SPENCER, A. J. M. 1980. Continuum Mechanics: 183, Longman. London.
35. BASSER, P. & C. PIERPAOLI. 1995. Elucidating tissue structure by diffusion tensor MRI. 900. SMR/ESMRMB, Nice, France.
36. CONTURO, T. E., R. C. MCKINSTRY, E. AKBUDAK & B. H. ROBINSON. 1996. Encoding of anisotropic diffusion with tetrahedral gradients: A general mathematical diffusion formalism and experimental results. Magn. Reson. Med. **35:** 399–412.

37. Pierpaoli, C. & P. J. Basser. 1996. Toward a quantitative assessment of diffusion anisotropy. Magn. Reson. Med. **36(6):** 893–906.
38. Pierpaoli, C., P. Jezzard, P. J. Basser, A. Barnett & G. Di Chiro. 1996. Diffusion tensor MR imaging of the human brain. Radiology. **201(3):** 637–648.
39. Pierpaoli, C. & P. J. Basser. 1996. New invariant "lattice" index achieves significant noise reduction in measuring diffusion anisotropy. SMR, 1326. Proceedings of the ISMRM, New York, NY.
40. Latour, L. 1995. London Workshop of Diffusion Imaging. London.
41. Nakada, T. & H. Matsuzawa. 1995. Three dimensional anisotropy magnetic resonance imaging of the rat nervous system. Neurosci. Res. **22:** 389–398.
42. Nakada, T., H. Matsuzawa & I. L. Kwee. 1994. Magnetic resonance axonography of the rat spinal cord. NeuroReport. **5(16):** 2053–2056.
43. Struik, D. J. 1961. Lectures on Classical Differential Geometry, 2nd ed. Dover Publications. New York, NY.
44. Peskin, C. 1975. Mathematical Aspects of Heart Physiology. Courant Institute of Mathematical Sciences. New York, NY.
45. Jezzard, P. & C. Pierpaoli. 1995. Diffusion mapping using interleaved spin echo and STEAM EPI with navigator echo correction, 903, SMR/ESMRMB Joint Meeting, Nice.

DISCUSSION

Question: In the diffusion tensor formulation that you referred to, a term that we will call "q" effectively introduces a spatial scaling in the measurement of the diffusion coefficient. It seems to me that that term might be an interesting parameter because in isotropic diffusion fields, there should be a scaling of the diffusion coefficient that reveals the size of the cell and could distinguish cases where fluid is transferred from inside to outside the cell in some swelling processes. Have you looked at that parameter?

Basser: There is another approach, which is called displacement imaging, that addresses that issue directly. You can measure the proton displacements using much shorter-duration diffusion gradients that are much larger than what we used in this study, and then estimate a conditional probability distribution of particles being at certain places at certain times. In our particular imaging application, owing to the use of long diffusion times and of imaging gradients, we don't have the ability to measure that probability distribution directly. We are also spatially averaging over a very large number of structures, which are not necessarily homogenous. So we are performing a spatial homogenization as well. So your question is on target, but it is very difficult to make these measurements using clinical scanners in a clinical environment.

Magnetic Resonance Microscopy in Basic Studies of Brain Structure and Function[a,b]

G. ALLAN JOHNSON, HELENE BENVENISTE, ROBERT T. ENGELHARDT, HUI QIU, AND LAURENCE W. HEDLUND

Center for In Vivo *Microscopy*
Duke University Medical Center
Durham, North Carolina 27710

INTRODUCTION

The inventors of magnetic resonance imaging (MRI) realized at the outset that the technology was scalable to the microscopic domain.[1,2] In its 20-year history, MRI has become an extraordinarily successful tool in the clinical arena, with research focused on human studies where resolution at ~1 mm is generally adequate. A small community of researchers has pursued the extension of MRI to magnetic resonance microscopy (MRM).[3,4] This paper will focus on (*a*) a definition of MRM; (*b*) a discussion of the essential technologies required for MRM; and (*c*) two specific applications of MRM in the study of brain structure and function.

THE DISTINCTION OF MRM FROM MRI

MRM is founded on the same fundamental principle as MRI, that is, the use of magnetic gradients to encode the signal derived in a nuclear magnetic resonance study—usually from hydrogen protons. In a typical two-dimensional MRI study, a gradient applied along the longitudinal (z) axis of the patient, for example, defines a "slice" that is selectively excited by the simultaneous application of a resonant radiofrequency (rf) pulse. Subsequent rf pulses and gradients are employed to generate and encode the signal in the selected slice, typically yielding a 256 × 256 digital array, with each element of the array representing the signal from a tissue volume (voxel) within the slice.

[a]This research was supported by NIH NCRR Grant No. P41 RR05959 and by a grant from Zeneca Pharmaceuticals.

[b]Address for correspondence: Elaine G. Fitzsimons, Center for *In Vivo* Microscopy, Box 3302, Duke University Medical Center, Durham, North Carolina 27710. Phone: (919)684-7758; fax: (919)684-7122; e-mail: egf@orion.mc.duke.edu

The resolution in an MR image must be defined on a volumetric basis. A standard clinical study, such as that shown in FIGURE 1a, employs a 5-mm-thick slice with an in-plane field of view of ~250 × 250 mm. Each discrete picture element (pixel) represents the signal from a 1 × 1 × 5 mm, that is, 5 mm^3, volume (voxel) of tissue. FIGURES 1b–1d are generated from a 3-D acquisition of a formalin-fixed specimen imaged at 9.4 Tesla (T). These

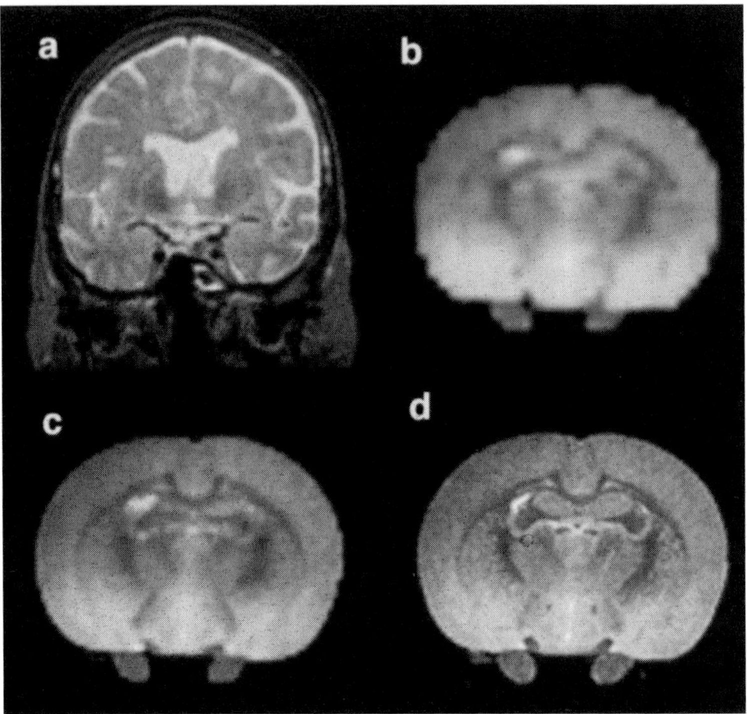

FIGURE 1. **(a)** standard clinical study (human) of a 5-mm slice with an in-plane field of view of ~250 × 250 mm. **(b)–(d)** formalin-fixed rat brain imaged at 9.4 T. **(b)** is a similar coronal plane at the same effective spatial resolution as **(a)**. **(c)** was acquired at 64× higher resolution (0.25 × 0.25 × 1.25 mm = 0.078 mm^3), but is still a poor depiction of the anatomy seen so clearly in **(d)** (.086 × .086 × .086 mm = .00064 mm^3), which is an ~8,000-times-higher resolution than the images in **(a)** and **(b)**.

images graphically demonstrate the consequences of limited resolution in defining the brain architecture in the significantly smaller rat brain. The "effective" resolution in each image is achieved by averaging adjacent pixels from the isotropic 3-D array to produce the desired voxel dimensions. The image in FIGURE 1b is a similar coronal plane at the same effective spatial resolution as that in the human image (FIGURE 1a). Figure 1c, acquired at

64-times-higher resolution (0.25 × 0.25 × 1.25 mm = 0.078 mm^3), is still a poor depiction of the anatomy seen more clearly in FIGURE 1d (.086 × .086 × .086 mm = .00064 mm^3), which is an ~8,000-times-higher resolution than the images in FIGURE 1a and 1b.

TECHNICAL CHALLENGES OF MRM

The increase in resolution in Figure 1d is accomplished only after overcoming several significant technical challenges. The largest challenge is limited signal. Magnetic resonance is a relatively insensitive technique deriving its signal from differences in two populations of protons, the higher and lower energy states defined by the magnetic field. But at 1.5 T, this difference is only ~5 protons out of every 10^6. There are four broad categories of technical solution to the sensitivity barrier: (*a*) more-sensitive radiofrequency (rf) coils; (*b*) operation at higher magnetic fields; (*c*) signal averaging with larger image arrays; and (*d*) design of more efficient encoding schemes.

The most direct method of improving the sensitivity is the design of more-sensitive rf coils. The rf coil is the antenna used to detect the generally very weak rf signal. By shrinking the coil volume, one moves this antenna closer to the source of the weak signal and limits the detection of extraneous thermal noise from other parts of the specimen. In MR microscopy, where the specimen volume is very small, the thermal noise from the specimen may sometimes be negligible. At this point, the thermal noise in the coil may, in fact, be the major noise source. Recently, Black *et al.* reduced this noise source considerably through the use of high-temperature superconducting receivers.[5]

Operation at higher magnetic fields provides a ready increase in sensitivity. The typical clinical fields of 1.5 T are achieved with large-bore magnets designed to accommodate human subjects. When the constraint of the large-bore diameter is removed, it is technically (and financially) possible to operate smaller-bore magnets at fields up to 11.4 T.[6] To the first order, the sensitivity in an MR imaging experiment will depend linearly on the field. Thus, one might expect to see an increase of 6–8 times resolution from operating at higher magnetic fields. But the solution is not as straightforward as that. Operation at higher magnetic fields changes the contrast between the tissues because the relaxation parameters, T1 (the spin-lattice relaxation time) and T2 (the spin-spin relaxation time) are field-dependent.[7,8] Moreover, a number of other effects (e.g., susceptibility effects) are also field-dependent.[9] The resulting change in sensitivity may not be as great as expected, the ability to define anatomical structure based upon differences in tissue contrast may be even less, and there may be an increase in artifacts due to susceptibility effects.

Finally, there has been substantial effort directed at improving the sensitivity through clever design of pulse sequences, the series of gradient and rf pulses applied to the specimen to generate and encode the MR signal.[3] The recovery of the magnetization between rf excitations and the decay of the signal once excited are governed by the spin-lattice relaxation time (T1) and spin-spin relaxation time (T2). Because these time constants are characteristics of the tissues, they determine not only the signal level, but also the contrast between tissues. Thus, the design of pulse sequences can have an impact on both the sensitivity and the contrast in the image.

APPLICATION OF MRM IN BRAIN FUNCTION

A number of laboratories use MR to study models of disease in small animals. The Center for *In Vivo* Microscopy, after years of addressing the challenges of physiologic support, motion, sensitivity and contrast, now routinely images animals weighing 40–400 gm in serial studies at microscopic resolution. Moseley *et al.* first demonstrated that a measure of the local diffusion coefficient of water is sensitive to the early onset of ischemia in the rat brain.[10] Benveniste *et al.* have demonstrated that during ischemia, subtle shifts in water occur from extracellular spaces, where the water is relatively mobile, to the intracellular compartments, where the diffusion coefficient is significantly lower.[11,12] Beaulieu *et al.* have described the fast spin-echo variant of diffusion-weighted encoding that allows a 3-D 64 × 256 × 256 acquisition in ~1 h with spatial resolution of 137 × 137 × 547 μm (~0.01 mm^3), or an ~500-times-higher resolution than a routine clinical study.[13] Hall *et al.* have extended the technique to a systematic study of a number of animals following the time course of the evolution of the ischemic volume.[14] FIGURE 2 shows images from one such study. FIGURES 2a and 2b show single slices of a Fisher 344 rat in which a middle cerebral artery was surgically

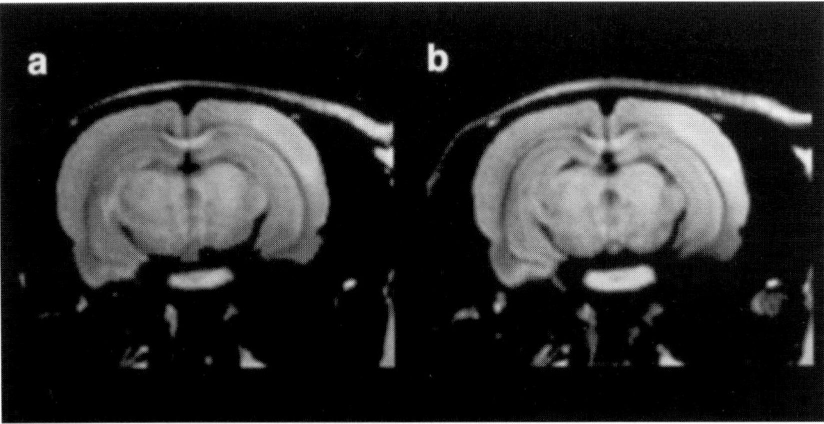

FIGURE 2. Single slices of a Fisher 344 rat in which a middle cerebral arterial occlusion has been surgically created acquired at 2 h **(a)** and 8 h **(b)** after the initial insult.

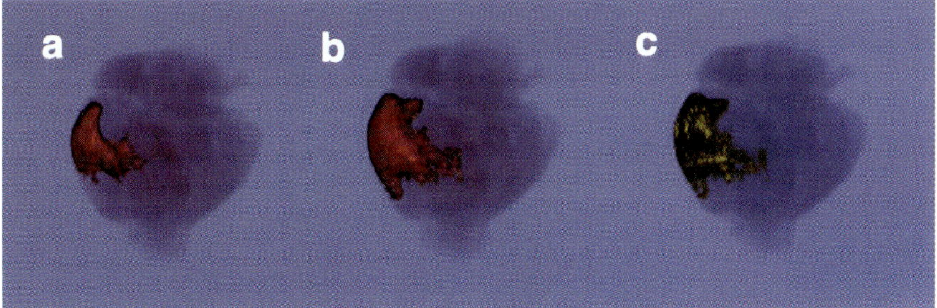

FIGURE 3. The volume of ischemic tissue in the same animal imaged ~2 h (**a**) and 8 h (**b**) after occlusion has been highlighted using a seeding method that identifies voxels on the basis of signal intensity and "connectivity." (**c**) shows the "difference" volume.

occluded. The individual two-dimensional images in FIGURES 2a and 2b are from 3-D acquisitions of 64 contiguous slices acquired ~2 h (*a*) and 8 h (*b*) after the occlusion. The spatial resolution is ~0.01 mm^3. It is possible to survey the same anatomy throughout the evolution of the ischemic response. It is clear in FIGURE 2b that the ischemic region has increased in the intervening time (~6 h) after the onset of ischemia. This has major consequences for drug discovery in that the animal can now act as its own control. The natural biological variability can be accommodated because it is now possible to measure the *change* in ischemic zones in the same animal.

The images in FIGURE 2 are selected slices from a volumetric set. Thus, it is possible to measure not just the area in a single slice, but also the volume of ischemic tissue in the whole brain. In FIGURES 3a and b, the volume of ischemic tissue in the same animal imaged ~2 h and 8 h after occlusion has been highlighted using a seeding method that identifies voxels on the basis of signal intensity and "connectivity." The images are volume-rendered on a high-end Silicon Graphics (SGI) workstation using VoxelView (Vital Images, Fairfield, IA).[15] The assumption is made that the ischemic volume is a contiguous set of voxels. Because the volume of each voxel is known, accurate 3-D morphometry is possible. While some ambiguity persists from the specific choice of threshold, the imaging instrument is stable to within 5% over the 6–8 h of a typical experiment, so the same threshold can be applied to both the early and late acquisition to monitor the change. Interestingly, both the volume and the signal intensity of the ischemic region change with time. Benveniste *et al.* have shown that the signal intensity of the ischemic volume continues to increase over an 8-hour period as the cells continue to swell.[11,12] The animal is left in the imager between the two acquisitions, and care is taken to stabilize it in the same position. The result is that the image sets are perfectly registered, allowing us to take a "difference" image, as shown in FIGURE 3c. Qiu *et al.* have recently demonstrated the use of these techniques in the evaluation of a glycine antagonist as a possible therapy for stroke.[16] The volume of the initial ischemic insult in control animals and treated animals at

2.5 h after surgery was similar. After 6 h, however, the stroke volume of the control animals increased by 15%, while the stroke volume of the treated animals decreased by 32%. Moreover, the percentage volume change for the treated animals was remarkably consistent. The combination of animal support, specialized rf coils, high-field imaging, and volume acquisition and analysis have yielded an extraordinary set of tools for routine drug study that should radically reduce the time, expense, and the number of animals required in such a study.

APPLICATION OF MRM TO STUDY BRAIN STRUCTURE

There are numerous examples of the application of MRM to study brain structure. We demonstrate here application for fixed specimens, an application we have labeled "MR histology." Histology is defined as the structure of tissue. In fixed specimens where biologic motion is no longer a barrier, it is possible to routinely obtain 3-D arrays with resolution of $\sim 20 \times 20 \times 20$ μm (0.000008 mm^3), that is, at a volume resolution some six orders of magnitude higher than a conventional clinical image. There are three unique advantages of MRM over conventional optical techniques: (*a*) MRM is nondestructive; (*b*) MRM offers unique "protons stains;" and (*c*) MRM is inherently three-dimensional.

The nondestructive nature of MRM presents several new opportunities for the histologist. FIGURE 4 demonstrates this with axial, coronal, and sagittal images from a "T2-weighted" acquisition from the same specimen "sliced" through three different planes. Because the slice is defined by the magnetic field gradients and not by a physical microtome, the specimen can be repeatedly imaged through multiple planes with varied acquisition schemes. The specimen was carefully fix-perfused with formalin glutaraldehyde. It was subsequently cast in an agarose gel to limit the susceptibility variation at the surface of the specimen. The images were acquired at 9.4 T using 3-D spin warp encoding with arrays of $256 \times 256 \times 512$, yielding isotropic resolution of 86 μm^3.

This particular scan employed a fast spin-echo sequence developed specifically for the high magnetic fields and strong gradients common for MRM.[17] The effective echo (TE) is 50 msec, which is significantly shorter than might be employed in a clinical setting, highlighting the fact that extension of our knowledge from the clinical domain into MRM is not always straightforward. The high fields and strong gradients used induce very rapid T2 decay in these specimens as spins diffuse through both the external gradients and internal gradients induced by microscopic susceptibility variations.

There are a number of "proton stains" available in MRM. We use the term "proton stain" to conceptually relate to the neuroscientist and pathologist the complex relaxation mechanisms that induce tissue-dependent contrast variations in MR histology. The mechanisms are understood at some level in the clinical arena. But for the high-field, strong-gradient, high-resolution situations in MRM, these mechanisms are not, at this point, fully understood. Nevertheless, like chemical stains, they can be exploited to differentiate varied structures in the brain. The stains can be endogenous, as in FIGURE 4, where contrast shows differences in the tissue water and how it is bound, or exogenous, that is, manipulated by some external chemistry.

FIGURE 5 shows an example of a stain developed for vascular imaging. The

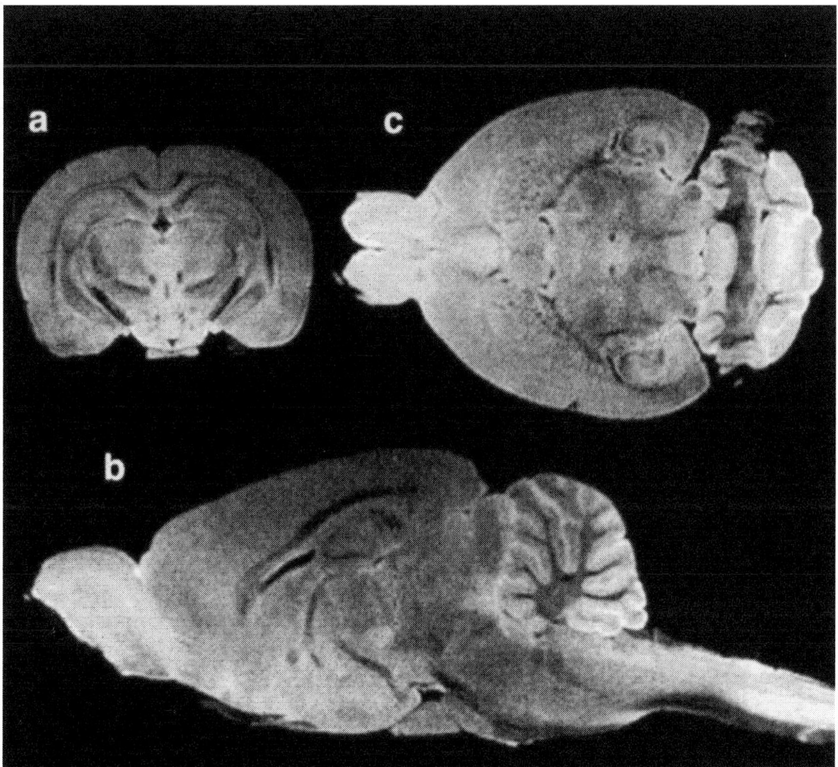

FIGURE 4. Three slices from the same volume image of fixed rat brain demonstrating the nondestructive nature of MRM. **(a)** is axial, **(b)** is sagittal, and **(c)** is coronal.

spin-lattice relaxation time, T1, has been altered in the vascular spaces by infusing those spaces with a gelatin containing gadolinium (Gd). The Gd is covalently bonded to bovine serum albumin to produce a large molecule that will not readily diffuse. The molecule is then dissolved in 3–5% gelatin that is infused into the vascular spaces following a warm infusion of saline immediately post mortem.[18] This figure is a volume-rendered image of a $256 \times 256 \times$

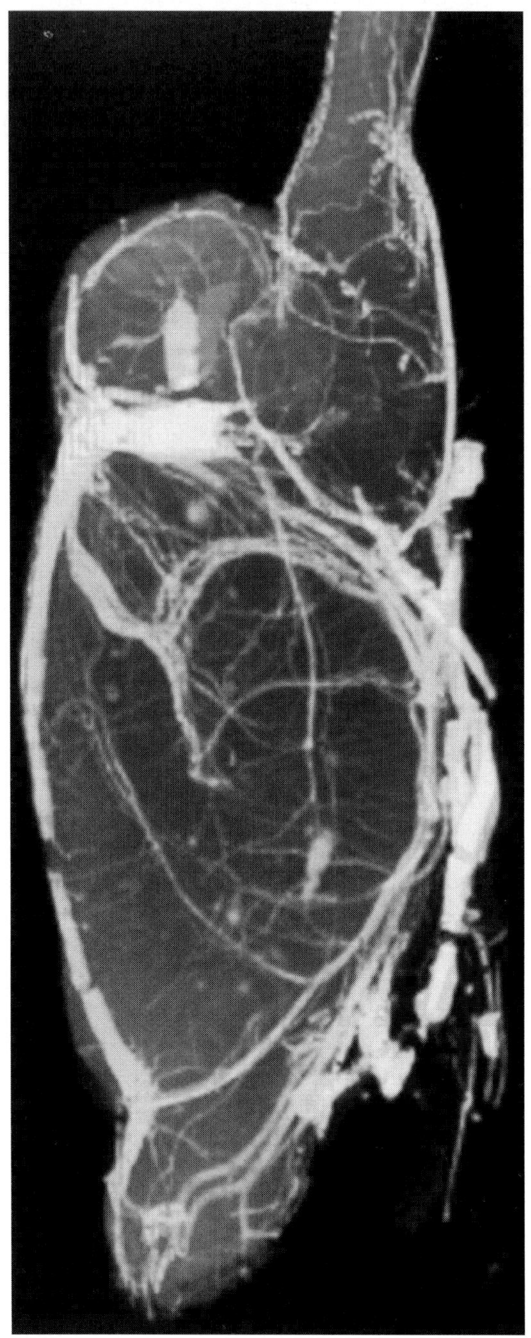

FIGURE 5. MR histology image of vasculature in a rat brain "stained" with gadolinium.

512 array. The rendering has been adjusted to highlight the "stained" vascular spaces.

CONCLUSION

Such a review cannot adequately cover all the potential applications of MR microscopy to the study of structure and function in the brain. The examples here have been chosen to span the range from *in vivo* to *ex vivo*. More recent advances in imaging strategies (such as more sensitive detectors, clever pulse sequences, and the use of implantable coils) will deliver increasing technical ability. As these techniques are refined, we fully expect the MR microscope to take its rightful place with traditional optical sectioning and electron microscopy in a complementary fashion for the study of brain structure and function.

REFERENCES

1. LAUTERBUR, P. C. 1973. Nature **242:** 190–191.
2. MANSFIELD, P. & P. K. GRANNELL. 1975. Phys. Rev. B. **12:** 3618.
3. CALLAGHAN, P. T. 1993. Principles of Nuclear Magnetic Resonance Microscopy. Oxford Science Publications. Oxford.
4. BLÜMICH, B. & W. KUHN, EDS. 1992. Magnetic Resonance Microscopy. VCH Verlagsgesellschaft. Weinhiem, FRG.
5. BLACK, R. D., T. A. EARLY, P. B. ROEMER, *ET AL.* 1993. Science **259:** 793–795.
6. BOWTELL, R., G. BROWN, P. GLOVER, M. MCJURY & P. MANSFIELD. 1990. Phil Trans. R. Soc. **A333:** 457.
7. DOCKERY, S. E., S. A. SUDDARTH & G. A. JOHNSON. 1989. Magn. Reson. Med. **11:** 182–192.
8. MALISCH, T. W., L. W. HEDLUND, S. A. SUDDARTH & G. A. JOHNSON. 1991. JMRI **1:** 301–305.
9. CALLAGHAN, P. T. 1990. J. Magn. Reson. **87:** 304–318.
10. MOSELEY, M. E., Y. COHEN & J. MONTOROVITCH *ET AL.* 1990. J. Magn. Reson. **14:** 330–345.
11. BENVENISTE, H., L. W. HEDLUND & G. A. JOHNSON. 1992. Stroke. **23:** 746–754.
12. BENVENISTE, H., L. HEDLUND & G. A. JOHNSON. 1991. Stroke. **22:** 259–268.
13. BEAULIEU, C. F., X. ZHOU, G. P. COFER & G. A. JOHNSON. 1993. Magn. Reson. Med. **30:** 201–206.
14. HALL, W., H. BENVENISTE, L. HEDLUND & G. JOHNSON. 1996. NeuroImage. In press.
15. DREBIN, R. A., L. CARPENTER & P. HANRAHAN. 1988. ACM Comput. Graphics **22:** 65–74.
16. QIU, H., L. HEDLUND, H. BENVENISTE, S. GEWALT & G. JOHNSON. 1996. Proc. SMR 4th Annual Scientific Meeting. New York, NY.
17. ZHOU, X., G. P. COFER, S. A. SUDDARTH & G. A. JOHNSON. 1993. Magn. Reson. Med. **30:** 60–67.
18. SMITH, B. R., G. A. JOHNSON, E. V. GROMAN & E. A. LINNEY. 1994. Proc. Nat. Acad. Sci. USA **91:** 3530–3533.

DISCUSSION

QUESTION: In ischemia and stroke there is a massive release of fatty acids that have a molecular weight on the order of 250 daltons. Can you pick up diffusion of fatty acids bound and unbound in the brain with any of these techniques?

JOHNSON: What sort of molar concentrations are we talking about?

RESPONSE: Micromolar concentration increases 10- to 50-fold.

JOHNSON: I will bow to my colleagues who were doing that work. Dr. van Zijl and others who do spectroscopy can probably answer that question. I think that you are bound by the sensitivity, but I would say that you are not going to see it at micromolar concentrations. You may see it as a consequence of how it changes some of the other things, but as has been pointed out several times, NMR is remarkably insensitive.

R. V. MULKERN: (*Children's Hospital, Boston, Mass.*): Changes in spectroscopy and stroke research have been reported.

Near-Infrared Imaging and Spectroscopy in Stroke Research: Lipoprotein Distribution and Disease[a]

R. J. DEMPSEY,[b,c] L. A. CASSIS,[b] D. G. DAVIS,[d]
AND R. A. LODDER[e]

[b]*College of Pharmacy, and*
[d]*Department of Pathology*
University of Kentucky Medical Center
Lexington, Kentucky 40536

INTRODUCTION

Stroke is a critical problem in the United States that affects more than 500,000 people annually. Research into the causes of stroke and testing of drug therapies to reduce ischemic and postischemic damage to the brain is hampered by an inability to continuously follow the physical and chemical events that occur during ischemia and reperfusion *in vivo*. Near-infrared (near-IR) spectrometry has recently been used to observe stroke-induced changes in the lipids and proteins of whole brain samples *in vitro* and *in vivo*.[1] The examination of whole brains was made possible by a combination of hardware and software techniques designed to make the sample presentation to the spectrometer more reproducible. Near-IR spectrophotometry of gerbil brain tissue discriminated between adult (3–4 months of age) and aged (18–20 months of age) brains as well as between brains exposed to 5 and 10 minutes of ischemia. The near-IR analytical method has many applications in aging and stroke research, including the noninvasive determination of age from brain spectra obtained transcranially, simultaneous multicomponent analysis of lipids and proteins, and quantification of stroke-induced edema. More recently, near-IR research has moved to the events preceding ischemic injury.

Arterial disease contributes to most of the deaths in the United States. Epidemiological studies performed over a period of years have indicated that reduction of blood cholesterol levels significantly reduces the risk of atherosclerosis, ischemia, myocardial infarction and death. For some time these data have been cited in experimental attempts to prevent arterial disease. One

[a]The clinical research reported in this paper was supported by funds from the NIH under Grants HL45143 and RR08242 and the American Heart Association (Kentucky Affiliate), and the computational research was supported by funds from the NSF under Grant CHE 9257998.

[c]Present address: Department of Neurosurgery, University of Wisconsin Clinical Science Center, 600 Highland Ave., H4/338, Madison, Wisconsin 53792-3232.

[e]Corresponding author. Phone: 606/257-9232; e-mail: Lodder@pop.uky.edu

study estimates that 60 million people, or 36% of all adults between the ages of 20 and 74, have cholesterol levels high enough to warrant medical advice and intervention.[2] A 1% reduction in plasma cholesterol concentration in individuals at risk for cardiovascular disease has been shown to reduce the risk of cardiac events in these individuals by approximately 2%. More recent data indicate that lowering cholesterol improves the condition of coronary arteries partially blocked by atherosclerotic lesions, actually effecting a regression of the disease process.[3] These data have been used to make a case for creating a target level for total blood cholesterol of 200 mg/dl,[4] a level below the average of the U.S. population.

The main carrier for cholesterol in the blood stream is low-density lipoprotein (LDL), which is the primary source of cholesterol deposits in the arteries at risk. Several studies have correlated an increase in serum LDL with an increased risk of atherosclerosis.[5] Evidence suggests that the oxidation of LDL may increase its involvement in atherosclerotic lesions. It is known that oxidatively modified LDL increases the lysolecithin content and increases its negative charge. The protein's density is increased and the content of polyunsaturated fatty acid is decreased, leading to the fragmentation of apolipoprotein B.[6] These changes lead to changes in the electrophoretic mobility and the aggregability of LDL as well as in the interaction of LDL with the arterial wall. The oxidized species is increasingly recognized by the acetylated LDL (scavenger) receptor on the macrophages and on the endothelial cells. Further, oxidized LDL is capable of vascular cell injury as well as the modification of cellular products of gene expression. The oxidation of LDL is hypothesized to occur through a free-radical mechanism.[7] The endogenously generated free radicals, in turn, may be related to continued generation of leukotrienes by a lypoxygenase mechanism.[8] Recent developments have suggested that the oxidation of LDL is a critical step in the acceleration of atherosclerosis to clinically significant levels.[5]

Oxidized LDL (oxLDL) also induces a monocyte binding activity in endothelial cells and is chemotactic to monocytes. OxLDL affects cytokine gene expression.[9] With the attraction of monocytes and their accumulation of oxidized LDL via the scavenger receptor pathway, foam cell formation is noted in the arterial wall.[5,9] The foam cell precursors to fatty streaks are hypothesized to arise from monocytes and macrophages, which migrate into the intima, although smooth muscle cell involvement is postulated as well.[5] The oxLDL may initially act as a cytotoxic agent, as shown in cell culture studies.[10]

The role of lipid oxidation in atherosclerosis has been inferred primarily by the examination of the naturally occurring and synthetic antioxidants. Ascorbic acid and bilirubin have been shown to be effective in protecting lipids from oxidative damage.[11] Alpha-tocopherol acetate (vitamin E) has been shown to be protective in the lipid profile of atherogenesis,[12] is active as an antioxidant,[13] and is believed to share the high-affinity receptor for LDL in cultures of fibroblasts.[14]

The lipophilic antioxidant probucol has been shown to decrease both the oxidation of lipoproteins as well as their cytotoxicity.[15] In addition to altering the oxidative modification of LDL, studies in Watanabe rabbits show that probucol pretreatment inhibits the degradation of LDL in fatty streaks. Probucol pretreatment significantly lowered the rate of atherosclerotic progression in such animals even when correcting for the lipid-lowering effects of probucol.[16,17] These data suggest that antioxidants may exert an effect by limiting the oxidized LDL component of atherosclerotic progression beyond that to be expected from lowering native LDL levels alone.

Stereotypic locations for atherosclerotic development have been identified and include the coronaries and carotid vessels.[18–22] The carotid arteries have been particularly accessible to noninvasive study due to their subcutaneous location and progressively better-understood role in the pathogenesis of cerebral ischemia and stroke.[20,22] In addition, noninvasive sonographic determination of atherosclerotic plaque present at the carotid bifurcation has been correlated with overall ischemic risk and systemic atherosclerosis, and suggests carotid atherosclerosis as a marker of overall atherosclerotic insult to vessels.[23]

While considerable interest has been placed on the geometry of the carotid arterial atherosclerotic plaques and their relationship to ischemia,[20,22] the actual biochemical composition of the plaque is of increasing importance. Approximately 30% of total fatty acids present in arterial walls lipids are readily oxidized.[21]

Reference methods for lipoprotein and apoprotein determinations in plaques involving ultracentrifugation are destructive of the sample, cumbersome, and/or expensive. Electrophoretic methods, immunofluorescence, and radioimmunoassays are far slower than a purely spectrometric method. Many times even radioimmunoassays have coefficients of variation as high as 5–10%.[24] The dynamic range and reproducibility of electrophoretic methods is even worse.[25] The cost of immunoreagents and the time required to complete an analysis are prohibitive for many screening applications. Radioimmunoassays are complicated even further by the need to handle radioactive compounds. None of these methods are well suited to preserve the spatial relationship of compounds in the plaque.

There is currently no accurate nondestructive *in vivo* reference assay for HDL, LDL, or apolipoproteins immobilized in the walls of living arteries in humans. Fiberoptic catheters have been used to locate atherosclerotic lesions, but most spectrometric techniques can do no more than distinguish lesions from healthy arterial tissue (i.e., a detailed breakdown of constituent proteins is not possible). Research currently under way in this laboratory employs InSb focal plane arrays (FPAs) and PtSi CCD near-IR video cameras and tunable light sources to identify lesions in living arteries of human patients and to map their chemical constituents in three spatial dimensions. Tunable light sources based on blackbody emission and tunable filters and monochromators, as well as a Nd:YAG-pumped KTP/OPO near-IR laser system, are used for different imaging experiments depending upon the light intensity required. Chemical analysis of lesions *in vivo* permits the kinetic study of atherogenesis and contributes to the understanding of lesion formation and growth. As new processes (e.g., oxidation of LDL) are identified as playing key roles in the initiation and progression of lesions, better treatment programs can be designed that focus on these mechanisms.

Near-IR spectroscopy has been used industrially for years in lipid analysis to determine saturation of unsaturated fatty acid esters.[26] More recently, near-IR spectrometry was used in our laboratories to examine lipids *in vitro* and *in vivo* in gerbil brains following experimentally induced stroke and to identify nine different saturated and unsaturated fatty acids found in the gerbil brain.[1] Near-IR spectrometry has also been used in our laboratories to analyze HDL, LDL, and cholesterol in the blood vessels of rats.[27] Additionally, near-IR spectroscopy has been used to determine fat content of commercial meat products.[28] Analytes including glucose, lactate, and many others have been determined simultaneously using near-IR spectrometry.[29] FT-near-IR imaging of lipid and protein in primate brain tissue has been described.[30] In humans, near-IR spectroscopy has been used noninvasively to analyze deoxyhemoglobin in blood and to determine whole body fat.[31,32] In our laboratories, near-IR imaging has been used in human stroke patients to locate atherosclerotic plaque by identifying and locating oxidized lipoprotein spectral signatures.[33] A major advantage of near-IR spectral analysis is its chemical imaging ability. Additionally, near-IR spectral imaging provides information on details of various internal structures including muscle, bone, and arteries.[34]

Near-IR methods are used in the following study to test the hypothesis that nondestructive spectrometric imaging of plaque lipoproteins relevant to atherosclerosis and stroke is as precise as protein extraction, ultracentrifugation, and gel electrophoresis. In the process, the analytical power of near-IR cameras and MPP (massively parallel processor) supercomputing is demonstrated.

EXPERIMENTAL METHODS

Lipoprotein Reference Analyses

LDL was isolated from fresh plasma ($<$24-hr-old) and tissue plaques of all endarterectomy patients according to the method of Havel.[35] A blood sample from each patient was withdrawn and plasma was isolated by centrifugation at 3,000*g* (4°C). For tissue plaque reference analysis, excised plaques were quickly rinsed in Kreb's physiological salt solution to remove adherent LDL and oxLDL before being frozen in liquid nitrogen. An aliquot of plasma or tissue extract was diluted with a 50 mM phosphate buffer containing the following preservatives (buffer A): 2.7 mM EDTA, 2 mM benzamidine, 10 μM probucol, 1 μM PPACK, 0.01% aprotonin, 0.008% chloramphenicol, and 0.008% gentamycin, 1 mM PMSF, 1 mM leupeptin, and 40 μM elastinal. For the tissue plaque extraction, plaque segments were cut into small pieces (~1 mm) in a cooled, nitrogen-purged glove box while under the de-gassed extraction buffer using a custom-made immersible tissue chopper. Minced tissue was then extracted overnight at 4°C under nitrogen using an orbital shaker (10 rpm) in 0.14 M NaCl/0.01 M phosphate buffer, pH 7.2, containing the preservatives as in buffer A. The extract was collected by low-speed centrifugation at 4°C, washed once with extraction buffer, and the supernatants were combined. The supernatant was transferred into 12-ml tubes, overlayered with 0.5 ml of water, and centrifuged at 100,000*g* for 30 min at 5°C. LDL (density, 1.019–1.063 g/ml) was isolated from plasma and plaque extracts by density gradient ultracentrifugation over a potassium bromide gradient at 200,000*g* (4 hours at 22°C). The LDL fraction (density of 1.019–1.063, determined by light illumination) was obtained and dialyzed overnight at 4°C against 0.14 M NaCl/0.01 M phosphate buffer (pH 7.4) containing 0.27 mM EDTA and 1 mM PMSF. After dialysis, the LDL fraction was sterile-filtered (0.45 μm) and stored under nitrogen at 4°C. Protein content was determined according to the 1971 method of Bradford. For comparison, commercial LDL (Sigma, St Louis, MO) and oxLDL (LDL oxidized in the presence of 10 μM copper sulfate at 37°C for 24 hr) were used as reference standards. A calibration curve was constructed for the near-IR spectra of freshly prepared ox-LDL to allow quantitative determination of oxLDL as well as to identify spectral peaks that correlate with oxLDL concentration.

Reference assays for plasma and tissue extracts consisted of SDS-PAGE[36] (index of alterations in electrophoretic mobility) and measurement of thiobarbituric acid–reactive substances (TBARS). Before electrophoresis, the samples were prepared in a buffer containing 0.063 M Tris-HCl, 2% SDS, 10% glycerol, 10 μM BHT, and 0.001% bromphenol blue (pH 6.8) and heated for 3 min in a boiling water bath. SDS-PAGE was performed using 4–12% gradient gels (100 V, 30 mA for 75 min; Protean 2 mini gel electrophoresis system, Biorad, Hercules, CA) in a running buffer containing 0.025 M Tris, 0.19 M glycine buffer, pH 8.3, containing 0.1% SDS. Coomassie brilliant blue or silver stains were used to visualize protein bands. Each stained gel containing extracted plaque lipoproteins was digitized using a Si CCD camera, and absorbance values were calculated for the bands in each lane. The bands on the gels were identified and quantified using molecular weight markers (broad range, Biorad, Hercules, CA), commercial LDL, and oxLDL standards on each gel. Additional details and illustrations of these methods are available on the World Wide Web at http://kerouac.pharm.uky.edu.

The *in vitro* near-IR scanning of excised plaques (for comparison with *in vivo* scans obtained in the operating room) was conducted in a nitrogen-purged glove box at 4°C. The optical window in the glove box was maintained at −20°C for the frozen plaques, which were scanned immediately before chopping and biochemical extraction).

Constructing Images from Near-IR Spectra

The BEST (bootstrap error-adjusted single-sample technique) calculates distances in multidimensional asymmetric nonparametric central 68% confidence intervals in spectral hyperspace (roughly equivalent to standard deviations). The BEST metric can be thought of as a "rubber yardstick" with a nail at the center (the multidimensional mean).[33] The stretch of the yardstick in one direction is therefore independent of the stretch in the other direction. This independence enables the BEST metric to describe odd shapes in spectral hyperspace (spectral-point clusters that are not multivariate-normal, like the calibration spectra of many biological systems). BEST distances can be correlated to sample composition to produce a quantitative lipoprotein calibration, or simply used to identify regions with lipoprotein distributions similar to plaque in a spectral image. The BEST automatically detects samples and situations unlike any encountered in the original calibration, making it more accurate in biomedical analysis than typical regression approaches to near-IR analysis. The BEST produces accurate distances even when the number of calibration samples is less than the number of wavelengths used in calibration, in contrast to other metrics that require matrix factorization. Unlike its predecessor, the BEAST,[37] the BEST retains the direction vector of a standard deviation in hyperspace throughout all calculations, an essential characteristic for multicomponent quantification of sample composition.

The BEST calculates the integral of a probability orbital in hyperspace by starting at the centroid of the orbital and working outward in all directions at a uniform rate. The *distance* between the center of a plaque orbital and a sample spectrum is *proportional to the concentration(s)* of the plaque constituent(s) responsible for the vector connecting the central and sample spectral points. The *direction of the vector identifies the constituent(s)* of the plaque. The BEST direction and distance are typically used to create color contour plots of the spatial distribution of lipoproteins.[33] In such plots, the contours are drawn at sequential distances in SDs, and RGB (red-green-blue) colors are used to denote class membership based on vector direction. The intensity of the color is proportional to the amount of substance present. Shades of blue are used to represent sample spectra similar to those already in the calibration set, while shades of red are used to represent sample spectra that contain the selected analyte. Shades of green are used to represent a second analyte or possible interfering effect. The BEST offers superior performance as an assimilation method (a method that progressively increases its analytical performance by incorporating previously unknown samples into its calibration). The calibration samples are analyzed by another reference method (such as those listed earlier) in the same manner that Beer's law is used to develop a conventional spectrophotometric calibration.

In the BEST, a population **P** in a hyperspace **R** represents the universe of possible spectrometric samples (the rows of **P** are the individual samples, while the columns are the independent information vectors, such as wavelengths or energies). **P*** is a discrete realization of **P** based on a calibration set **T**, which has the same dimensions as **P*** and is chosen only once from **P** to represent as nearly as possible all the variations present in **P**.

P* is calculated using a bootstrap process by an operation $\kappa(\mathbf{T})$, and **P*** has parameters **B** and **C**, where $\mathbf{C} = E(\mathbf{P})$ and **B** is the Monte Carlo approximation to the bootstrap distribution. The expectation value, E( ), of **P** is the center of **P**, and **C** is a row vector with as many elements as there are columns in **P**.

Each new sample spectrum **X** is analyzed by an operation $\psi(\mathbf{T},\mathbf{B},\mathbf{X},\mathbf{C})$,[27] which projects a

$$\left\{\sigma \left| \frac{\int_0^{\sigma}\left(\int_R^{\mathbf{P}^*} \rightarrow \overrightarrow{cx}\right)}{\int_R^{\mathbf{P}^*} \rightarrow \overrightarrow{cx}} = 0.68\right.\right\} \quad \textbf{(Eq. 1)} \qquad (c - c_T) \rightarrow \overrightarrow{cx} \quad \textbf{(Eq. 2)}$$

discrete representation of the probability density of **P** in hyperspace by many-one mapping onto the vector connecting **C** and **X**. **X** and **C** have identical dimensions. The directional standard deviation (SD) σ is found from the projected probability density in Eq. 1. The integral over the hyperspace **R** is calculated from the center of **P** outward. The calculation of a skew adjusted σ is based on a comparison of the expectation value $\mathbf{C} = E(\mathbf{P})$ and $\mathbf{C}_T = \text{med}(\mathbf{T})$, the median of **T** in hyperspace (with the same dimensions as **C**) projected on the hyperline connecting **C** and **X** in Eq. 2.

The result of the corrected projection is an asymmetric σ that provides two measures of the standard deviation along the hyperline connecting **C** and **X**.

$$\left\{\overleftarrow{+\sigma} \left| \frac{\int_0^{+\sigma}\left(\int_R^{\mathbf{P}^*} \rightarrow \overrightarrow{cx}\right)}{\int_R^{\mathbf{P}^*} \rightarrow \overrightarrow{cx}} = 0.34\right.\right\} \quad \textbf{(Eq. 3)}$$

$$\left\{\overrightarrow{-\sigma} \left| \frac{\int_0^{-\sigma}\left(\int_R^{\mathbf{P}^*} \rightarrow \overrightarrow{cx}\right)}{\int_R^{\mathbf{P}^*} \rightarrow \overrightarrow{cx}} = 0.34\right.\right\} \quad \textbf{(Eq. 4)}$$

Eq. 3 is in the direction of **X** in hyperspace, and Eq. 4 is in the opposite direction along the hyperline connecting **C** and **X**. Skew-adjusted SDs can be used to calculate mean distances between spectra of different samples.

The use of these equations in both *quantitative* and *qualitative analysis* of plaque provides a number of advantages over all other methods of analysis:

1. No analytical assumptions are required to make the problem solvable. Other chemometric methods assume that no discriminating variable (wavelength) is a linear combination of other discriminating variables,

that the covariance matrices for all spectral groups are approximately equal, and that each group is drawn from a population that is normally distributed on the discriminating variables. None of these assumptions are usually true and violations of these assumptions increase the likelihood of producing incorrect quantitative and qualitative analytical results.

2. This nonparametric assimilation method can be used with *full spectra* of samples, which often include a thousand or more variables that describe each sample. The large global memory on the newest supercomputers has made possible the manipulation of images involving tens of thousands of spectra at thousands of wavelengths. No wavelength selection procedures or data compression techniques, such as principal-axis transformation or Fourier transformation, are required by this assimilation method in order to analyze complete spectra. Collinearity in the discriminating variables (wavelengths) does not degrade the results. (Collinearity disturbs conventional matrix techniques like the Mahalanobis method, which relies on matrix inversion or factorization to produce a distance in SDs.)
3. The vector **CX** in the assimilation method identifies the sample components. The metric is calculated by a *highly parallel code* that can be *distributed across as many processors as are available,* and can be used in computerized searches of spectral libraries for qualitative analysis of plaque samples. The length of the vector is proportional to the concentrations of the plaque constituents. Thus, quantitative analytical capabilities are also provided by the same assimilation method, which can still be distributed across as many processors as are available.
4. The BEST metric not only is more accurate and precise than the Mahalanobis metric (the metric commonly used in near-IR spectrometry), but also is often calculated more rapidly as well. The matrix inversion required by the Mahalanobis metric is usually accomplished by algorithms whose complexity (in terms of number of operations required) increases as the number of wavelengths cubed. In contrast, *the complexity of the BEST metric increases linearly* with the number of wavelengths.

The assimilation model developed by the BEST can be compressed, if desired, with eigenvalue/eigenvector or singular value decomposition procedures to conserve memory, and can be converted into a hash table and hash function by calculating the distance and direction from the center of the calibration set to each of the replicates, and used on laboratory PCs.

Supercomputer

The supercomputer used to run the BEST is a 4 hypernode (32 processor) Convex Exemplar SPP1200 system with 7 Gigabytes of memory and 80

Gigabytes of disk storage. The unit processor in the Exemplar SPP1200/XA is Hewlett-Packard's PA-RISC 7200 processor with 240 MFLOPS peak performance. The SPP1200/XA can have up to 16 hypernodes, for a total of 128 processors, with a peak performance of 30.7 GFLOPS.

Carotid Ultrasound Duplex Scanning

All patients were studied with carotid ultrasound duplex scanning utilizing a Hoffrel Duplex Scanner with a 7.5 MHz scanning probe. Frequency distribution, disruption in flow column, and the geometry of any atherosclerotic plaque were recorded. Geometry measurements of the plaque included residual lumen of vessel, maximum thickness of plaque, and percentage of stenosis as compared to normal carotid artery lumen. All measurements were recorded preoperatively and within 3 months postoperatively for assessment of completeness of plaque removal and evidence of carotid restenosis. Both carotid and vertebral arteries were assessed. Carotids arteries were studied in two planes. Frequency analysis was correlated to angiographic and intraoperative findings. The primary data point was the maximum thickness of intraarterial plaque measured to within 0.1 mm at the level of the carotid bifurcation flow divider.

Carotid Endarterectomy

All patients were preoperatively evaluated for medical suitability after obtaining cardiac and medical clearance and operative consent. Carotid endarterectomy was carried out with the patient under general anesthesia. Operations were done unilaterally under EEC and continuous arterial monitoring. Selective placement of intravascular shunting was done at the discretion of the surgeon. Atherosclerotic plaque was removed with the guidance of a Zeiss operating microscope to maintain a meticulous media plane of dissection. Plaque was removed from the distal centimeter of the common carotid artery and the dissection extended distally in the internal carotid artery for the full extent of the plaque. Microscopic inspection of the remaining vessel was carried out for breaks in the wall or any evidence of a residual intimal flap or atherosclerotic plaque. Plaque was then removed and rapidly frozen for analytical and near-IR assessment. Arteries were closed with running 6.0 suture proline with microscopic placement of sutures. Ultrasound assessment of postoperative integrity was carried out during the postoperative period of study.

In vivo *Near-IR Imaging*

Two to four light sources were employed for spectrometric imaging to reduce shadows and achieve the best possible S/N. Both a near-infrared camera (InSb focal plane array or PtSi CCD) and a visible-light camera (Si CCD) were located outside the sterile field, approximately 1 m from the patient. The near-IR and visible-light cameras were operated side-by-side. Images were obtained transarterially as soon as the vessels were exposed (before shunting or opening the vessel for endarterectomy). The number of wavelengths recorded in the images was determined by available time: 8 sec of signal integration were used at each wavelength (the frame rate was 51.44 frames/sec), and spectral images were collected at each wavelength with the near-IR light sources off and again with them on to correct for the presence of other lights in the room and for blackbody photon emission from the sample. The total time allotted for imaging in a normal patient is 7–8 min. BEST contour plots were used to depict the near-IR results. FIGURE 1 shows a visible-light image of the exposed carotid bifurcation in one of the patients. FIGURE 2 is the corresponding near-IR contour plot; the white box inset in the figure surrounds the location of the plaque inside the artery.

Whenever near-IR cameras were used to collect spectra, two spherical silicon dioxide reflectance standards (one high-reflectance and one low-reflectance) were placed in each image to control for variations in light intensity and direction. Images collected on different days and with the light sources in different locations were made comparable by adjusting the gain and offset by multiplicative scatter correction on the images so the intensities on the standards were identical. The specular reflectance on the standards was used to pinpoint the locations of the light sources and to provide a means to calibrate reflected intensity from wet surfaces in tissue samples. Diffuse reflectance from the curved surfaces of the two standards was used to calibrate shaded areas and sloping surfaces in the images.

RESULTS AND DISCUSSION

Results of Ultracentrifugation and Gel Electrophoresis Measurement of Extracted Plaque Proteins

The SDS-PAGE of LDL and oxLDL have been published.[33] In the present study, extracted plaque lipoproteins were monitored on the gels from 8 to 200 kD in 2-kD increments by capturing images of the gels on a CCD camera. FIGURE 3 shows a few of the significant correlations (*f* test on model residuals, $p = 0.05$) between the gel data and the medical histories of the patients ($n_c = 29$, $n_v = 29$). Other significant correlations noted have been previously described.[33] The white bars in the figure show the value of the Pearson correlation coefficient and the black bars show the percentage of the total spectral variation accounted for by the principal components showing the correlation. Coronary artery disease (CAD) and bypass grafts (CABG) have similar correlations and contributions to variation. FIGURE 4a–d shows the relative contribution of the lipoproteins in the gel to the observed correlations. (These contributions were calculated by inverse principal axis transformation. The *y*-axis on the gels was z-scored, so the average gel appears as a flat line centered at zero through the graph. The actual average gel for the set of patients appears as FIGURE 5, and represents the content of the mean spectrum of the area inside the inset box in FIGURE 2). The difference between the gels of plaques in patients with CAD and CABG and the gels of plaques in patients

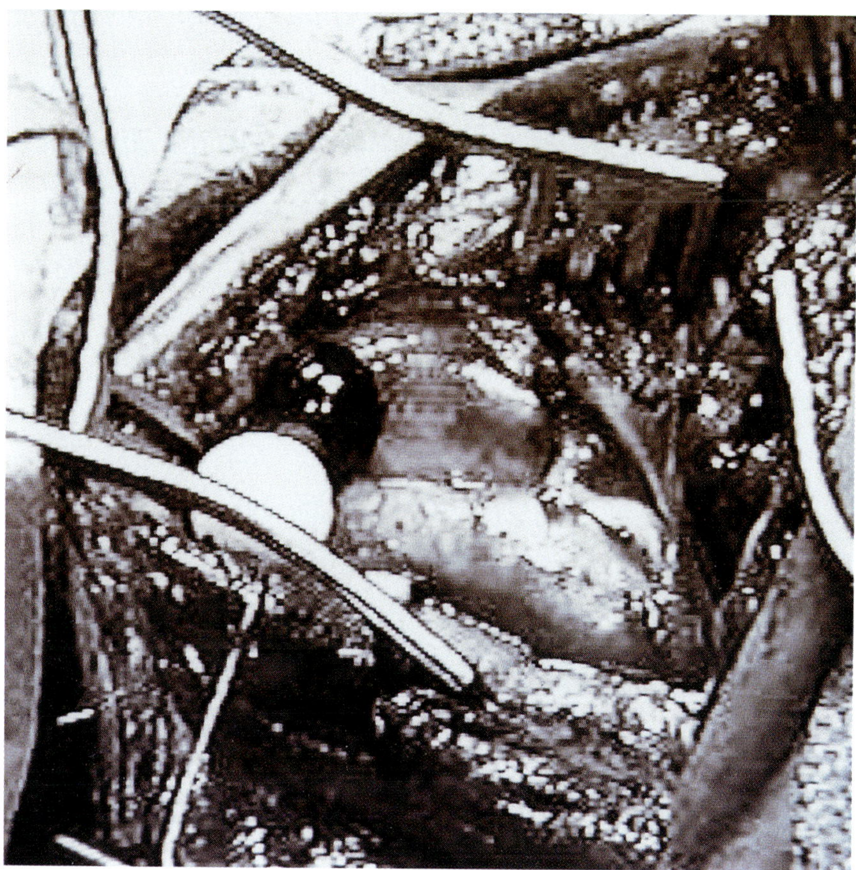

FIGURE 1. A visible-light image of a human carotid bifurcation exposed at the beginning of endarterectomy. The carotid artery is located at about 4 o'clock relative to the black and white sterile reflectance standards. The top two reflections in the black reflectance standard are the surgical lights, which are equipped with cold filters and emit little near-IR light. The two smaller reflections beneath the surgical light reflections are the tungsten sources for the near-IR camera. Images are collected at each wavelength with the near-IR sources on and off to enable correction for sample blackbody emission in the near-IR and for other light sources in the room.

without these conditions is the difference between the solid and the dashed lines, respectively. While the CAD and CABG patients overall had less protein than average in the 24–200 kD range in their plaques, the plaques were slightly enhanced in their content of the proteins at 16, 28–38, and 66 kD. A

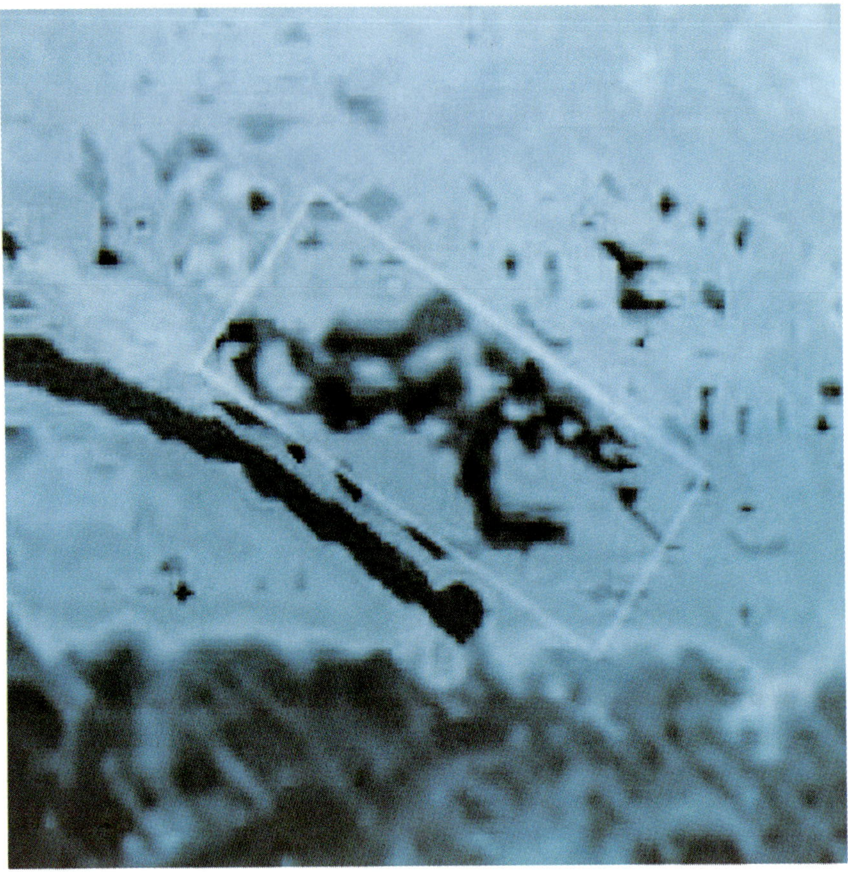

FIGURE 2. A probability-density contour map of the carotid artery seen in FIGURE 1. The density contours (in SDs) are calculated from near-IR spectra using the BEST algorithm. A crosshair can be positioned anywhere on a contour map and used to select full spectra for analysis, to calculate a chemical composition at the selected location, or to give a distance from the calibration samples in multidimensional BEST SDs.

smaller enrichment of the proteins at 84, 96, and 125–140 kD was also observed. The gels of patients experiencing speech problems showed a similar overall pattern, with a slightly different band region from 30–40 kD. The pattern of proteins in progression from CAD to CABG to stroke and speech problems to major surgery (such as bypass grafts or previous carotid endarterectomy on the opposite side) suggests free radical/oxidation reactions that break the proteins into smaller and smaller fragments, causing an overall *increase* in the proteins <24 kD and an overall *decrease* in proteins >24 kD. The finding that proteins of mass ~130 kD (and to a lesser extent, 100 kD) correlated positively with increasing severity of disease symptoms suggests that these proteins may be more-stable byproducts of free-radical reactions. Alternatively, the 100- and 130-kD proteins may be specific protein involved in plaque growth or correlated disease processes. A medical history of previous major surgery was also associated with a reduction in the amount of larger proteins in the plaque and an increase in the amount of smaller proteins. The crossover point was about 45 kD, and the peak features at 66 and 130 kD were reminiscent of those in the LDL standard samples.[33]

There were also strong correlations between the proteins in the plaque and examination of the plaque by pathologists. FIGURE 6 shows a few of the significant correlations between the gels and pathology reports. Other significant correlations noted are given in Dempsey.[33] Microhemorrhage (FIG. 7a) and microulceration[33] produced the strongest correlations to protein content, and these correlations accounted for major fractions of the total variation in the gels. The most visible protein feature of microhemorrhage involved the proteins at 130 kD. Overall, the loss of proteins in the patient plaques was similar to that seen in the cases of medical histories of CAD, CABG, and major surgery.

The presence of necrosis in the plaque (FIG. 7b) in the report of the pathologists' microscopic examination of the plaque correlated significantly

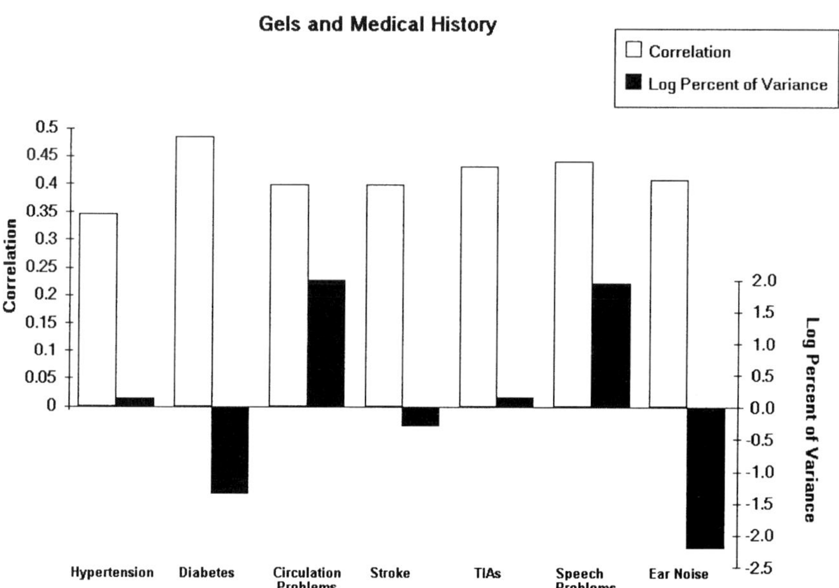

FIGURE 3. Some of the significant correlations ($n_c = 29$, $n_v = 29$, all bars $p < 0.05$) between linear combinations of lipoproteins in carotid plaques and patients' medical histories are shown in the *white bars*. The lipoproteins were determined by extraction, ultracentrifugation, and denaturing gel electrophoresis. The variation shown in the *black bars* is calculated from principal component analysis of sample lanes in gel images.

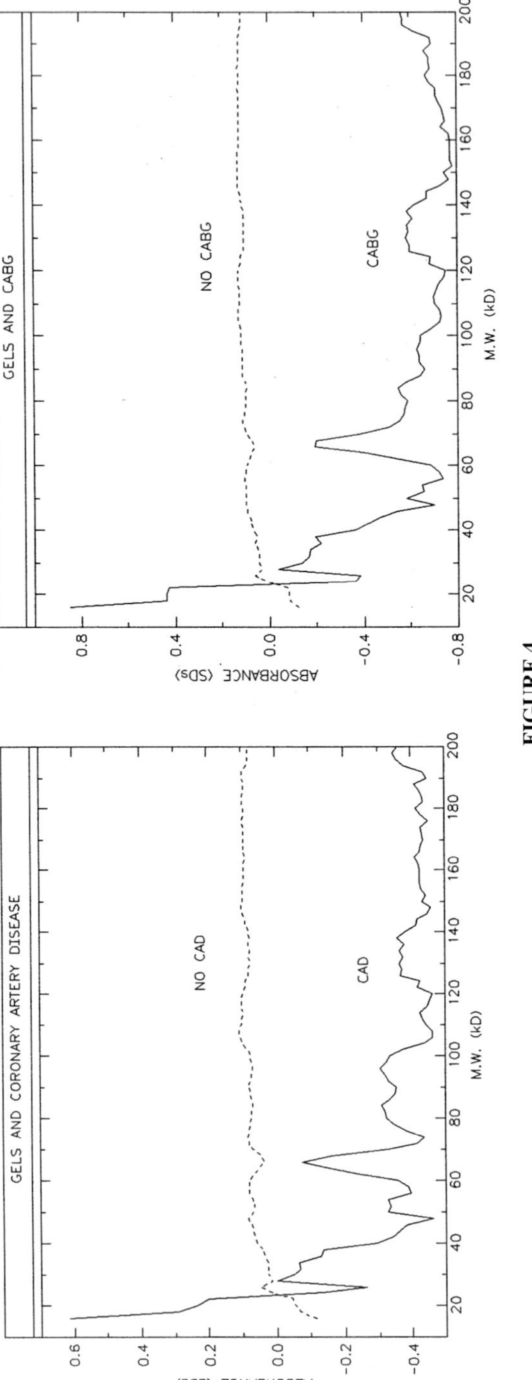
GELS AND CORONARY ARTERY DISEASE
NO CAD
CAD
ABSORBANCE (SDs)
M.W. (kD)
0.6
0.4
0.2
0.0
-0.2
-0.4
20
40
60
80
100
120
140
160
180
200
GELS AND CABG
NO CABG
CABG
ABSORBANCE (SDs)
M.W. (kD)
0.8
0.4
0.0
-0.4
-0.8

FIGURE 4

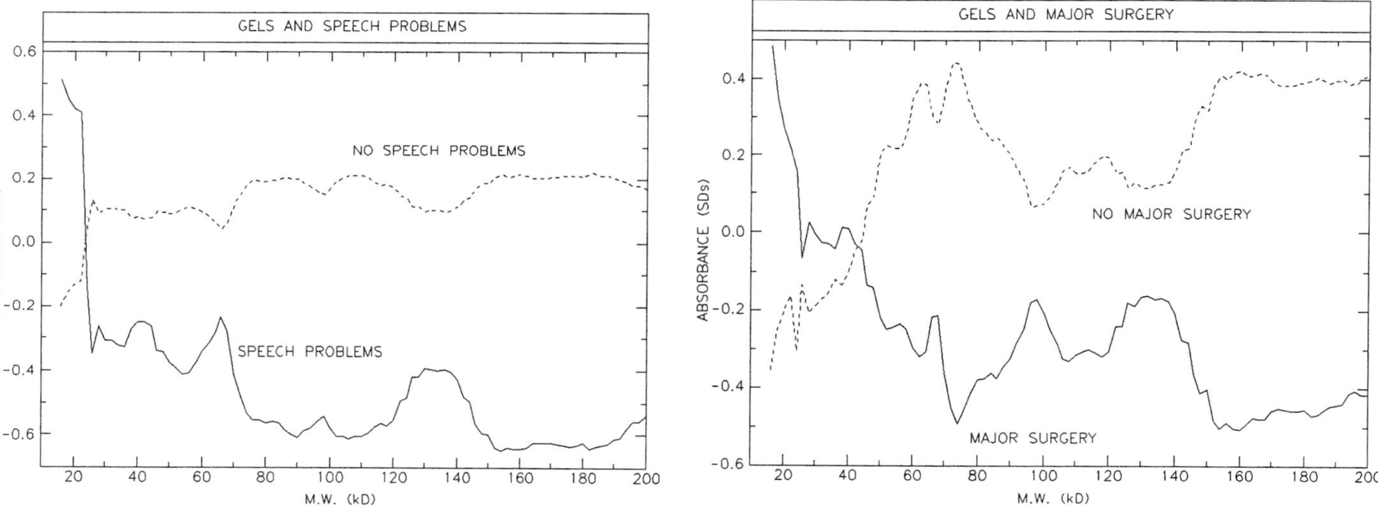

FIGURE 4. Inverse principal axis transformation reveals the linear combination of lipoproteins that correlate to each record in the medical histories. The data were z-scored, so a flat line at y-axis = 0 represents the average gel appearance (shown in FIGURE 5). A progression in lipoprotein peaks parallels the increasing severity of atherosclerotic disease.

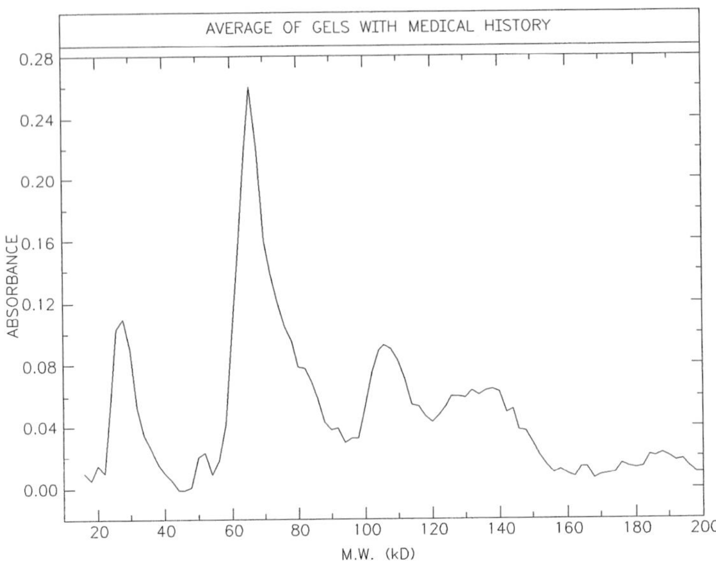

FIGURE 5. The actual average gel absorbance bands from all of the patients from whom complete medical histories are available.

to certain proteins in the plaque. A major protein feature in necrosis was an increase in the amount of proteins with masses 38 kD and 85 kD, and from a 50-kD-wide band centered at 125–130 kD. These proteins were also easily identifiable features in patients with medical histories of CAD, CABG, and major surgery. The severity of disease appeared to be a function of the concentration of these proteins in the plaque. Specifically, the peaks were larger in size in the patients in which CAD has progressed to the point that a bypass graft was necessary.

Results of Near-IR Spectrometry of Carotid Plaque

Near-IR spectra correlated significantly (*f* test, $p = 0.05, n_c = 23, n_v = 21$) to the concentration of most of the 93 protein molecular weights monitored by gel electrophoresis (protein peaks at 20, 162, and 180 kD were the only exceptions). In other words, the appearance of a gel of extracted and centrifuged plaque lipoproteins could be calculated from nondestructive near-IR spectrometry of the whole plaque. The correlation was strongest in the proteins that produce the largest peaks in the electrophoresis. Near-IR spectra are generally far less noisy and have a much larger linear dynamic range than gel electrophoresis (up to 6 orders of magnitude for near-IR spectrometry, compared to perhaps 2 for gel electrophoresis). In fact, gel electrophoresis is used as a calibration method for near-IR spectrometry only because it is widely employed, fairly well understood, and permits quantification of a large number of proteins in a sample simultaneously. The eventual replacement of gel techniques with near-IR ones will not only speed the process of plaque analysis but will make it more precise as well.

Quantification of proteins in plaque by near-IR spectrometry compared favorably to values obtained by ultracentrifugation and gel electrophoresis when these separation methods were used for calibration and validation. A single near-IR spectrum of each plaque was run through an assimilation model to simultaneously predict the concentration of each of the ten protein peaks selected from the gels. The calibration model (FIG. 8) was designed with bias = 0 so all error appears as RSD (black bars). The results were about as accurate as quantification by gel electrophoresis itself. The fact that the error did not depend upon the magnitude of the near-IR signal (white bars), combined with the fact that error was a little higher at the ends of the gel, suggests that the gel electrophoresis was the limiting error source.

Inverse principal axis transformation of near-IR spectra permitted calculation of the approximate spectrum of each protein in its natural plaque matrix. The spectrum of the 128-kD protein (FIG. 9) showed increasing absorbance with increasing concentration at 1750 and 2310 nm, which suggested that the protein was a lipoprotein or had substantial lipophilic character. A similar

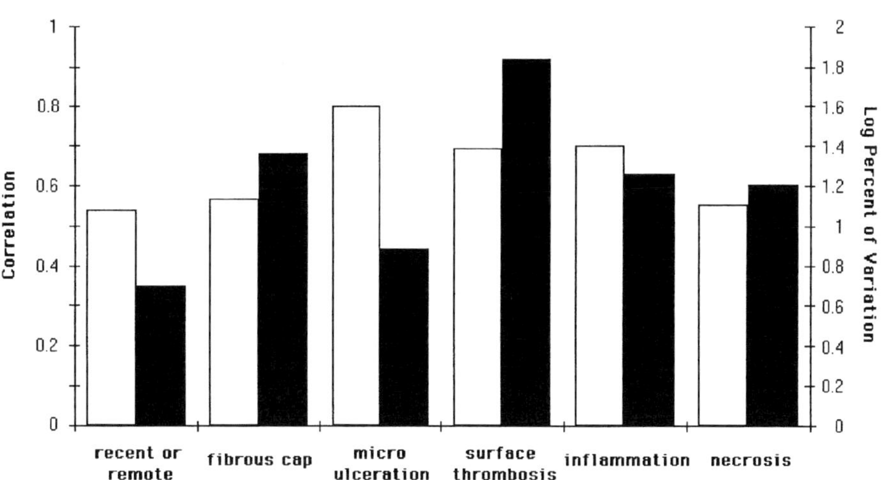

FIGURE 6. Some of the significant correlations ($n_c = 34$, $n_v = 34$, all bars $p < 0.05$) between linear combinations of lipoproteins in carotid plaques and plaque pathology reports are shown in the *white bars*. The lipoproteins were determined by extraction, ultracentrifugation, and denaturing gel electrophoresis. The variation shown in the *black bars* is calculated from principal component analysis of sample lanes in gel images.

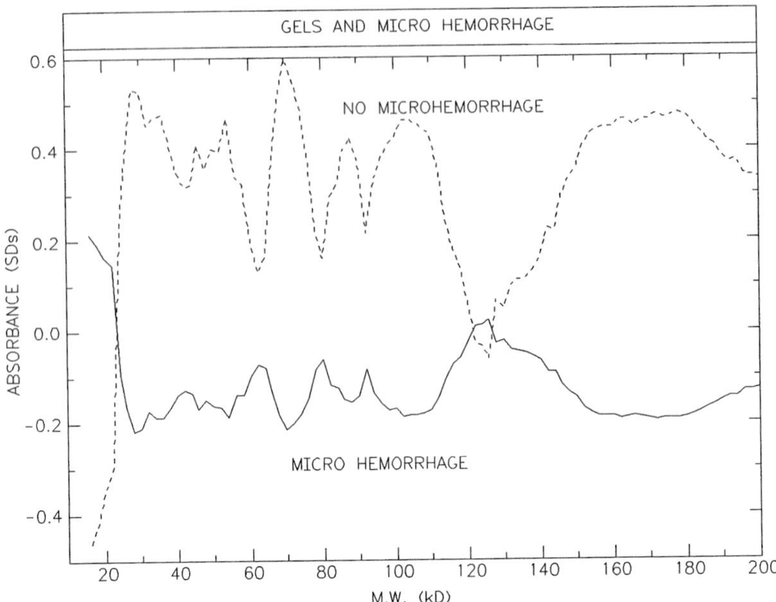

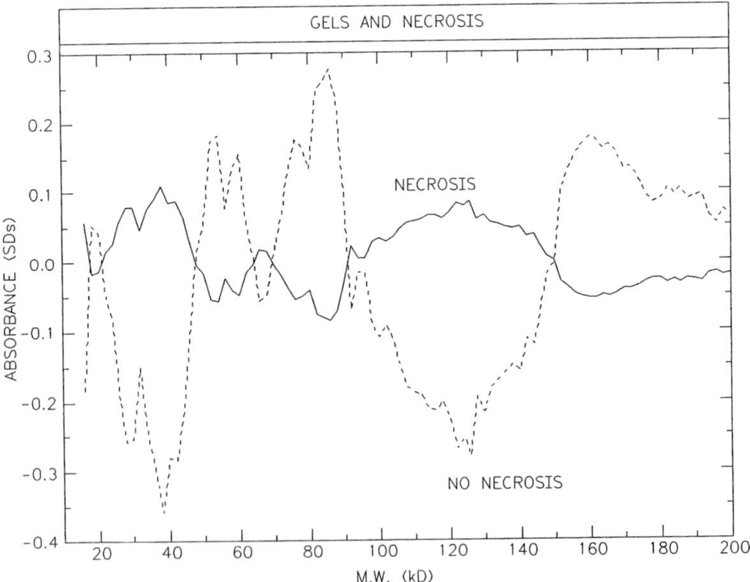

FIGURE 7. Inverse principal axis transformation reveals the linear combination of lipoproteins that correlate to characteristics in the plaque pathology reports. The data were z-scored, so a flat line at y-axis $= 0$ represents the average gel appearance.

spectral pattern was noted for the other proteins, with the exception of the 40-kD protein, which did not appear to possess lipophilic character.

CONCLUSIONS

Near-IR spectrometry has recently been used to observe stroke-induced changes in the lipids and proteins of whole-brain samples *in vitro* and gerbil brains *in vivo.* In this study, near-IR spectrometric imaging was used to examine events in blood vessels that might precede ischemic brain injury in humans. Near-IR imaging methods were shown to provide spatially resolved nondestructive analysis of plaque lipoproteins relevant to atherosclerosis and stroke at least as precise as ultracentrifugation and gel electrophoresis. In the

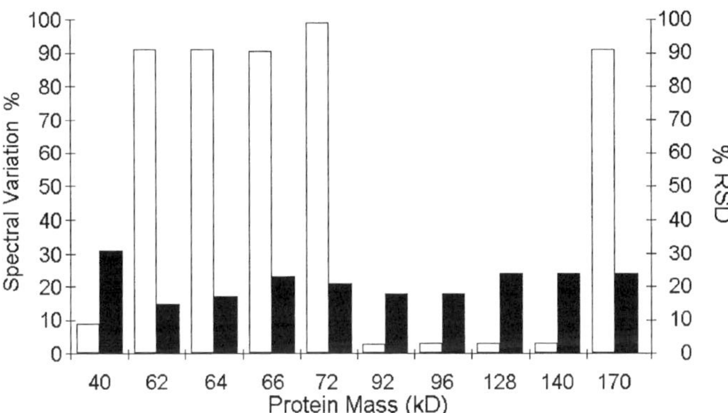

FIGURE 8. The measurement precision for 10 lipoproteins determined simultaneously in carotid plaque by near-IR spectrometry (n_c = 23 calibration plaques, n_v = 21 validation plaques). The precision of near-IR spectrometry appears to be limited by the extraction/ultracentrifugation/gel electrophoresis reference method.

process, the analytical power of near-IR imaging cameras and MPP (massively parallel processor) supercomputing was demonstrated. These spectrometric techniques permit enormous quantities of data on the protein and lipid composition of carotid plaque to be obtained quickly with high S/N, and make the testing of hypotheses about atherogenesis and the progression of disease easy and nondestructive. The eventual extension of this technology to noninvasive transcutaneous laser measurements in patients should increase greatly our understanding of the disease process, and may even make possible a rational assignment of symptomatic patients to drug and/or surgical interventions.

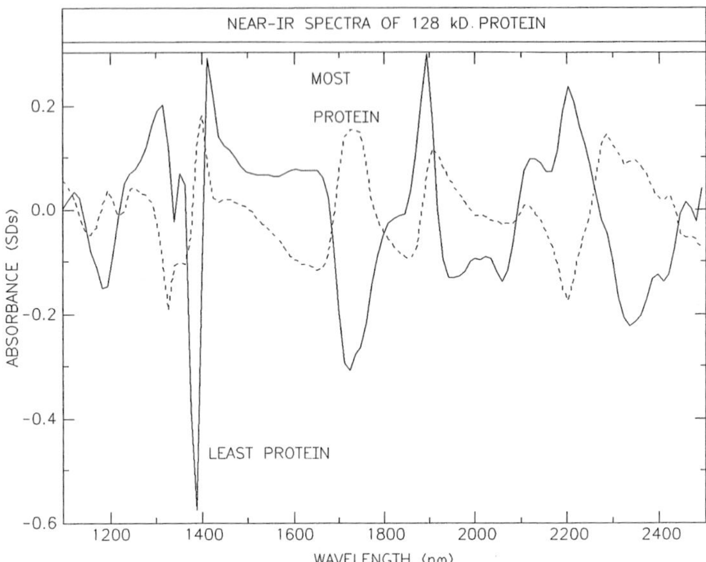

FIGURE 9. The near-IR spectra of lipoproteins in plaques can be calculated by inverse principal axis transformation. In all of the plaques examined, the plaque with the least amount of the 128-kD protein is shown by the *solid line,* while the plaque with the largest amount of the 128 kD protein is shown by the *dashed line.*

REFERENCES

1. Carney, J. M., R. A. Lodder, *et al.* 1993. Anal. Chem., **65:** 1305–1313.
2. Sempos, C. *et al.* 1989. J. Am. Med. Assoc. **262:** 45–52.
3. Blankenhorn, D. H. *et al.* 1987. J. Am. Med. Assoc. **257:** 3233–3240.
4. McManus, B. M. *et al.* 1989. J. Am. Med. Assoc. **262:** 83–88.
5. Esterbauer, H., *et al.* 1990. Chemical Res. Toxicol. **3:** 77–92.
6. Steinberg, D., *et al.* 1989. N. Engl. J. Med. **320:** 915–924.
7. Sato, K., E. Niki & H. Shimasaki. 1990. Arch. Biochem. Biophys. **279:** 402–405.
8. Sun, A. Y. 1972. Biochim. Biophys. Acta **266:** 350–360.
9. Chisolm, G. M. 1991. Clin. Cardiol. **14:** I 25–30.
10. Hessler, J. R., D. W. Morel, L. J. Lewis & G. M. Chisolm. 1983. Arteriosclerosis **3:** 215–222.
11. Frei, B., R. Stocker & B. N. Ames. 1988. Proc. Natl. Acad. Sci. USA **85:** 9748–9752.
12. Paul, J., N. J. Bai & C. L. Devi. 1989. Int. J. Vit. Nutr. Res. **59:** 35–39.
13. Burton, G. W. & M. G. Traber. 1990. Vitamin E. Annu. Rev. Nutr. **10:** 357–382.
14. Esterbauer, H., M. Dieber-Rotheneder, C. Streigl & G. Waeg. 1991. Am. J. Clin. Nutr. **53:** 314S–21S.
15. Chilsolm, G. M. III & D. W. Morel. 1988. Am. J. Cardiol. **62:** 20B–26B.
16. Steinberg, D., S. Parthasarathy & T. E. Carew. 1988. Am. J. Cardiol. **62:** 6B–12B.
17. Carew, T. E., D. C. Schwenke & D. Steinberg. 1987. Proc. Natl. Acad. Sci. USA **84:** 7725–7729.
18. Bassiouny, H. S., H. Davis, N. Massawa, B. L. Gewertz, S. Glagov & C. K. Zarins. 1989. Vasc. Surg. **9:** 202–212.
19. Dutch TIA Trial Study Group. 1991. N. Engl. J. Med. **325:** 1261–1266.

20. NORTH AMERICAN SYMPTOMATIC CAROTID ENDARTERECTOMY TRIAL COLLABORATORS. 1991. N. Engl. J. Med. **325:** 445–453.
21. HARMAN, D. 1984. *In* Free Radicals in Molecular Biology, Aging, and Disease. D. Armstrong *et al.,* Ed: 1–41. Raven Press. New York.
22. MAYBERG, M. R., S. E. WILSON, F. YATSU, D. C. WEISS, L. MESSINA, L. A. HERSHEY, C. COLLING, ESKRIDGE, D. DEYKIN & H. R. WINN. 1991. JAMA **266:** 3289–3294.
23. DEMPSEY, R. J., A. L. DIANA & R. MOORE. 1990. Neurosurgery **27:** 343–348.
24. GINSBERG, H. N. *et al.* 1990. N. Engl. J. Med. **322:** 574–579.
25. JORGENSON, J. W. 1986. Anal. Chem. **58:** 743A–760A.
26. WETZEL, D. 1983. Anal. Chem. **55:** 1165A.
27. CASSIS, L. A. & R. A. LODDER. 1993. Anal. Chem. **65:** 1247–1256.
28. WOLD, J. P., J. KRANE & L. KRANE. 1996. J. Food. Sci. **61(1):** 74.
29. CHUNG, H., M. A. ARNOLD, M. RHIEL & D. W. MURHAMMER. 1996. Appl. Spectrosc. **50:** 270–276.
30. LEWIS, E. N., A. M. GORBACH, C. MARCOTT & I. W. LEVIN. 1996. Appl. Spectrosc. **50:** 263–269.
31. CONWAY, J., K. NORRIS & C. BODWELL. 1984. Amer. J. Clin. Nutr. **40:** 1123.
32. OZAKI, Y., T. MATSUNAGE & T. MIURA. 1992. Appl. Spect. **46:** 180–182.
33. DEMPSEY, R. J., D. G. DAVIS, R. G. BUICE, JR. & R. A. LODDER. 1996. Appl. Spectrosc. **50:** 18A–34A.
34. VANDEVAN, M., T. FRENCH, J. FISHKIN & F. GRATTON. 1991. Biophys. J. **59:** 167a.
35. HAVEL, L. J., H. A. EDER & J. H. BROGDON. 1955. J. Clin. Invest. **34:** 1345–1353.
36. YLA-HERTTUALA, S., W. PALINSKI & M. E. ROSENFELD. 1989. J. Clin. Invest. **84:** 1086–1095.
37. LODDER, R. A. & G. M. HIEFTJE. 1988. Appl. Spectrosc. **42:** 1351–1365.

Strategies of Visual Perception Suggested by Optically Imaged Patterns of Functional Architecture in Monkey Visual Cortex

GARY BLASDEL[a]

Department of Neurobiology
Harvard Medical School
200 Longwood Avenue
Boston, Massachusetts 02115

INTRODUCTION

"Seeing" begins in the retina. Patterns of light, refracted by the optics of each eye, are first transduced by photoreceptor cells at the back of each retina into two-dimensional arrays that are then relayed through a second layer, consisting of *bipolar neurons,* to a third layer of *retinal ganglion cells,* whose axons form the optic nerve(s) that carry information out of each eye. They carry it centrally, through the optic tracts to the lateral geniculate nuclei (LGN) that are located on each side of the thalamus. In the LGN, six separate and aligned layers of neurons receive this information in parallel before passing most of it along to the input layers of the primary visual cortex (a.k.a., V1, Area 17, and striate cortex). From there the information passes radially to one or more layers before arriving at one or more arrays of output neurons that project to other cortical areas.

In many ways it is simplest to think of this system, the retino–geniculo–striate system, as a sequence of discrete transforms taking place between successive and relatively independent representations of visual space. The process is easiest to visualize in the retina, where the overwhelmingly two-dimensional arrangement is obvious. As this information passes centrally, from photoreceptors to bipolar cells, it is acted upon by wide-ranging networks of *horizontal cells,* located in the *outer plexiform layer,* that generate the first *center–surround* receptive fields. As it progresses centrally, from bipolar to ganglion cell layers, it is modified yet again by *amacrine cells,* which shape the physiological properties of retinal ganglion cells even further before allowing this information to proceed to the LGN.

[a]Phone: (617) 432-3053; fax (617) 432-1892; e-mail: gblasdel@warren.med.harvard.edu

REDUCING REDUNDANCY IN THE VISUAL FIELD

The effects of these serial transforms are easiest to comprehend in the context of lateral redundancy of information and the need to reduce it. This is done by pooling laterally redundant, or correlated, information to glean more accurate information about sparsely distributed but much more pertinent events. A simple example can be seen in the familiar center–surround receptive fields of the retina. These are characterized by On or Off responses to light in their centers that are antagonized rather completely by comparable amounts of light in their doughnut-shaped surrounds. As a direct consequence of center–surround interactions, retinal and LGN neurons respond weakly, if at all, to diffuse illumination, or even to gradually changing illumination. Yet they respond enthusiastically to any luminance discontinuities (i.e., edges), especially ones that move in the visual field. Information about average luminance, which may be described as laterally correlated or redundant, is thereby ignored, while information about luminance differences (between center and surround) is amplified and passed along.

The strategy of removing laterally redundant luminance information in many ways resembles the algorithms used by fax machines, which optimize transmission over lines of limited bandwidth by ignoring blank regions on a piece of paper and transmitting only information about the transitions encountered at the edges of alphanumeric characters. In addition to achieving impressive compression ratios of 100:1 or 1000:1, this strategy facilitates subsequent tasks, like scene segmentation and feature abstraction, by vastly reducing the quantity of useless information passed along.

This strategy continues in the LGN and striate cortex. However, due to the evolving arrangement of visual representations, the consequences of center–surround interactions change. While there may be photographically correct representations in the retina, there are none in the LGN. Consequently, center–surround operations must lead to something else, the nature of which can be inferred from the relative absence of luminance information, which has been pooled and decorrelated to highlight the discontinuities produced by edges. Center–surround LGN interactions therefore pool laterally distributed information about edges, reducing or concentrating it if they can. The effect can be seen from the behavior of LGN neurons, which are much more sensitive to moving edges in their surrounds than they are to comparable levels of diffuse light.[1]

Another type of redundancy reduction can be seen in the pooling of information from both eyes into a single coherent representation. Although this information is maintained separately in the LGN and the first input layers of V1, it converges rapidly thereafter onto single cells at the very next stage. As this happens and information from the two eyes is pooled to improve resolution, signal/noise ratios, and so on, minor differences related to stereoscopic depth perception are extracted, concentrated, and retained in greatly compressed form.

In summary, therefore, center–surround interactions primarily appear to reduce the redundancy of laterally distributed information. As new aspects are unmasked, redundancies in their distributions are reduced as well. In retina the most redundant information lies in the correlated levels of light registered at adjacent locations. Once this redundancy has been eliminated, the redundancy of edges prevails. And to the extent that edge densities are correlated and can be calculated (as one might expect from the "smoothness" of edge-rich visual textures), this redundancy can be reduced or eliminated as well. Because edges entail more than one degree of freedom, however, the task is more complicated than the removal of correlated luminance information that can be described by one (if color is included, slightly more than one) variable, and consequently must be achieved in several discrete steps. These begin in the LGN (possibly even in the retina) and continue through the first area of primary visual cortex onto which LGN cells project. By pooling and removing laterally redundant information, which is correlated and therefore recoverable later on, these operations appear to shift attention to the sparser events and to perceptually much more important properties arising from the reflectance properties of actual objects in physical space.

BINOCULARITY AND ORIENTATION SELECTIVITY

Simultaneous with the convergence of information from the two eyes onto single cells, there is an emergence of neurons selective for the orientation of contours in the visual field (see FIG. 1). Because the convergence is usually not complete (in V1, in any case), there is a selectivity for one eye (that may encode depth in the form of near and far disparities—see LeVay and Voigt[2]) that organizes in 0.5-mm-wide cortical slabs, known as "ocular-dominance" columns or ocular-dominance slabs because neurons within each one are dominated by one or the other eye.

FIGURE 1. Organizational schemes for ocular dominance and orientation preferences, deduced from microelectrode penetrations.[3,4] **(a)** Ocular dominance bands from tangential sections of a monkey's right occipital lobe, visualized by the reduced silver method of Liesegang LeVay *et al.*[2] Alternate bands have been inked in. (From Hubel and Freeman.[19]) **(b)** Hubel and Wiesel's results[3,4] for electrode penetrations conducted perpendicular and parallel to the cortical surface. For perpendicular penetrations, the preferred orientation remains constant (except in layers 4a and 4c, where the selectivity for orientation is weak or absent). For lateral penetrations, the preferred orientation rotates continuously for distances of 0.5 to 1.0 mm. **(c)** "Ice-Cube" model of striate cortex, proposed by Hubel and Wiesel.[3,4] This model has four principal components: (1) regions preferring one eye or one orientation project vertically between pia and white matter, and accordingly take on the appearance of slabs; (2) slabs representing the two eyes lie parallel to one another; (3) slabs representing different orientations lie parallel to one another; and (4) the two sets of slabs (representing the two eyes and different orientations) intersect at a consistent angle. Doubt was cast on this last component by experiments with the metabolic marker, 2-deoxyglucose (2DG), that showed 2DG labeled "iso-orientation" bands intersecting ocular dominance bands at many different angles (Hubel *et al.*[20]). These illustrations are redrawn from those appearing in Hubel and Wiesel.[4,19]

What is most intriguing about the emergence of orientation selectivity and binocularity (and the associated encoding of depth, and ocular-dominance columns) is that both properties develop at approximately the same stage, appearing simultaneously between the input and output layers of striate cortex. Most likely arising from the network interactions of cortical neurons,

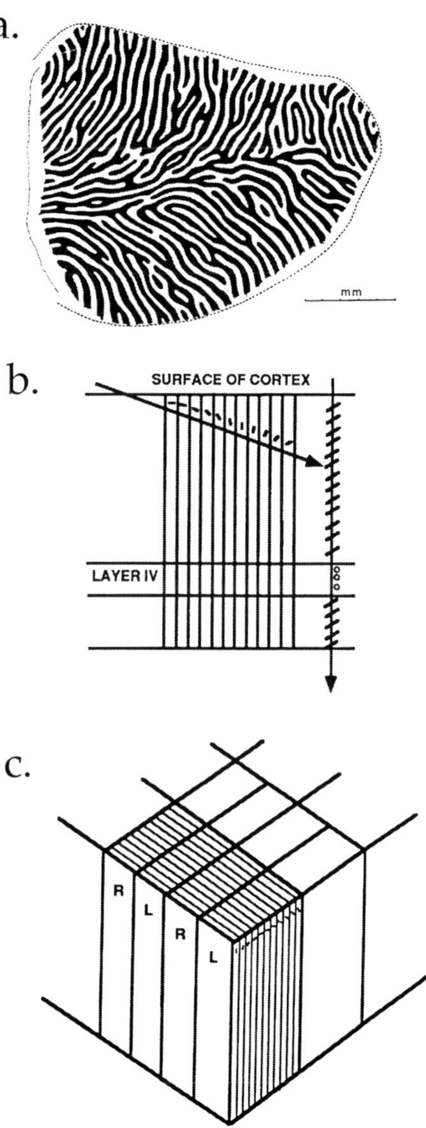

FIGURE 1

these response properties are by far their best known physiological characteristics. Presumably, the lateral arrangements of neurons selective for a particular eye or orientation speak volumes about the strategies taken by cortex in processing and solving information gathered about the external world.

The importance of orientation selectivity and ocular dominance also seems apparent from the continuity with which they are mapped laterally, in ways that preserve neighborhood relationships, for orientation and eye dominance, at the expense of information about local retinotopic position, which is obliterated. As a consequence of these transformations, lateral movements through the upper layers are accompanied by smooth, virtually linear transitions in ocular dominance and preferred orientation, superimposed on decidedly discontinuous jumps in the positions of receptive fields over distances smaller than 1–2 mm^2 (see also FIG. 1b, 1c). The local continuity of orientation preference and ocular dominance may therefore be said to preëmpt the continuity of position, at least in the upper (output) laminae of primary visual cortex.

Because of these and related observations, the lateral grouping of response properties is obviously relevant to visual information processing, and the relevance has been apparent for some time.[3,4] At the very least, these functional topographies generate the latest "images" on which subsequent center–surround operations might be based. Because information is not distributed as luminance maps, however, the consequences of such operations differ and are virtually indecipherable unless the input images are known.

In spite of their obvious importance, however, these patterns proved remarkably difficult to map and analyze for the following reasons: (1) physiological response properties are not usually obvious from known anatomical structures (e.g., somata, neurites, distributions of enzyme, etc.), and (2) until recently, such response properties could only be gleaned painstakingly, by inserting microelectrodes (one at a time, and with considerable difficulty) into discrete sites in the brain. Due to the difficulty of such recordings, analyses involving more than a few sites, or a few tens of sites at most, were rarely if ever achieved. Accordingly, the spatial resolution of such electrode analyses never reached the threshold for detecting patterns.

One early technique for overcoming these difficulties entailed the use of a radioactively labeled sugar (2-deoxyglucose), which was injected during selective stimulation, in hopes of visualizing patterns of neurons made active at the time. While simple in concept, this technique suffered from a critical flaw in that it could be used only *once* on any given area, which meant that comparisons and controls were difficult or impossible obtain. Not only was it impossible to perform controls (by comparing, for example, the patterns generated by the presence and absence of stimuli in the same tissue), it also was impossible to compare responses to different stimuli, on which the definitions of most response properties (e.g., orientation selectivity, ocular dominance, etc.) are based.

DIFFERENTIAL VIDEO IMAGING

A way around these difficulties was provided by small changes in reflectance that have been known for some time to accompany changes in neural activity. Penfield,[5] for example, noticed that regions of cortex became visibly darker during seizures, due to a number of factors, including engorgement of blood vessels and active cell swelling as seizure activity progressed. Due to the recent appearance of affordable imaging technologies (e.g., television cameras, image processors, computers, etc.) that were capable of detecting very faint changes (as small as 0.01%, or 500 times smaller than can be seen by the human eye), it later proved possible to visualize the changes induced by normal (nonpathological) activity as well.[6] Eleven years after these initial studies, it is now practical to map activity in any cortical region that can be seen, with resolutions limited only by the wavelength of light and the imaging technologies employed (which typically offer samples of a quarter of a million points or more). In terms of functional architectures, where the physical dimensions of neurons become a factor, activities in regions finer than 100 μm have become routine.[6–11]

Our primary apparatus for doing this is illustrated in FIGURE 2, where light from a quartz halogen lamp is shown to be filtered and focused on the end of a fiber-optic conduit that carries it to our imaging microscope. Monochromatic light (720 nm $\pm$ 20 nm) is then projected from this source onto the surface of cortex, which has been exposed by reflecting the dura, and which is protected by a pressurized glass plate. During all of our initial experiments, and some of our current ones, a voltage-sensitive dye was superfused over the cortical surface to amplify contrast and augment the responses that could be seen.

The temporal sequence of events can be seen from the photodiode recordings depicted in FIGURE 2b. As one can see, there is a baseline achieved prior to stimulation that changes abruptly with short latency to a monotonic increase in absorption as vertical grating stimuli are made to drift across the animal's visual field. After a small glitch there is a similar response produced by horizontal lines, presumably because the cortical area monitored is large enough to contain vertical and horizontal orientation columns (see below).

The actual events responsible for these changes are poorly understood at best, but are thought to include a host of events with implications for transparency (e.g., membrane depolarization, potassium release, glial cell hyperpolarization, and swelling, followed by the dilation of capillary beds in response to local metabolic demand) that develop in response to sustained cortical activity. By staining the cortex with a voltage-sensitive dye, moreover, one can render the signals even stronger due to visual transduction of membrane potential, particularly in glial cells, producing signals of similar polarity. As an added benefit, it appears that most dyes increase the contrast of intrinsic changes in reflectance that develop in response to cell swelling, potassium scattering, and so on.

Once the cortex has been rendered accessible (by removing the overlying

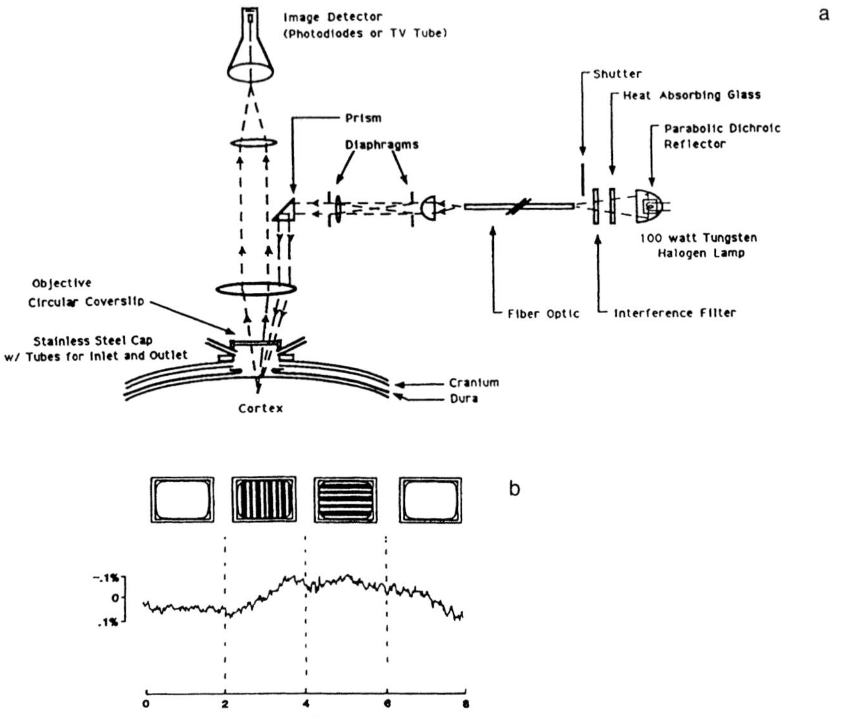

FIGURE 2. Illustration of optical recording in monkey striate cortex. **(a)** Experimental arrangement for monitoring optical signals. A 25-mm disk of bone was removed with a trephine and replaced with a threaded stainless-steel ring, cemented to the skull. A round glass coverslip, secured to a second threaded ring, was screwed into this chamber to provide a clear view of the cortex (with dura reflected). Stainless-steel inlet and outlet ports allowed dye solutions (NK2367 in ~0.1% balanced salt solution) to be introduced and removed. Light from a 100-W tungsten halogen light was directed through a heat filter and interference filter (720 nm, ±20 nm, Omega Optical, Brattleboro, Vermont), mounted in a filter wheel, onto the end of a 0.25-in. fiber-optic cable, which was used to eliminate vibrations. Light at the other end of this cable was collimated and directed through a diaphragm, which lay in a plane of point sources that was focused through the edge of a 50-mm objective onto the cortex. Reflected light was collected by the same objective lens and focused by a projection lens on an image sensor that consisted either of a 2 × 2-mm photodiode array or a Newvicon-based television camera (COHU 5300). **(b)** Averaged optical signal from a single photodiode that measured light from a 100-μm patch of cortex as it responded to 10 presentations of visual stimuli. Each presentation consisted of four episodes, lasting 2 seconds apiece: (1) a blank screen, followed by (2) a vertical drifting grating, followed by (3) a horizontal drifting grating, followed by (4) a blank screen. As one can see from this signal, there is a sudden inflection less than 200 ms after the onset of the vertical grating, much faster than one would expect from intrinsic signals (Grinvald *et al.*[21]). The signal increases steadily during vertical stimulation, undergoes a small glitch with the transition from vertical to horizontal, and returns to baseline when the horizontal grating is removed. Sequential presentations were synchronized to both the electrocardiogram and the respiration to minimize movement artifacts, as suggested previously by Orbach *et al.*[22] (Reprinted with permission from Blasdel and Salama.[6])

scalp, cranium, and meninges) and immobile under a thin plate of glass, it is possible to image cortical preferences for a number of visual stimuli by averaging video frames while the animal views one stimulus and subtracting the result from another average obtained while the animal views another, complementary, stimulus. By comparing responses to the right and left eyes, for example, it is possible to produce images of regions dominated by each one, which because of the ocular-dominance slabs appear as dark and light bands. Similarly, by comparing responses to orthogonal orientations, it is possible to visualize preferences for orientation.

Two examples appear in FIGURE 3, where images of the cortical vasculature are shown in FIGURE 3a and 3b for comparison. While the dense covering of superficial blood vessels, apparent in FIGURE 3a (because of the strong absorption of green light, by hemoglobin), might appear to present problems, these blood vessels are transparent, for all intents and purposes, to light at wavelengths longer than 700 nm. As one can see in FIGURE 3b, the same blood vessels that stand out prominently when imaged under 540-nm light are difficult or impossible to detect, due to the weak absorption by hemoglobin of 720-nm light. This is the image that is seen by the camera, and that is averaged and compared for small changes in reflectance induced by visual stimulation.

The small difference in absorption induced by left and right eye stimulation would be too small (by a factor of 100) to see by eye, but when done repeatedly and averaged over 1000–2000 frames (to improve the ratio of signal to noise), an image of ocular dominance bands is obtained (FIG. 3c). If instead of comparing responses to each of these two eyes, one compares responses to orthogonal orientations, an image of orientation-sensitive zones is seen instead (FIG. 3d). FIGURE 4a through 4h show the results of such comparisons, from the same cortical region, to stimulation by orthogonally oriented contours, at eight different orientations, in increments of 22.5°. As one can see, the activity relative to the small ×, which is located over the center of a vertical preferring iso-orientation columns, changes continuously in relation to the orientation of stimulus contours in the visual field.

During our efforts to hone this technique, since its introduction 11 years ago,[6] it has become apparent that the very best images are obtained by maintaining everything as constant as possible, including visual stimulus parameters (e.g., contrast, type of stimuli, velocity of motion, etc.), except for one that is modulated systematically in phase with frame averaging. To the extent this can be done successfully, this approach allows one to isolate changes associated (because they are brought about in phase) with the variable being manipulated. Hence, the best images of ocular dominance are obtained by keeping all stimulus variables as constant as possible, except for the eye receiving input, which is alternated in phase with positive and negative frame collection. Similarly, the purest images of orientation are obtained by keeping everything (in this case, including ocularity) as constant as possible, while the dominant orientation of stimulus contours is modulated

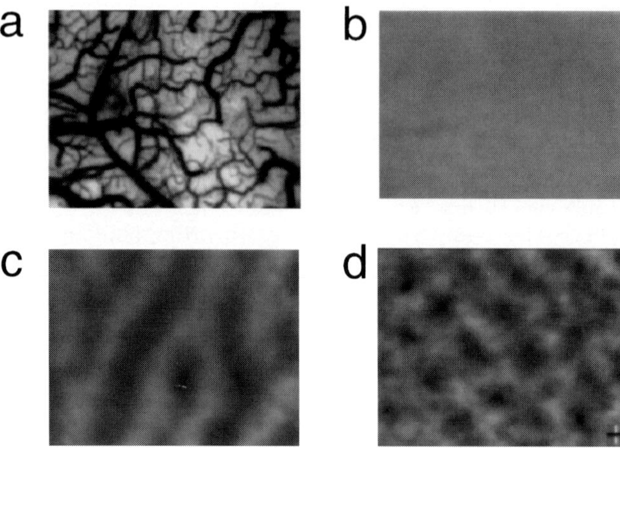

FIGURE 3. Visualization of ocular dominance bands. **(a)** When striate cortex is viewed under green light, the vasculature appears prominent because hemoglobin absorbs strongly at this wavelength. **(b)** Hemoglobin does not absorb strongly at the longer wavelength used to monitor activity, however, and consequently, the same vasculature is much less noticeable when viewed under monochromatic light at 720 ± 20 nm. Moreover, from the image in **(c)**, where the ocular dominance of cortical tissue is visualized underneath most of the vasculature, it becomes clear that blood vessels smaller than 150 μm are virtually transparent to light at this wavelength. **(c)** Differential image of ocular dominance bands obtained by averaging two images of cortex separately, while the right and left eyes were stimulated alternately, and subtracting the image acquired during left-eye stimulation from that acquired during right-eye stimulation. The degree of left- and right-eye preference is indicated by lightness in the image; regions lighter than neutral preferred the left eye, while regions darker than neutral preferred the right. This image has been averaged laterally by binning and convolution (to improve the signal/noise ratio), and normalized. Note the independence of this pattern from that formed by blood vessels in **(a)**. **(d)** Differential image of orientation, revealed by subtracting images of cortex responding to horizontal (indicated by *white bar* in lower right-hand corner) from averaged images of it responding to vertical (indicated by *dark bar*). *Dark and light regions* indicate relative preference for vertical and horizontal orientations. (Reprinted with permission from Blasdel.[9])

FIGURE 4. Differential images of orientation achieved at high magnification with *eight* different pairs of orthogonal contours. The horizontal axis in each frame corresponds to 4.4 mm. As in FIGURES 3 and 4, all images were acquired with orthogonal pairs of contours moving bilaterally at 1.5°/sec. Dark and light values in each frame reflect preferences for each of two orthogonal contours, which are indicated by *dark and light bars* in the lower right-hand corner, and which are rotated by 22.5° in successive frames. Therefore, these images reflect response differences for 0°–90°, 22.5°–112.5°, 45°–135°, 67.5°–157.5°, 90°–0°, 112.5°–22.5°, 135°–45°, and 157.5°–67.5°. (Reprinted with permission from Blasdel.[10])

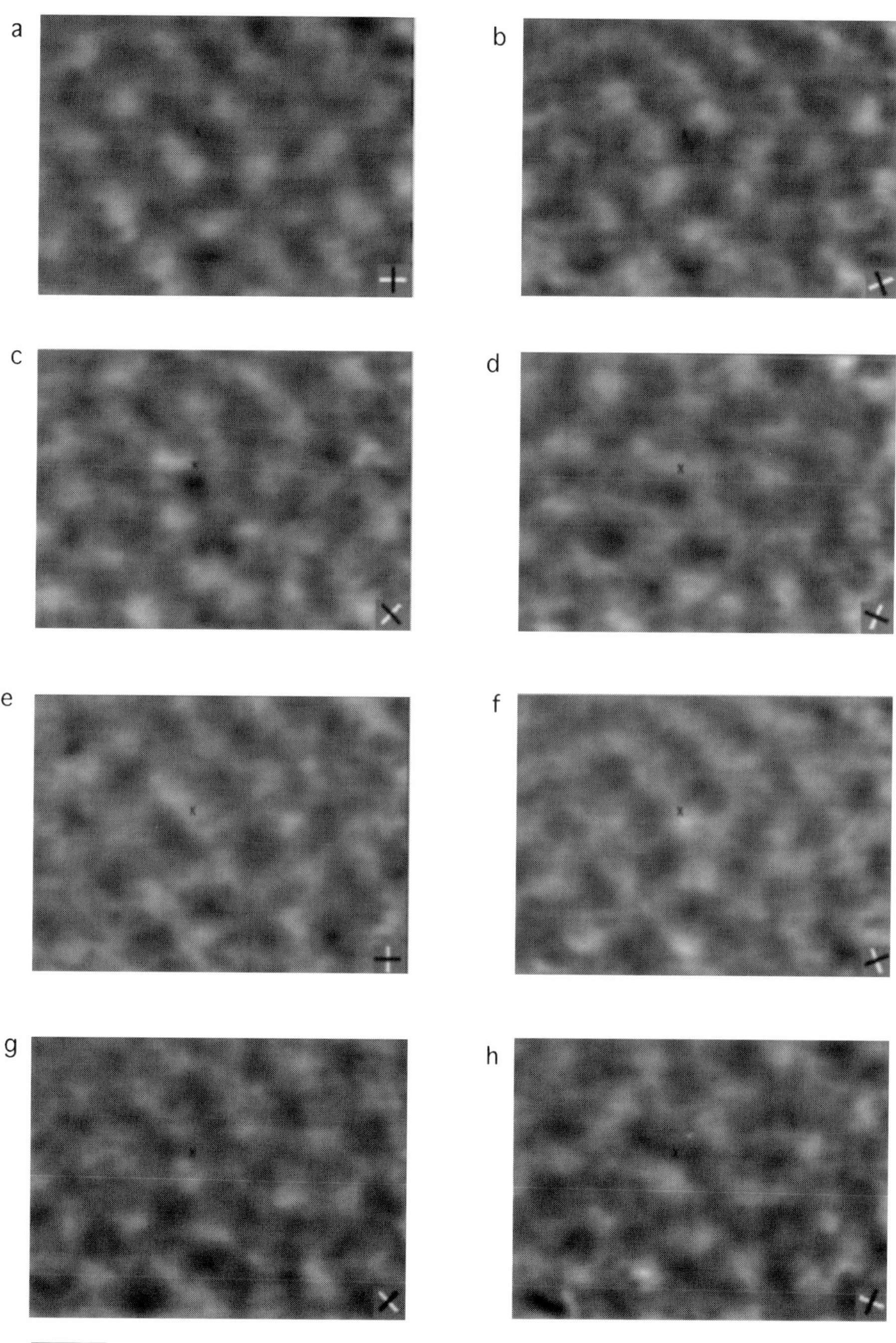

FIGURE 4

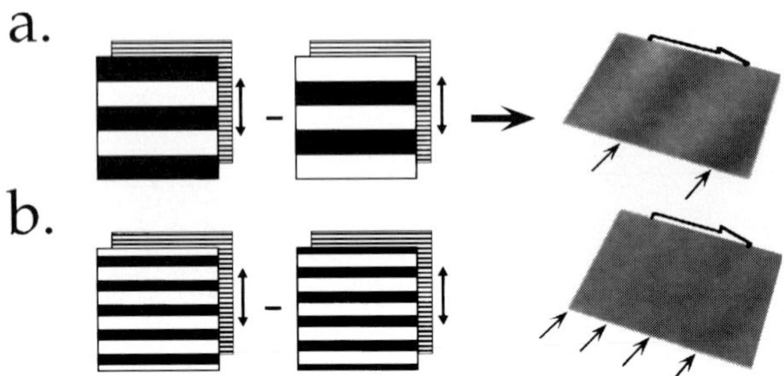

FIGURE 5. **(a)** Differential images of horizontal strips in space, spaced 1.2° apart, visualized by masking a moving grating alternately by complementary masks on alternate trials. **(b)** When the interval between stripes is halved, the interval between cortical bands is halved as well.

between one primary orientation and its orthogonal in phase with positive and negative frame collection.

The principle even works if the variable being modulated pertains to spatial location. By alternately stimulating complementary ribbonlike regions of visual space, it is possible to visualize the representations of these regions on the cortical surface. As illustrated in FIGURE 5, one does this by stimulating complementary regions of space while positive and negative (to be subtracted) frames are averaged. The cortical regions activated in and out of phase with stimulation then appear dark and light, respectively. In the case of vertically oriented ribbons of space, the activated cortical regions take on the appearance of dark and light bands running parallel to the V1/V2 border (which represents the vertical meridian in visual space). In the case of horizontally oriented stimulus zones, the induced bands run at right angles to the V1/V2 border (indicated in FIG. 5 by the open arrow directed toward the fovea), as one would expect. The cortical patterns induced by four different orientations of complementary stimuli appear in FIGURE 6, where they have been inverted and rotated to bring the cortical maps of visual space into alignment with the visual field. As one can see, the patterns achieved from the same cortical region are strikingly aligned with the stimulus regions used to make them, curving and dilating slightly along the trajectories one would expect from changes in cortical magnification and the known representations of visual space on the cortical surface.

FIGURE 6. The patterns of bands produced in one cortical location by ribbons of complementary stimulation at four different orientations. In each example, the cortical patterns have been rotated and inverted to bring the position of the V1/V2 border into correspondence with the vertical meridian of the visual field (which it represents).

V1 / V2

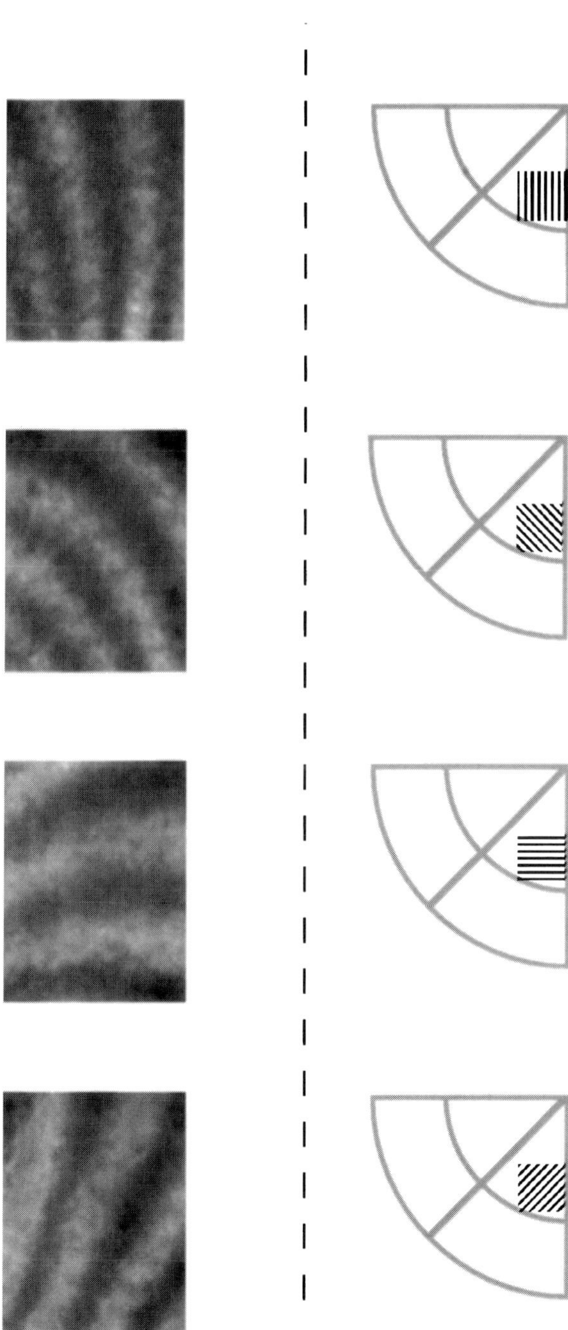

FIGURE 6

INSIGHTS INTO THE FUNCTIONAL ORGANIZATION OF OPTICALLY IMAGED PATTERNS OF ORIENTATION SELECTIVITY

As one might note from the images in FIGURE 4, the various gray values at any particular location reveal which of two orthogonal test orientations (indicated in the lower right-hand corner of each frame) excited it the most, as well as by approximately how much. They do not indicate which orientation was *optimal,* however, since this information can be inferred only by comparing the responses generated by several different orientation pairs. Because this information is contained within all the images, collectively, it can be extracted by combining their data vectorially (see Blasdel[10] for further details) and displaying it in polar form. FIGURE 7a, for example, which was computed in this way, illustrates the orientations (indicated by color, with red and green denoting horizontal and vertical, and blue and yellow indicating left and right oblique) that actually were preferred in each part of cortex, as deduced from the differential images in FIGURE 4. FIGURE 7b indicates the degree of selectivity and/or responsiveness apparent at each location.

As one can see, the observed organization of orientation preferences differs significantly from that predicted earlier (see FIG. 1c) since iso-orientation domains (those preferring the same orientation) extend no farther than 0.5–1.0 mm in any lateral direction. Regular changes in orientation that might be modeled by sets of slabs are also confined to stretches 0.5–1.0 mm across, giving these linear zones a two-dimensional patchlike appearance. One must keep in mind, though, that even though Hubel and Wiesel's[4,43,44] inference of parallel iso-orientation slabs fails at scales larger than 0.5 mm, it does remarkably well at the scales smaller than 0.5 mm that would have prevailed during microelectrode recordings. If one confines one's attention to regions 0.5–1.0 mm across, for example, the suggestion of parallel iso-orientation slabs is pronounced. And within these zones orientation preferences definitely change in linear sequences along one axis while remaining constant along the other.[4,43,44] Only over much longer distances do more complicated patterns emerge.

The failure of orientation preferences to change linearly over distances longer than 0.5 mm could be attributed to biological imperfection. However, if this were the case, one would expect the disruptions to occur at random intervals. As one can see in FIGURE 8a, where the linear zones are illustrated separately, this is not the case. These structures, and the interruptions between them, occur at regular intervals, which suggest that the linearity of orientation preferences is periodic as well. The regions that include singularities and fractures—the ones that disrupt and break up the continuity of the "linear zones"—appear separately in FIGURE 8b, where it is apparent that even though they cover territory, they nevertheless distribute complete representations of orientation at similar intervals (due to the convergence of iso-orientation contours and their resulting higher density).

From this relatively simple analysis, it is possible to conclude that orientation preferences organize according to one of *at least* two competing schemes—a linear one, confined to patches 0.5–1.0 mm across, where orientation preferences change linearly along one axis (remaining constant

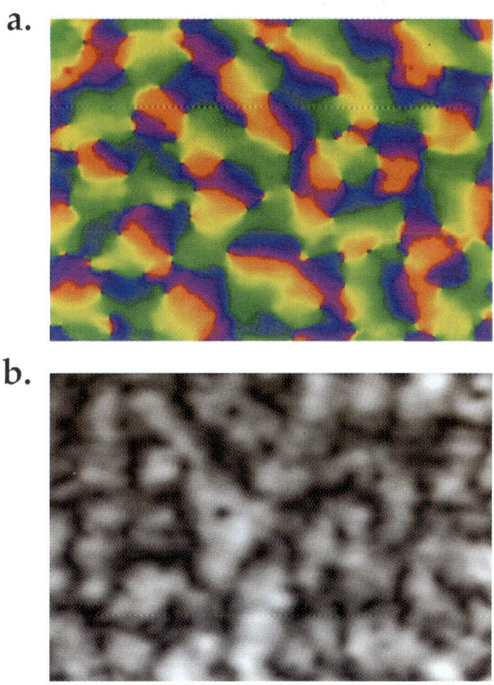

FIGURE 7. The differential images in FIGURE 4 can be combined vectorially to yield maps of orientation preference and selectivity, which are illustrated by two different images in **(a)** and **(b)** of this figure. Because orientation preferences change cyclically, they cannot be illustrated by gray levels. One way around this is to illustrate them in color, with opponent colors representing orthogonal orientations (e.g., *red* and *green* indicate horizontal and vertical, while *blue* and *yellow* indicate left and right oblique, respectively), as done in **(a)**. A different strategy is used in FIGURE 8a. **(b)** The second part of this figure, illustrated in black and white, indicates the degree of selectivity for orientation, with *black* and *white* indicating the lowest and highest selectivity, respectively.

along the other), and (2) a discontinuous one, where orientation preferences change continuously around singularities that may take the form of lines or points. The linear scheme predominates in two-dimensional patches 0.5–1.0 mm across, while the disruptions of singularities are confined to zero and one-dimensional domains, where all orientation preferences converge.

a.

b.

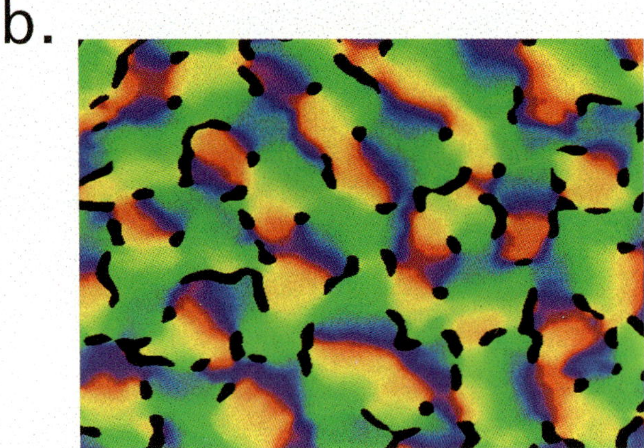

c.

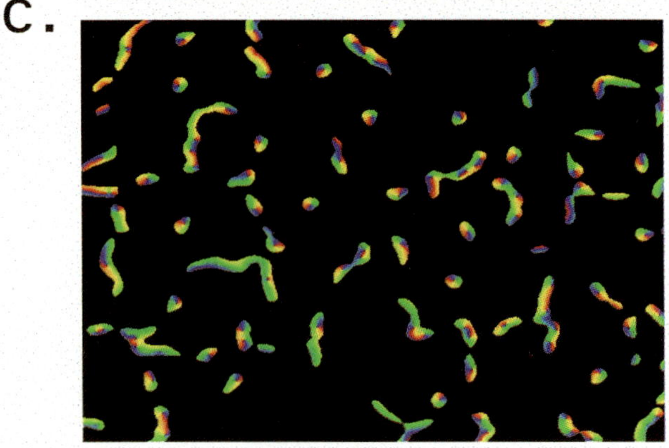

FIGURE 8

GEOMETRY OF ORIENTATION AND OCULAR DOMINANCE

As Hubel and Wiesel recognized initially,[4,43,44] it could be desirable for the observed organizations of ocular dominance and orientation to have a precise geometrical relationship, with one possibility (illustrated in FIG. 1c) being that slabs associated with each organization intersect at right angles. Such intersections would make sense for many different reasons, one of which might be the economy of wiring as the connections needed to generate different orientation preferences converge. For similar reasons, an orthogonal relationship between ocular dominance and orientation slabs might be expected to reduce interference between two periodic organizations.

Experiments with the metabolic marker 2-deoxyglucose appeared to cast doubt on this possibility at first, because the iso-orientation contours inferred from these experiments appeared to intersect ocular-dominance boundaries at all angles. When it subsequently became clear, however, that the iso-orientation domains indicated by 2-deoxyglucose are ambiguous and misleading for many reasons[12] (see also Blasdel[9,10] for discussion), the possibility of an orthogonal relationship between orientation and ocular-dominance slabs returned.

Because responses to numerous orientations can be determined and compared with optical imaging, however, accurate maps of orientation preference can be obtained (and verified, as they have been on numerous occasions). When these are then compared with patterns of ocular dominance, numerous correlations emerge. At the simplest level, the discontinuous zones—fractures and singularities—clearly correlate with the centers of ocular dominance columns.[6–10,13] And consequently, the linear zones between them straddle the "borders" of ocular dominance columns. Within these *linear zones,* it is also clear that the aligned slabs of iso-orientation and ocular dominance intersect at angles of approximately 90°.[10,13–15] The overall arrangement is illustrated in FIGURE 9, where fine

---

FIGURE 8. **(a)** As described in FIGURE 7a, the use of different schemes to illustrate orientation preferences and selectivities have different drawbacks. The scheme used in FIGURE 7a, for example, has the drawback that the selectivity for orientation at any particular location (which varies as well) tends to get ignored. This is not a problem with the approach used previously, as shown here, where the orientation preferred at any location is indicated by a *short line,* with the degree of selectivity indicated by its length. In **(b)** one sees the distribution of orientation preferences in the continuous patches, where they change linearly but slowly. Regions of rapid change, corresponding to the indicated regions in **(c)**, have been blacked out. Even though orientation is defined precisely, and linearly, representations of all orientations cover large areas, at least 700 μm across. Consequently, the neurons in these zones, with average 250–350-μm-wide dendritic fields, would receive information over a range of only ~60°. In **(c)** one sees the converse, where the linear zones have been blacked out, leaving the regions surrounding zero and one-dimensional singularities intact. As one can see, all orientation preferences converge at these sites, giving them complete representations of all orientations, even though they cover a disproportionately small percentage of the total cortical area. (Reprinted with permission from Blasdel.[10])

white lines are used to indicate iso-orientation contours (regions of constant color), and fine black lines indicate the edges of ocular-dominance columns.

Although the organization of ocular dominance in striate cortex can be described as one consisting of "slabs,"[16] the concept is misleading since it suggests discontinuous transitions at borders between slabs that extend through all layers. As one can see in FIGURE 10, this is true only in layer 4c; in

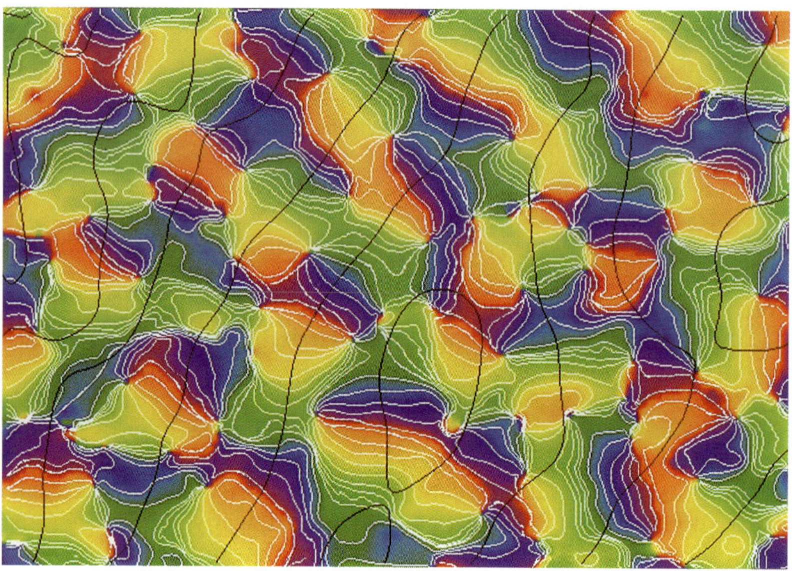

FIGURE 9. Geometric relationship between ocular dominance and orientation slabs. The edges of ocular dominance bands (see Blasdel[9,10]), are indicated by *fine black lines* in this figure, while the trajectories of iso-orientation contours are indicated by *fine white lines*. As one can see, the white lines appear most highly aligned near the fine black lines, due to pronounced correlation between linear zones and edges of ocular dominance columns, where most of the white lines intersect black lines at angles of approximately 90° (as suggested originally by Hubel and Wiesel[3,4]). As a consequence, orientation preferences have a marked tendency to change linearly along axes parallel to the ocular dominance slabs, and to remain constant along axes that are perpendicular. For reasons outlined in the text and in Blasdel,[10] it is likely that retinotopic position is mapped linearly along the iso-orientation domains extending between the centers of adjacent ocular dominance columns. (Adapted from Obermayer and Blasdel.[15])

other layers the lateral transition of ocular-dominance values is actually quite continuous. In fact, it is virtually linear across regions where the borders of ocular dominance slabs are usually illustrated, and least linear in between—in the centers of the slabs. Keeping this in mind, the organization of orientation preferences described previously implies three things: (1) that *linear zones* lie exactly where they need to be located to receive balanced information from both eyes, about one part of visual space, (2) that ocular dominance

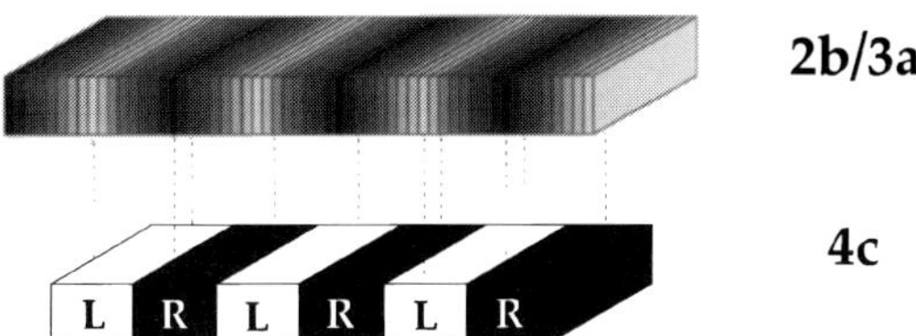

FIGURE 10. Binary ocular-dominance slabs exist only in layer 4c of monkey striate cortex, where geniculate afferents terminate and where cells respond to only one eye. Outside layer 4c, in layers where orientation selectivity is prominent, binocularity also must be taken into account, which means that the ocular dominance of these layers must be illustrated differently. In this figure, ocular dominance is illustrated in binary fashion in layer 4c, with *black* and *white slabs* reflecting exclusive responses to the right and left eyes, and with many gradations of ocular dominance above. From this illustration it is clear that ocular dominance shifts continuously, between extremes of right- and left-eye dominance that lie in register with the centers of right- and left-eye slabs in layer 4c.

is mapped linearly, along with orientation preference, in the linear zones, and (3) that within each *linear zone* the gradients of orientation preference and ocular dominance intersect at right angles. Because of the linear mapping of position in each ocular dominance band (in layer 4c), moreover, the gradients of ocular dominance in the upper layers represent gradients of position in layer 4c, which means that gradients of orientation preference and receptive field position, represented by afferents from layer 4c, intersect at right angles as well.

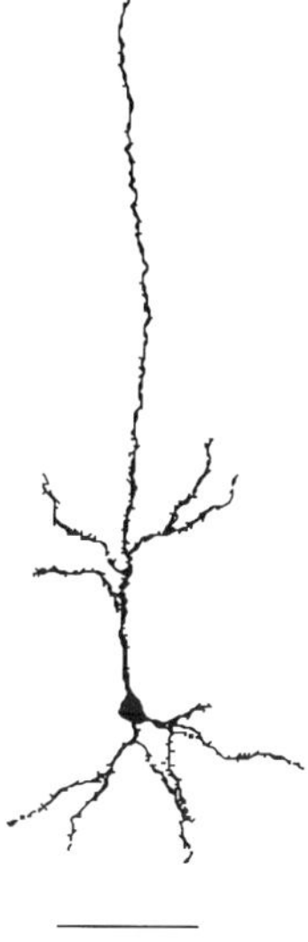

FIGURE 11. Example of typical upper layer pyramidal cell in monkey striate cortex. As one can see from the *scale bar,* which indicates 100 μm, the dendritic fields of these cells extend approximately 200 μm across, filling cylindrical volumes, with marked regularity. (Reprinted with permission from Lund.[23])

MORPHOLOGICAL CONSTRAINTS OF UPPER-LAYER NEURONS

While the precise significance of the preceding arrangement remains to be established, there is one intriguing insight offered by the dimensions of pyramidal neurons in upper layers. Not only are these cells responsible for the maps of orientation preference that are observed, they are also the cells most likely to use this information. If conventional neuroanatomical concepts hold, these cells are likely to receive this information on their dendritic arbors, which means that the surprisingly regular distribution of these arbors in the upper layers,[17] each of which fills a roughly cylindrical volume 200–300 µm across (see FIG. 11), may be extraordinarily significant.

Given that upper-layer pyramidal neurons provide the primary outputs to subsequent cortical areas, the spread of their dendritic fields should constrain the flow of information. For a cell lying in a linear zone, for example, where

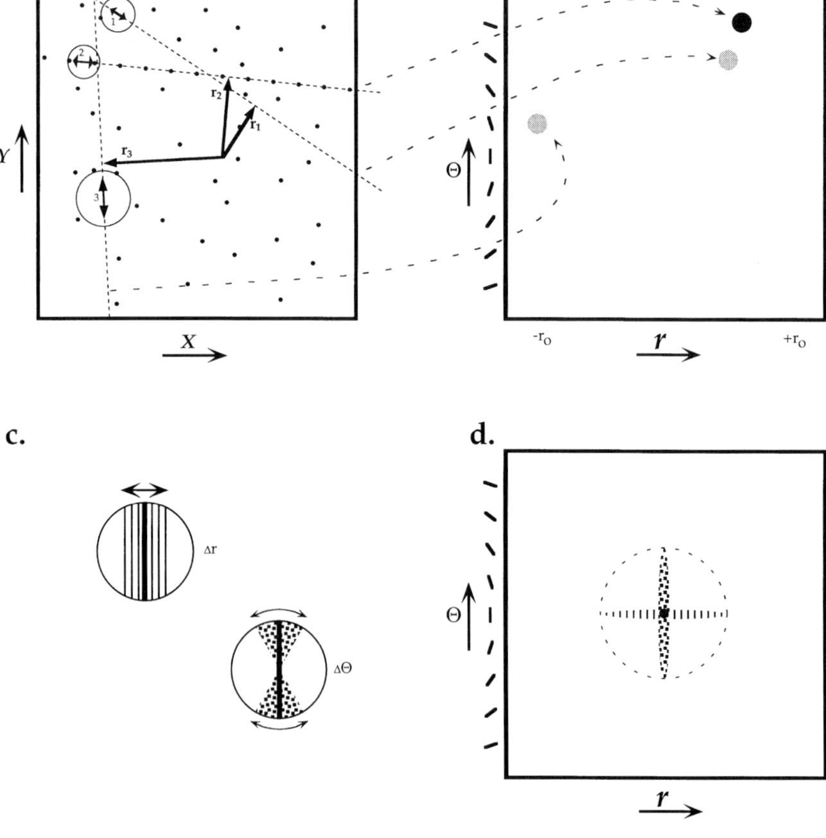

FIGURE 12

orientation preferences change slowly (requiring 700 μm to rotate through 180°), a dendritic field 200–300 μm in diameter cannot sample more than half the possible orientations. Moreover, since these cells are highly selective for orientation, information about orientations outside this range is probably not available. As a consequence, these cells are not suited to the comparison of edges over a broad range of orientations. They would be poor candidates indeed for analyzing textures that are often distinguished by different densities of edges at orthogonal orientations. Due to their exquisite selectivity for the orientation of a single edge, however, a cell in these zones should excel at the detection and characterization of boundary contours within its range. One possible way in which this might occur is illustrated by (but not confined to) the Hough transform in FIGURE 12.

The reciprocal problem is encountered by neurons near singularities. Because all orientation preferences converge at these locations (see FIGS. 8c and 13), any cell lying within 100 μm of a singularity should receive some information about all orientations, making it a good candidate for texture discrimination, though the poor orientation selectivity apparent within these zones must degrade the accuracy with which the orientation of any particular edge can be determined. In other words, these cells pay a price in the precision with which they can encode orientation.

FIGURE 12. One way in which the linear zones might facilitate the detection and encoding of boundary contours is indicated by the Hough transform (Hough[24]), a special case of the radon transform described by Schwartz,[25] which was invented to automate the detection of particle tracks in bubble chambers. Since the task at hand resembles that of contour detection in noisy visual environments (Ballard and Brown[26]), and since orientation is mapped linearly with respect to distance in Hough space as well as in striate cortex, it provides a compelling metaphor for the operations likely to be carried out in striate cortex. **(a)** The problem, illustrated in this section, is to distinguish between bubbles in a straight line, which may indicate a particle track, and those occurring randomly. The transform works by taking the position of each bubble and comparing it with that of its nearest neighbor to find the orientation and displacement of an infinitely long (*dotted*) line passing through both locations. These values specify a unique location in a new "Hough" space **(b)** where orientation and position are mapped linearly along orthogonal axes. Three sample pairs are indicated by filled *circles* in this section, where the infinitely long lines running through them are indicated by *dotted lines* corresponding to distinct locations in **(b)**. **(b)** When this operation is performed iteratively, on every point in the image, values build up rapidly at Hough coordinates corresponding to particle tracks because the bubbles associated with them lie along the same infinitely long lines. It is obvious in **(a)**, for example, that bubbles corresponding to **r2** are much more numerous than those corresponding to **r1** or **r3**, and that consequently they give rise to a larger value (indicated by a *darker dot*) in **(b)**. **(c)** The power of this transform derives from the *linearity* of maps for orientation and position. Because of this, positional uncertainty (indicated by *vertical hatching*, **upper left aperture**) leads to scatter about the horizontal axis (see **(d)**), while orientational uncertainty (indicated by *stippling*, **lower right aperture**) registers as scatter about vertical. **(d)** Since orientation and position axes are orthogonal, however, values arising from a degraded contour cluster around a central point representing the best possible fit for the observed contour. What has happened, therefore, is that single contours are represented as single points rather than one-dimensional strings of points. (Reprinted with permission from Blasdel.[10])

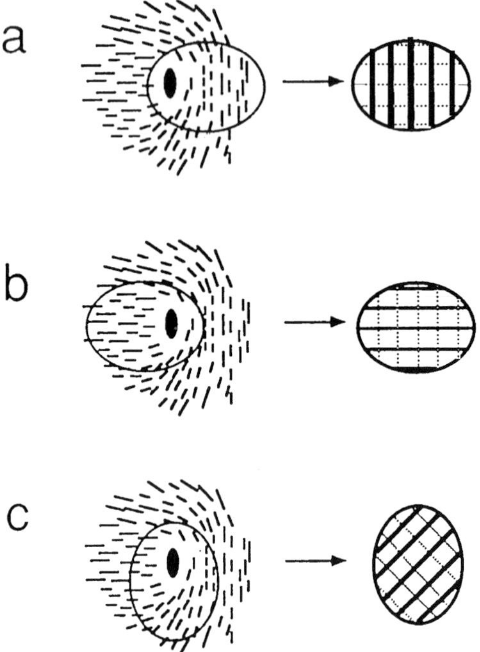

FIGURE 13. This figure illustrates one possible implementation of *texture space* near singularities. Because the dendritic fields of most cortical neurons are constrained within uniform zones 250–350 μm across (or narrower), the spectrum of orientations impinging on each cell may well depend on those available within each zone. If this is the case, the unique arrangements of orientation preferences around singularities may generate continuous maps of edge density (with special emphasis on edges that are perpendicular) in populations of postsynaptic cells. Consider the tight loop of orientation preferences around the positive singularity above. Dendritic fields enclosing this singularity can be expected to receive some information about all orientations. But those displaced toward the right **(a)** receive more inputs preferring horizontal than vertical, which could impose a preference for higher densities of horizontal edges in two-dimensional textures (keep in mind that the selectivities for orientation and position are both reduced). Similarly, the dendritic fields illustrated in **(b)** and **(c)** might be expected to receive more inputs for vertical and left oblique, implying preferences for higher densities of edges at these orientations (as opposed to others). In this simple fashion, a continuous coarse coding of all possible textures might be achieved for one part of visual space, with the advantage that *most similar textures* are represented by *nearest neighbors.* (Reprinted with permission from Blasdel.[10])

Singularities are particularly intriguing in regard to texture discrimination. Due to the fact that each one arises from the continuous rotation of orientation preferences through precisely 180°, for one trip around, regions on opposite sides always prefer orthogonal orientations. As illustrated in FIGURE 13, this type of organization could facilitate the discrimination of surface textures in the visual field. Since textures and color are associated mostly with "surfaces" in the context of visual perception, this possibility is further strengthened by the correlation between singularities and cytochrome oxidase blobs, where many color-sensitive cells are found.[18]

HYPOTHESIS SUGGESTED BY OPTICALLY DETERMINED MAPS

The hypothesis implied by these results is actually quite simple: one of many problems encountered by the visual system is the discrimination between different types of edge—for example, between edges denoting boundary contours and textures, or even between edges denoting different textures. An extreme example is illustrated in FIGURE 14, where a single line defines a rectangle. Where it appears alone it is seen unambiguously as part of a boundary contour—similar to a door, for example. Where it is flanked by similar lines, however, it dissolves into a "surface" of vertical lines.

How are these two very different types of edge to be discriminated when they arise from luminance distributions (e.g., black lines) that are basically identical? To be sure, there are many global ways of solving this problem, such as template matching. Very few of these are possible at the striate cortical level, however, where global information is not available (at least not quickly) because receptive fields are so small, causing each cell to see the world through an aperture a fraction of a degree across (for foveal and parafoveal vision).

If striate cells are to make any progress on this problem at all, therefore, they must do so on the basis of local information, which is available mostly from the lateral redundancy of visual events. A simple rule therefore might go as follows: (1) an edge that appears in isolation is most likely a boundary contour (see FIG. 15), while (2) an edge that appears in the company of

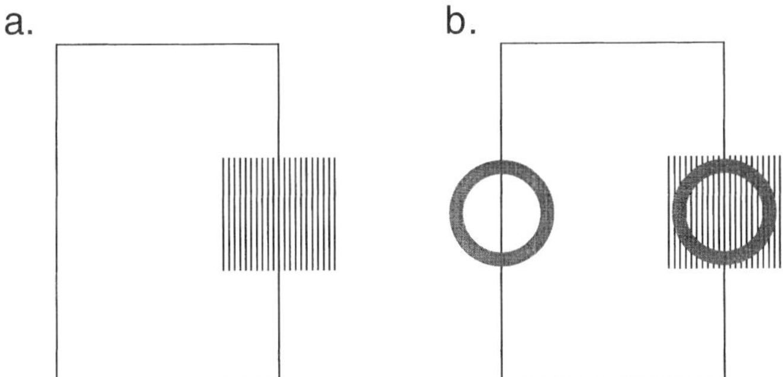

FIGURE 14. Illustration of boundary contour and surface texture generated by the same *thin black lines*. As one can see in **(a)**, where this line appears in isolation, forming a rectangle, it is seen unambiguously as part of an boundary contour (Cohen and Grossberg[27]). Where it is flanked by similar lines, however, it is seen (also unambiguously) as part of a surface texture. If cortical cells were to distinguish between these two distributions, as suggested in the text, they would have to do so on the basis of local information (indicated by the *circles* in **(b)**, since their receptive fields are quite small.

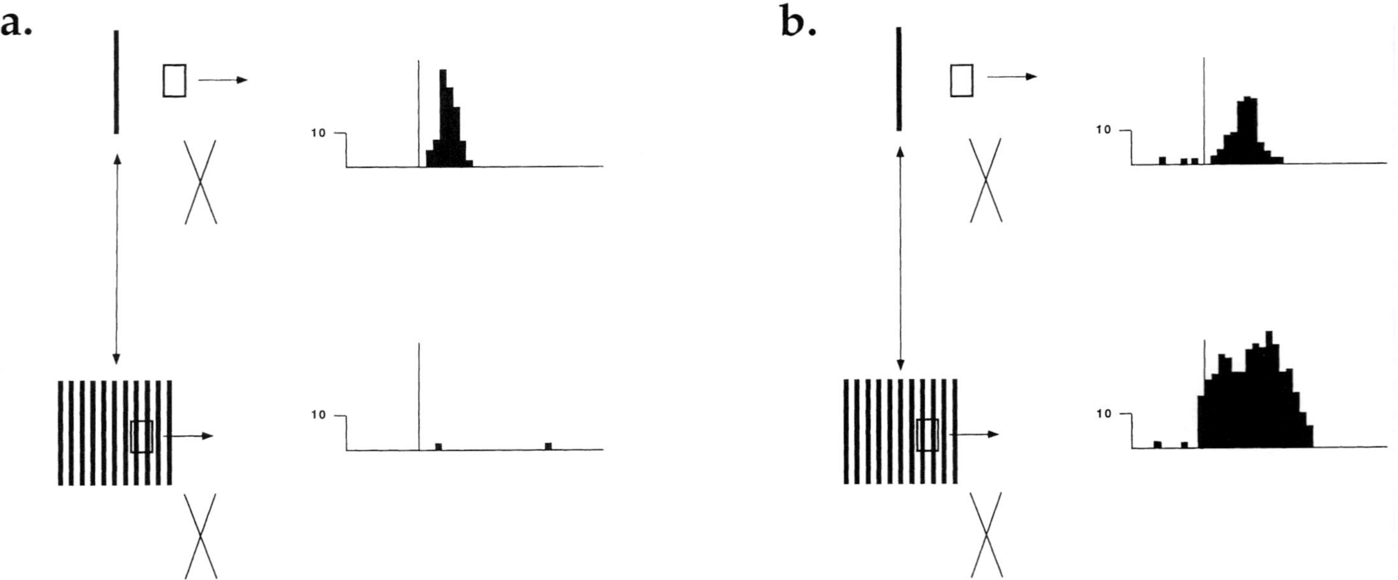

FIGURE 15. This figure depicts poststimulus histograms determined for two neurons located **(a)** in the middle of a linear zone, and **(b)** within 100 μm of a singularity. Both cells were recorded within 500 μm of the surface of striate cortex. As one can see in the poststimulus-time histograms on the left, the cell recorded in the middle of a linear responded selectively to *single bars* and was inhibited by *gratings,* similar to the "bar cells" reported previously by Schiller *et al.,*[28] and, more recently, by Born and Tootell[29] and von der Heydt *et al.*[30] "Bar" selectivity also characterized the responses of four other cells recorded at laterally displaced sites within the same linear zone. All cells recorded near singularities, however, displayed a marked preference for gratings, as can be seen from the poststimulus-time histogram for the cell depicted in **(b),** on the right. These cells, which resemble the "grating cells" of von der Heydt *et al.,*[30] all lay within 100 μm of an orientation singularity, which means they also resided in cytochrome-oxidase-rich areas that (according to the hypothesis of this article) may specialize in the detection of "surfaces" in the visual world (see Blasdel[10] for further discussion).

similar flanking edges, especially if they are periodic, is most likely a surface (see FIG. 15b). In other words, the distinction is based on the statistics of spatial distribution: edges that distribute in one and two dimensions are most likely to arise from boundary contours and surfaces, respectively. The two-dimensional distribution of surface textures is even more apparent in the more common event of edges overlapping at different orientations. With such rules, one can hypothesize that it is possible to distinguish between likely edges and surfaces on the basis of local criteria. And while decisions like this may not hold up later on at the global level (and hence may need to be overridden), they could establish a bias, or tentative solution, that favors one interpretation over the other and thereby facilitates the task of scene segmentation in subsequent cortical areas—a task that is difficult, to say the least. If this is indeed the case, striate cortex could easily justify its occupation of such a large portion of the *entire* neocortex—a proportion that runs as high as 20% in some Old World primates.

REFERENCES

1. MARROCCO, R. T., J. W. MCCLURKIN & R. A. YOUNG. 1982. Spatial summation and conduction latency classification of cells in the lateral geniculate nucleus of macaques. J. Neurosci. **2**(9): 1275–1291.
2. LEVAY, S. & T. VOIGT. 1988. Ocular Dominance and disparity coding in cat visual cortex. Visual Neurosci. **1:** 395–414.
3. HUBEL, D. H. & T. N. WIESEL. 1974. Uniformity of monkey striate cortex. A parallel relationship between field size, scatter and magnification factor. J. Comp. Neurol. **158:** 295–306.
4. HUBEL, D. H. & T. N. WIESEL. 1974. Sequence regularity and geometry of orientation columns in the monkey striate cortex. J. Comp. Neurol. **158:** 267–293.
5. PENFIELD, W. 1933. The evidence for a cerebral vascular mechanism in epilepsy. Ann Intern. Med. **7:** 303–310.
6. BLASDEL, G. G. & G. SALAMA. 1986. Voltage-sensitive dyes reveals a modular organization in the monkey striate cortex. Nature **321:** 579–585.
7. BLASDEL, G. G. 1989. Topography of visual function as shown with voltage sensitive dyes. *In* Sensory Systems in the Mammalian Brain, J. S. Lund, Ed.
8. BLASDEL, G. G. 1989. Visualization of neuronal activity in monkey striate cortex. Annu. Rev. Physiol. **51:** 561–581.
9. BLASDEL, G. G. 1992. Differential imaging of ocular dominance and orientation selectivity in monkey striate cortex. J. Neurosci. **12**(8): 3115–3138.
10. BLASDEL, G. G. 1992. Orientation selectivity, preference and continuity in monkey striate cortex. J. Neurosci. **12**(8): 3139–3161.
11. TS'O, D. Y., R. D. FROSTIG & E. E. LIEKE. 1990. Functional organization of primate visual cortex revealed by high resolution optical imaging. Science **249:** 417–420.
12. HORTON, J. C. & D. H. HUBEL. 1980. Regular patchy distribution of cytochrome oxidase staining in primary visual cortex of macaque monkey. Nature **292:** 762–764.
13. BARTFELD, E. & A. GRINVALD. 1992. Relationships between orientation-preference pinwheels, cytochrome oxidase blobs, and ocular-dominance columns in primate striate cortex. Proc. Natl. Acad. Sci. USA **89:** 11905–11909.
14. OBERMAYER, K., H. RITTER & N. K. SCHULTEN. 1992. A model for the development of the spatial structure of retinotopic maps and orientation columns. IEICET Fine **75A:** 537–545.
15. OBERMAYER, K. & G. G. BLASDEL. 1993. Geometry of orientation and ocular dominance columns in monkey striate cortex. J. Neurosci. **13:** 4114–4129.

16. HUBEL, D. H. & T. N. WIESEL. 1972. Laminar and columnar distribution of geniculo-cortical fibers in the macaque monkey. J. Comp. Neurol. **146:** 421–450.
17. LUND, J. S. & T. YOSHIOKA. 1991. Local circuit neurons of macaque monkey striate cortex: III. Neurons of laminae 4B, 4A, and 3B. J. Comp. Neurol. **311:** 234–258.
18. LIVINGSTONE, M. S. & D. H. HUBEL. 1984. Anatomy and physiology of a color system in the primate visual cortex. J. Neurosci. **4:** 309–356.
19. HUBEL, D. H. & D. C. FREEMAN. 1977. Short communications: Projection into the visual field of ocular dominance columns in macaque monkey. Brain Res. **122:** 336–343.
20. HUBEL, D. H., T. N. WIESEL & M. P. STRYKER. 1978. Anatomical demonstration of orientation columns in macaque monkey. J. Comp. Neurol. **177:** 361–380.
21. GRINVALD, A., E. LIEKE, R. P. FROSTIG, C. GILBERT & R. M. WIESE. 1986. Functional architecture of cortex revealed by optical imaging of intrinsic signals. Nature **324:** 351–364.
22. ORBACH, H. S., L. B. COHEN & A. GRINVALD. 1985. Optical mapping of electrical activity in rat somatosensory and visual cortex. J. Neurosci. **5:** 1886–1895.
23. LUND, J. S. 1973. Organization of neurons in the visual cortex, area 17, of the monkey (*Macaca mulatta*). J. Comp. Neurol. **147:** 445–496.
24. HOUGH, P. V. C. 1962. Method and means for recognizing complex patterns. U.S. Patent #3069654. U. S. Patent Office. Washington, DC.
25. SCHWARTZ, E. L. 1984. Anatomical and physiological correlates of visual computation from striate to infero-temporal cortex. IEEE Trans. Syst. Man, Cybern. **SMC-14**(2): 257–291.
26. BALLARD, D. H. & C. M. BROWN. 1982. Computer Vision. Prentice-Hall. Englewood Cliffs, NJ.
27. COHEN, M. A. & S. GROSSBERG. 1984. Neural dynamics of brightness perception: Features, boundaries, diffusion and resonance. Percept. Psychophys. **36**(5): 428–456.
28. SCHILLER, P. H., B. L. FINLAY & S. F. VOLMAN. 1976. Quantitative studies of single-cell properties in monkey striate cortex. III. Spatial frequency. J. Neurophysiol. **39:** 1334–1351.
29. BORN, R. T. & R. B. H. TOOTELL. 1991. Single unit and 2-deoxyglucose studies of side inhibition in macaque striate cortex. Proc. Natl. Acad. Sci. USA **88:** 7066–7077.
30. VON DER HEYDT, R. V. D., E. PETERHANS & M. R. DURSTELER. 1992. Periodic-pattern-selective cells in monkey visual cortex. J. Neurosci. **12**(4): 1416–1434.
31. ALBRECHT, D. G., R. L. DE VALOIS & L. G. THORELL. 1980. Visual cortical neurons: Are bars or gratings the optimal stimuli? Science **207:** 88–90.
32. CAMPBELL, F. W. & J. G. ROBSON. 1968. Application of Fourier analysis to the visibility of gratings. J. Physiol. (Lond.) **197:** 551–556.
33. DE VALOIS, R. L., D. G. ALBRECHT & L. G. THORELL. 1982. Spatial frequency selectivity of cells in macaque visual cortex. Vision Res. **22:** 545–559.
34. HUBEL, D. H. & T. N. WIESEL. 1962. Receptive fields, binocular interaction and functional architecture of monkey striate cortex. J. Physiol. (Lond.) **160:** 106–154.
35. KULIKOWSKI, J. J. & P. O. BISHOP. 1981. Fourier analysis and spatial representation in the visual cortex. Experientia **37:** 160–163.
36. MORRONE, M. C., D. C. BURR & L. MAFFEI. 1982. Functional implications of cross-orientation inhibition of cortical visual cells. I. Neurophysiological evidence. Proc. R. Soc. Lond. [Biol.] **216:** 335–354.
37. MOVSHON, J. A., I. D. THOMPSON & D. J. TOLHURST. 1978. Spatial summation in the receptive fields of simple cells in the cat's striate cortex. J. Physiol. (Lond.) **283:** 53–77.
38. MOVSHON, J. A., I. D. THOMPSON & D. J. TOLHURST. 1978. Receptive field organization of complex cells in the cat's striate cortex. J. Physiol. (Lond.) **283:** 79–99.
39. OBERMAYER, K., H. RITTER & K. SCHULTEN. 1990. Large-scale simulations of self-organizing neural networks on parallel computers: Application to biological modeling. Parallel Comput. **14:** 381–404.
40. OBERMAYER, K., H. RITTER & K. SCHULTEN. 1990. A principle for the formation of the spatial structure of cortical feature maps. Proc. Natl. Acad. Sci. USA **87:** 8345–8349.
41. POLLEN, D. A. & S. F. RONNER. 1982. Spatial computation performed by simple and complex cells in the visual cortex of the cat. Vision Res. **22:** 101–111.

42. WILSON, H. R., D. LEVI, L. MAFFEI, J. ROVAMO & R. L. DE VALOIS. 1989. The perception of form: Retina to striate cortex. *In* Visual Perception: The Neurophysiological Foundations, L. Spillman & J. S. Werner, Eds.: 231–272. Academic Press. New York, NY.
43. HUBEL, D. H., T. N. WIESEL & S. LEVAY. 1977. Plasticity of ocular dominance columns in monkey striate cortex. Phil. Trans. R. Soc. Lond. B **278:** 377–409.
44. HUBEL, D. H. & T. N. WIESEL. 1977. Functional architecture of macaque monkey visual cortex. Ferrier Lecture. Proc. R. Soc. Lond. B **198:** 1–59.

DISCUSSION

QUESTION: Is it possible that you can bypass the retina at some point in the future—or is that too much science fiction?—and contemplate that you can induce vision by stimulating the proper set of neurons in the patterns that you described?

BLASDEL: Well, this has already been done. I think Giles Brindley did it first, with patients who were blind due to ocular problems but whose visual cortex was intact. When they were stimulated with microelectrode arrays, inserted surgically in V1, these patients saw star-like points of light that Brindley called "phosphenes." Since the phosphenes occurred at retinotopically mapped locations, geometric patterns could be seen—sufficient to represent recognizable alphanumeric characters, for example. The trouble was that none of the richness that normally characterizes visual perception—like textures, color, compelling contours, and depth—was there; only points in space. But, in answer to what I think was the intent of your question, information from the maps we are obtaining might one day be exploited, in conjunction with something like the silicon array Jim Bower was describing, to make it possible to stimulate subdivisions within cortex to recreate compelling images of color, texture, contours, and depth at appropriate retinotopic locations, thereby creating much more vivid images that might then be processed by subsequent cortical areas as though they originated in V1. I don't think this is out of the question at all, provided the technology becomes available to stimulate repeatedly and atraumatically at high enough resolution. To emulate the processing power of striate cortex, with its half a billion neurons, it would furthermore be necessary to develop some sort of portable microprocessor equivalent in processing power to approximately 10–100 Cray Computers. So this might not happen for some time.

Near-field Scanning Optical Microscopy and Near-field Confocal Optical Spectroscopy: Emerging Techniques in Biology[a]

SILVIO P. MARCHESE-RAGONA[b] AND PHILIP G. HAYDON[c]

Laboratory of Cellular Signaling
Department of Zoology and Genetics
Room 339 Science II
Iowa State University
Ames, Iowa 50011

INTRODUCTION

Near-field scanning optical microscopy (NSOM) is a scanning probe technique that utilizes a subwavelength light source in close proximity to the surface of a sample to generate optical images with a lateral optical resolution below the diffraction limit. The concept of NSOM predates its more familiar cousins by six decades. It was first considered theoretically in 1928 by Synge,[1] and first demonstrated with microwave radiation in 1972 by Ash and Nicholls.[2] However, due to experimental difficulties it was not until 1984, and the advent of STM, that it was possible to demonstrate the technique using visible light.[3]

The essential elements for a NSOM are (1) a subwavelength light source, which is generally a single-mode optical fiber coated with aluminum, except for a 20–100-nm aperture at the apex; (2) a feedback mechanism that allows the tip to remain a fixed distance from the surface of the specimen, as the specimen is scanned relative to the probe; (3) a raster mechanism for scanning the sample in x and y for image formation; and (4) a photosensor (usually a PMT or photon counter) with associated filters and analyzers.

INSTRUMENTATION

The system used in our laboratory is shown in FIGURE 1. The NSOM is mounted on a Nikon Diaphot inverted microscope. The sample is scanned on a piezo-driven xyz stage with a maximum xy scan range of 18 μm and a

[a]This work was supported by grants from the ISU Laboratory of Cellular Signaling, the National Institutes of Health, the McKnight Foundation, and TopoMetrix.

[b]Present address: Chapman Instruments, 175 Research Boulevard, Rochester, New York 14623.

[c]Corresponding author. Phone: (515) 294-6097; fax: (515) 294-6097; e-mail: pghaydon@iastate.edu

z-range of 3.2 μm. We use a shear-force feedback mechanism to allow the probe to maintain a fixed distance above the sample during a scan. The shear-force feedback mechanism consists of a fiber oscillating at its resonant frequency using a dither piezo coupled to the fiber mount. The resonant frequency is generally between 50 and 200 kHz, depending on the length of the fiber, shorter fibers generally having the higher frequency. As the resonating probe approaches to within a few nanometers of the surface of the sample, shear forces act on the probe causing a drop in dither amplitude and a corresponding phase lag in the dither motion with respect to the signal

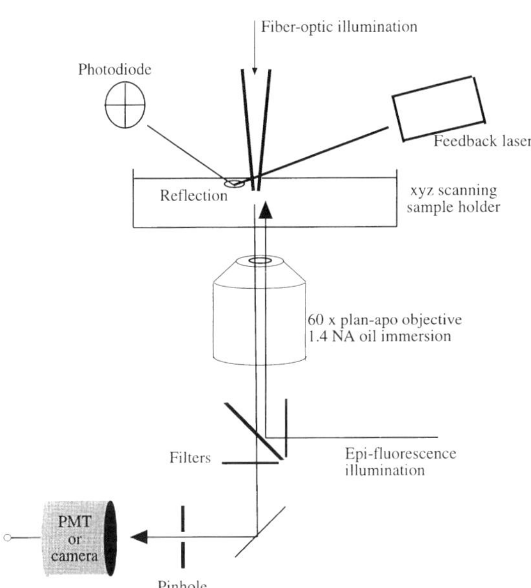

FIGURE 1. Equipment configuration.

generator. The shear-force sensing optics are also contained in the NSOM head. The sensing optics consist of a laser diode (wavelength 670 nm) focused to within 5–30 μm of the apex of the fiber at a shallow angle, producing a shadow of the probe that bisects the laser light on the sample. The reflection of this bisected illumination falls onto a split photodiode that is sensitive to perturbations in the dither amplitude and phase shift of the resonating fiber. By locking into a specific phase lag, we are able to maintain a fixed sample-probe separation by regulating the height of the sample during scanning. Thus, by controlling the sample height, the near-field fiber can remain stationary and in the focal plane of the objective lens. This mechanism of sample scanning produces a near-field image and a corresponding topographic image.

FABRICATION OF NEAR-FIELD PROBES

Subwavelength apertures are produced at the apex of a drawn single-mode fiber. The fabrication of the aperture is essentially a two-step procedure. First, the optical fiber is heated and drawn to a fine taper using a laser-based micropipette puller. Second, aluminum is evaporated onto the sides of the optical fiber to prevent leakage of light through the sides of the fiber. The aluminum is angle evaporated onto the fiber while the fiber is rotated about its long axis with the tip of the fiber facing away from the evaporation source. This configuration allows the sides of the fiber to be coated, while allowing the apex of the tip to be uncoated to function as the subwavelength aperture.

The taper of the drawn fiber and the radius of curvature at the end of the pulled fiber can be regulated during the tip-pulling procedure by varying the pulling parameters[4] (Sutter Instrument Co., personal communication). The eventual shape of the tip depends on a combination of the following five variables: the heat applied to the fiber (H); the length of fiber heated (F); the velocity at which the laser is turned off (V); the delay time for the onset of the hard pull (D); and the pulling force (P). Using a Sutter P-2000 micropipette puller, with the values of $H = 325$, $F = 0$, $V = 20$, $D = 125$, and by varying P between 75 and 200, we were able to control the overall shape of the tip in a predictable manner (FIG. 2). Lower values of P generally resulted in a relatively short, conical taper length, with a corresponding large radius of curvature; whereas, high values of P tended to result in longer taper lengths with a low radius of curvature at the end. Low P values of 75 or less often resulted in abnormalities at the end of tip, as shown in FIGURE 2(c). The shape and frequency of the abnormalities were unpredictable, but are thought to be due to excessive heating of the fiber that occurred during the weak pull phase. Before the pulled fibers are coated with aluminum, each fiber is coupled to a laser and inspected under an optical microscope. Only fibers that show a single light source at the end are selected for coating. Fibers that showed multiple light sources or a single light source distal to the tip of the fiber were discarded. Fibers are glued into capillary mounts (FIG. 3a) and are stored until used. FIGURE 3(b) shows a 50-nm aperture at the apex of an aluminum-coated pulled optical fiber.

IMAGING CONDITIONS

The shear-force feedback mechanism maintains the tip-sample separation of several nanometers. To maintain this constant separation and prevent the tip

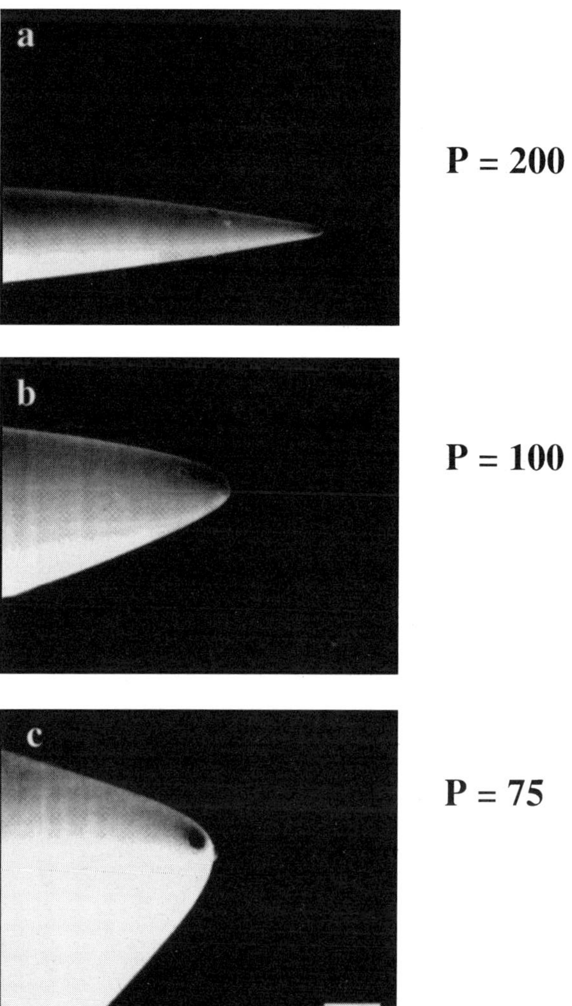

FIGURE 2. Different near-field tip geometry produced by altering the pull (P) value of the Sutter P-2000 micropepette puller. The *scale bar* represents 500 nm.

from being damaged by "crashing" into the sample, diligent precautions need to be taken. The two major precautions are vibration isolation and optimization of the z feedback loop. To reduce vibration, our instrument is mounted on a vibration isolation table. All necessary placement and manipulation of filters, apertures, and shutters are performed prior to attaining feedback. Once feedback is attained, a repetitive topographic line scan is performed so that the z piezo responsiveness can be optimized. In general, samples with abrupt

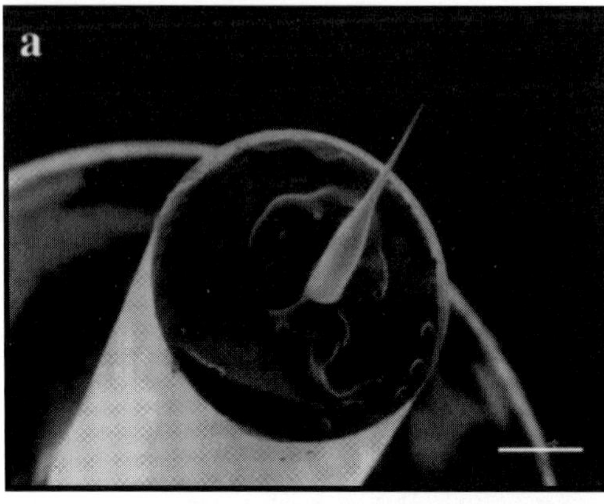

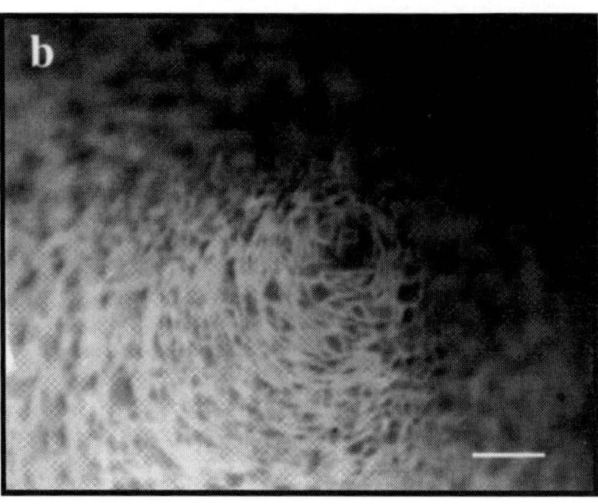

FIGURE 3. **(a)** A near-field probe glued into a capillary mount and ready for use. The *scale bar* represents 1.0 mm. **(b)** the subwavelength aperture at the apex of an aluminum-coated near-field probe. The *scale bar* represents 200 nm.

changes in topography need high gains and lower scan speeds than samples with a more gradual change in topography.

Once the system is in feedback and scanning mode, the tip can be damaged by the mechanical vibrations of opening a camera shutter or changing a filter cube. Damage to the tip is readily discernible by an increase in the amount of light being emitted from the tip by at least an order of magnitude and a corresponding loss of optical resolution. Both of these phenomena can be attributed to an increase in the size of the aperture. In most case, the topographic resolution is also reduced. However, occasionally a tip crash that results in the loss of optical resolution can sometimes result in an increased topographic resolution (data not shown). Our interpretation of these observations is that the tip breaks at an angle or is jagged; consequently, the tip that is profiling the surface is finer than before and would result in an increase in topographic resolution, while the larger optical aperture reduces the optical resolution.

IMAGE ANALYSIS

The shear-force feedback mechanism generates a topographic image at the same time that the optical image is being generated. FIGURE 4 depicts a topographic and NSOM image of a standard test sample provided by TopoMetrix (Santa Clara, Calif.). The sample consists of metal islands on a glass substrate arranged in a hexagonal pattern. The contrast in the topographic image is a function of z-height—the taller the topographic features, the brighter they appear, whereas in the corresponding NSOM image, contrast is a function of transmitted light intensity. A comparison of the images shows that the raised metal islands seen in the topographic scan appear dark in the NSOM image. The subdiffraction optical resolution is most discernible by examining the intensity profile in the NSOM image (FIG. 5). The highest resolution features that can be resolved on the line profile are 25 nm. While the spacing between maximum and minimum intensity (boundary between glass and metal island) is 60 nm, the FWHM spacing for areas of high transmittance is 90 nm. FIGURE 6 shows a superposition of the topographic and NSOM line profiles. A comparison of the line profiles shows that where the topography is greatest—the metal islands—the transmitted intensity is lowest. The simplest interpretation of these results is that adsorption of light is the predominant factor affecting lateral optical resolution for this type of

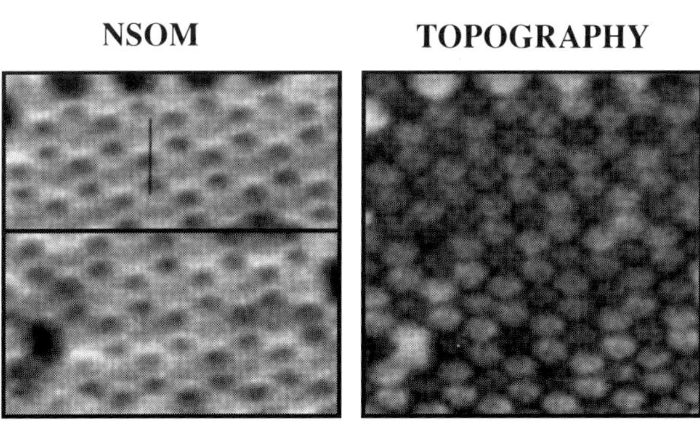

700 nm

FIGURE 4. The NSOM image and the corresponding topographic image of a standard sample. The *vertical line* drawn on the NSOM image is depicted as an intensity profile in FIGURE 5. The *horizontal line* drawn on the NSOM corresponds to an intensity profile depicted in FIGURE 6 with the corresponding topographic profile superimposed.

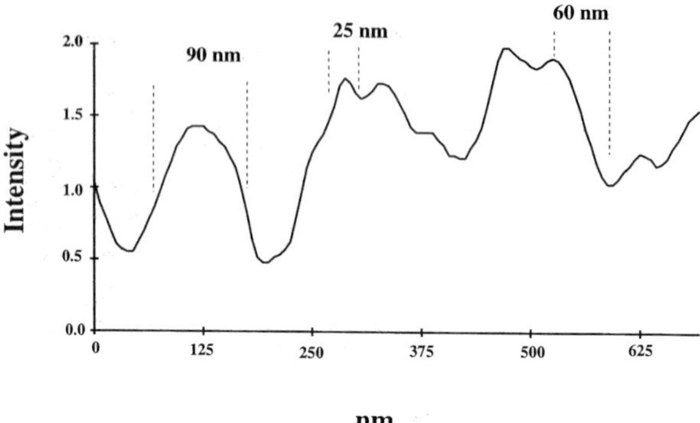

FIGURE 5. Intensity profile of the NSOM image depicted in FIGURE 4. The line shows 3 resolution measurements. The highest resolution features are on the order of 25 nm, whereas the distance between minimum and maximum intensity is around 60 nm, and the FWHM measurement for features exhibiting high intensity is around 90 nm.

sample. An excellent paper on NSOM image interpretation is provided by Valaskovic *et al.*[5]

If one examines an image with abrupt, large changes in topography, the NSOM image is not so easy to interpret. FIGURE 7 is a 450-nm-thick cross section of muscle prepared for conventional electron microscopy that has been etched with ethanoic NaOH for 5 minutes. In both the topographic and

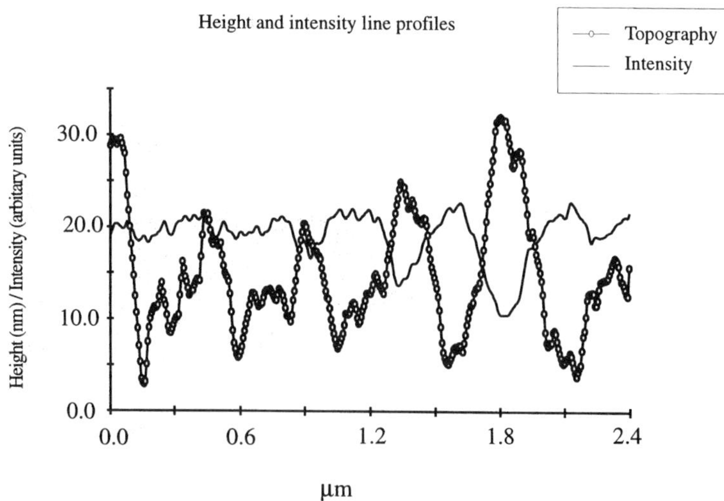

FIGURE 6. Comparison of NSOM and topographic line profiles for the images in FIGURE 4. The comparison shows that the highest features in the topographic image correspond to lower transmitted intensity in the NSOM image. The simplest interpretation of these results is that light adsorption is the predominant contrast mechanism affecting lateral optical resolution for this type of sample.

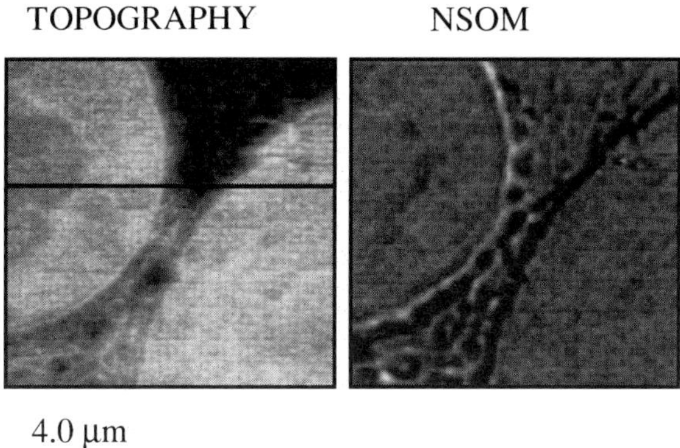

FIGURE 7. Topographic and NSOM image of an etched thin section of muscle tissue. In both the topographic and NSOM image, the muscle can be seen and the myofibrils discerned. The *horizontal line* drawn across the image detones the region from which the height and intensity profiles are plotted in FIGURE 8.

NSOM images, the muscle fiber can be seen and the myofibrils discerned. An examination of superimposed topographic and NSOM line profiles (FIG. 8) shows that the correlation between topography and transmitted intensity is not as straightforward as it was in FIGURE 6. While the intensity of the transmitted signal does generally increase when the sample becomes thinner, there are regions where the intensity does not readily correlate with the topography, as denoted by the asterisk.

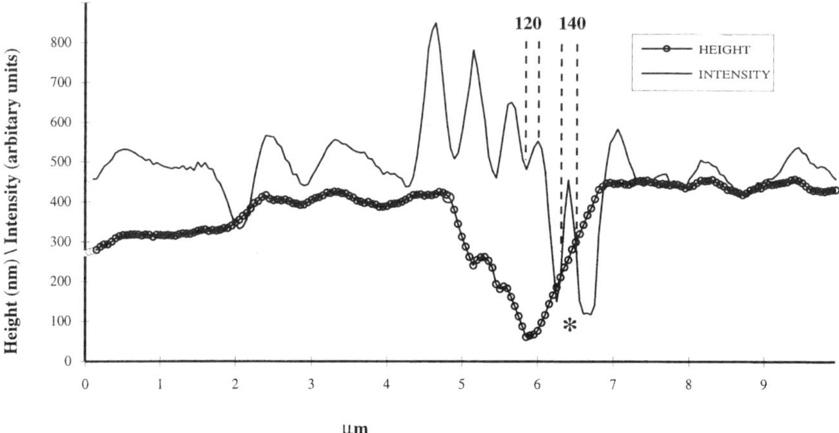

FIGURE 8. Comparison of the topographic profile and intensity profile of the images depicted in FIGURE 7. The comparison shows that in general the intensity increases as the topography decreases. However there are areas of increased transmission that cannot be readily reconciled with topographic features, as denoted by the *asterisk*.

NSOM OF LIVING SYSTEMS

The near-field technique has been demonstrated to be most applicable for the analysis of surfaces with no abrupt topographic changes. The challenge in biology is how to apply this technique to samples that are relatively thick, wet,

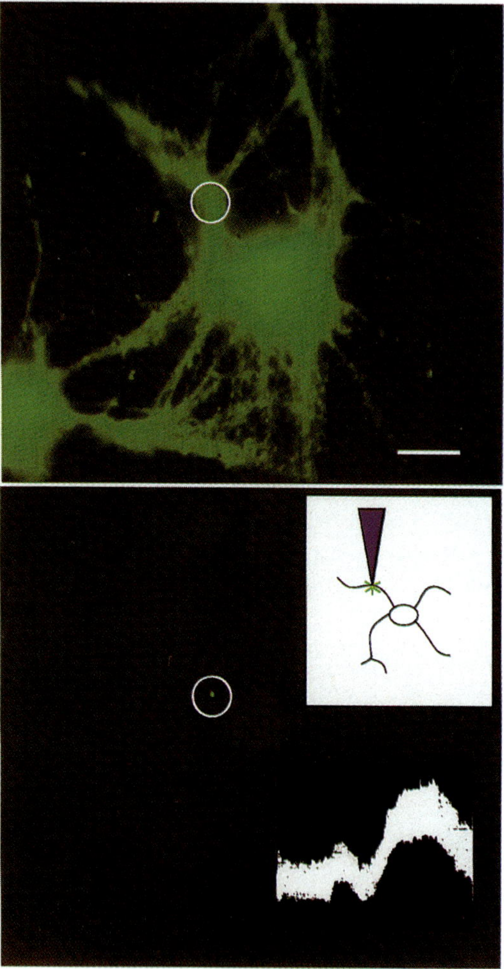

FIGURE 9. The **top panel** shows an epi-fluorescence image of a hippocampal neuron loaded with fluo-3, whereas the **lower panel** shows the same region illuminated by a near-field probe with the epi-fluorescence turned off. The *scale bar* represents 5.0 µm. Only a small region of the cell beneath the probe is excited and fluoresces. The local illumination of the cell by the near-field probes is schematically depicted in the **upper insert of the lower panel.** Using near-field illumination, we have been able to perform point spectroscopy, and observe the effects of increased fluorescence intensity caused by depolarization of the neuron resulting in a Ca^{2++} influx **(lower insert in lower panel).** The time duration of the trace is 15 seconds.

soft, and translucent. We have taken the first step in this direction by using a near-field spectroscopic technique on living astrocytes and neurons.[6] We have been able to demonstrate that the near-field probes can be placed in contact with a living cell without any apparent damage to the cell being observed. We used cultured cortical astrocytes, loaded with the fluorescent calcium indicator fluo-3, as test specimens, and found that we could routinely place the probe on the cell without causing damage. We were able to monitor fluorescence intensity as a function of z-separation between the tip and the cell. As the probe approached the cell, the fluorescence signal increased to a maximum upon contact with the cell (FIG. 9). Advancing the tip further, causing the cell to deform under the pressure of the tip, resulted in a decreased fluorescent intensity. However, when the tip was retracted the intensity once again increased to its previous maximum value, and then decreased as the tip pulled away from the cell. The top panel in FIGURE 9 shows an epi-fluorescence image of a neuronal cell loaded with the calcium-sensitive indicator fluo-3, whereas the bottom panel shows the same area with near-field illumination. By using this technique to illuminate a small area of the cell immediately below the plasma membrane, we have been able to perform point spectroscopy and measure rapid changes in fluorescence intensity after depolarization of the neuron using 50 mM KCl. One such change is depicted in the lower insert of the lower panel of FIGURE 9. The trace shows fluorescence intensity change over a 15-s period. Especially noticeable is the two-component nature evident in the trace. One possible explanation of this is that we are observing rapid changes in calcium immediately under the plasma membrane, followed by a delayed, volume-averaged response of the whole cell. The enhanced resolution in the near-field technique is only achievable when the sample being illuminated is within the immediate vicinity of the near-field aperture. By contacting the cell with the probe, we caused fluorescence to occur in both the near field and the far field. The far-field illumination resulted in an overall degradation of our optical resolution. Using optical principles borrowed from confocal microscopy, we incorporated a confocal pinhole. When used in conjunction with a near-field probe, we were able to significantly increase our near-field to far-field ratio. We anticipate that using near-field confocal optical spectroscopy (NCOS), it might be possible to study signal transduction events, such as vesicle fusion and the kinetics of individual ion channels.

ACKNOWLEDGMENTS

The authors are grateful to the following people: Steffan Kammer of TopoMetrix for providing the images and raw data for FIGURE 4. Clark Lindgren and Dennis Emery for the preparation of the thin-sectioned material depicted in FIGURE 7. Bruce Wagner for the SEM images of the pulled optical fibers depicted in FIGURES 2 and 3.

REFERENCES

1. SYNGE, E. H. 1928. A suggested method for extending microscope resolution into the ultra microscopic region. Philos. Mag. **6:** 356–362.
2. ASH, E. A. & G. NICHOLLS. 1972. Super-resolution aperture scanning microscope. Nature **237:** 510–512.
3. POHL, D. W., W. DENK & M. LANZ. 1984. Optical stethoscopy. Image recording with resolution λ/20. Phys. Lett. **44:** 651–653.
4. VALASKOVIC, G. A., M. HOLTON & G. H. MORRISON. 1995. Parameter control, characterization and optimization in the fabrication of optical fiber near-field probes. Appl. Opt. **34:** 1215–1228.
5. VALASKOVIC, G. A., M. HOLTON & G. H. MORRISON. 1995. Image contrast of dielectric specimens in transmission mode near-field scanning optical microscopy: Imaging properties and tip artefacts. J. Microsc. **179:** 29–54.
6. HAYDON, P. G., S. P. MARCHESE-RAGONA, T. BASARSKY, M. SZULCZEWSKI & MCCLOSKEY. 1996. Near-field confocal optical spectroscopy (NCOS): Subdiffraction optical resolution for dynamic imaging of biological specimens. J. Microsc. **182:** 208–216.

DISCUSSION

QUESTION: I was wondering whether, using this technique of looking at particular cells, it is possible to hold them long enough to look at the results of what appears to be a calcium influx. For a long time now the theory of excitotoxicity stated that cells die because of the influx of calcium along with other ions. I wonder if you could hold them long enough to see the eventual results of this calcium influx?

MARCHESE-RAGONA: The true answer to your question is that (a) I would think that maybe you can, but (b) I've never done it or tried it, so I can't give a definite answer. But these are fairly recent results, and I think this is just beginning. At this point, I think it would be fair to say, I'm not actually sure what's possible. In fact, I spent most of my time perfecting the technique and only recently have been thinking about the experiments to do with it.

QUESTION: Can you give us an idea, in practical terms, how long it takes to scan a sample?

MARCHESE-RAGONA: The answer is based on how many pixels you want in your image, but I'll give you a ballpark figure. It may take a few minutes to scan a 2-μm by 2-μm area with 500 pixels of resolution with very little topography. If you have some topography or quite a lot of abrupt changes in topography, then you have to scan at a significantly slower speed. This is because, as the probe is scanning along, if you scan slower, your ZPA has more time to retract the tip.

QUESTION: In the fluorescence mode, clearly one of the advantages of the near-field microscopy is the spacial resolution, so you're limited essentially to see membranes.

MARCHESE-RAGONA: Yes, in this particular case.

QUESTION: If a 20-nm resolution is true in every membrane when you label with fluorescence probe, you usually have very few fluorescence molecules in the field of view, so the fluctuation intensity should be very, very large. Actually, you should be able to tell from the fluctuation intensity what the volume of illumination is.

MARCHESE-RAGONA: Yes, that is if you're just illuminating the membrane. The cell was full of fluorescent indicator in this case.

QUESTION: Suppose you have a total of a few molecules?

MARCHESE-RAGONA: Then one should be able to actually get a very small volume fluorescing.

QUESTION: One thing you did not talk about is the force applied to the specimen by these two scanning probe microscopies. In the figure you showed of the atomic force microscope on a fairly thin lamellapodia of cells, we could see that the plasma membrane is pushed down tightly over the cytoskeleton, so what you were really mapping is the cytoskeleton, not the native cell shape. This same problem applies and I hope you will talk about this regarding the near-field optical microscopy because Newton's law applies, and the forces that you use to bend that optical fiber to find out how far above the surface you are are forces on the specimen. Wouldn't you think about the sizes of those forces?

MARCHESE-RAGONA: Absolutely, but I didn't talk about it because I only had 35 minutes to talk. In fact, the force resolution of the AFM work is less than 3 piconewtons. In the image I showed, you saw the cytoskeletal structure because one of the microscopes was pressing down on the surface of the cells. Otherwise you wouldn't have seen those. In fact, the actual forces you're applying there are probably on the order of several nanonewtons. In fact, it's also a function of the tip radius of curvature. I have additional slides where I've used different tip geometries for imaging cells. This is really quite interesting because some of the best images published have been taken with very sharp tips. The images look really superb because they've punctured the cell, the cytoplasm flowed out of the cell, and the membranes simply collapsed on the structures in there. In fact, I have some slides where I can see the cell and I don't see much structure in the cell because I'm not pressing very hard on it. But a lot of attention has to be paid to the forces, though I think that's a strength of the technique. By paying attention to the forces, one can do a lot more with the cell. For example, if you put antibodies on the tip and you go in to actually bond two receptor sites on the surface, you can use the force resolution of this technique to actually determine location of receptor ligand sites. So I think the forces in here and the different tip geometries and how you press on the cell are actually advantages of the technique.

Automated Light Microscopy for the Study of the Brain: Cellular and Molecular Dynamics, Development, and Tumorigenesis[a]

D. L. TAYLOR, K. BURTON, R. L. DEBIASIO,
K. A. GIULIANO, A. H. GOUGH, T. LEONARDO,
J. A. POLLOCK, AND D. L. FARKAS[b]

Center for Light Microscope Imaging and Biotechnology
Carnegie Mellon University
Pittsburgh, Pennsylvania 15213

INTRODUCTION

The impressive advances in technology within the last few decades have had a major impact on the field of microscopy. This is particularly true of biological light microscopy, where research has benefited from a convergence of developments in fields as diverse as electronics, optics, molecular biology, computer science, robotics, and reagent chemistry.[1,2] The integration of these developments has provided a dynamic research tool that puts within reach the elucidation of key mechanisms of biological functions, by noninvasive, high-resolution, quantitative monitoring of living cells, tissues, and organisms.[3] By adding optical and electrical micromanipulation techniques, one can simultaneously measure and modify cell physiology.[4,5]

One can hardly think of a research field for which such possibilities are more exciting than the study of the brain, where these tools now permit analysis from the subcellular to the fully functional level. Research initiated about a century ago by Santiago Ramón y Cajal and his contemporaries showed that the nervous system is made up of individual cells interconnected and functioning by virtue of the structure of the neural networks.[6] He was able to make these astounding interpretations by capitalizing on new techniques for staining tissue developed in his day by Camillo Golgi and new technology invented by Carl Zeiss, that improved the light microscope. Today, another renaissance in our understanding of the nervous system is occurring, again due to new methods for staining and new technologies for optical imaging and visualization of events as they occur in cells and tissues. We can now peer into

[a]This work was supported by NSF Science and Technology Center Grant MCB-8920118, NSF Grant BIR-9217091, and the Pittsburgh Foundation, Copeland Fund (K.A.G.).

[b]Corresponding author. Phone: (412) 268-6460; fax: (412) 268-6571; e-mail: farkas+@cmu.edu

the depth of a tissue or complex network with improved light penetration or image an individual cell with enhanced axial resolution. By applying these new capabilities to the investigation of the nervous system, we have already seen breakthroughs in our understanding of neural morphology, development, and the functional activity of neurons and networks. The ability to directly study functional differences between normal and genetically mutant or diseased states, as well as the details of tumorigenesis are clearly among the most exciting applications of these methods.[7]

In this review, we describe the instrumentation and molecular reagents that underlie the rebirth of light microscopy as an important *new* tool for the dissection of brain development, function, and disease. We then present examples of this exciting live-cell technology by describing its application to the cellular and molecular events involved in the development of the *Drosophila* visual system and in human primary brain tumorigenesis. Finally, we take a look forward to the continued evolution of advanced light microscopic imaging and its impact, not only on mapping brain function at the molecular level, but on biology, biotechnology, and medicine in general.

MULTIMODE MICROSCOPY AND THE AUTOMATED INTERACTIVE MICROSCOPE

It is a well known but often overlooked fact that the ability to successfully perform an experiment is not solely dependent on the microscope, but that the reagents and peripheral devices play a major role as well. Fluorescence-based light microscopy coupled with electronic imaging, for example, has dramatically extended the kinds of observations and experiments that biologists can perform on living cells, tissues, developing organisms, and whole animals. It is now possible to treat biological systems as "living cuvettes" and to use fluorescent reagents and protein biosensors to explore the chemical and molecular dynamics of the ions, metabolites, macromolecules, and organelles involved in basic cell functions such as locomotion and division, as well as in interactions between populations of neurons and cellular immunology. Other techniques have been developed that allow the investigator to place in cells and tissues, chemically blocked ("caged") molecules that can be released or activated ("uncaged") by a pulse of light (photolysis).[4] Therefore, a variety of reagents can be released at carefully controlled times and locations within the specimen. To take maximum advantage of this wide array of reagents however, requires sophisticated light microscope imaging instrumentation. In addition, instrumental factors, such as the choice of optical filters, must be optimized not only for the individual fluorophores used, but also to take into account the combination of fluorophores in the sample.[8] Peripheral components, such as an environmental chamber for the maintenance of cell viability, must also be designed for Koehler illumination, laminar liquid flow, and precise temperature control.[9] The multimode microscope and the automated interactive microscope (AIM) represent two generations of integrated microscope workstations designed around these concepts.

Multimode: The Concept and the Microscope

Multimode microscopy refers to the systematic application of several optical imaging modes, such as multiwavelength fluorescence, differential interference contrast (DIC), and reflection interference contrast, to the investigation of a single biological specimen on a single automated microscope workstation. Significant problems related to sample or population variability are thus addressed. More important, however, the complementary data acquired in the individual modes combines synergistically to provide enhanced structural and functional information, down to the molecular level. A multimode microscope workstation must be highly automated ("robotic"), with precise motion, timing, and specimen manipulation controls managed by advanced software, to enable parallel monitoring of many selected (spatially or spectrally) sample regions, thus increasing data yields from a single experiment. For example, the dynamics of cell shape, organellar movement, and cytoskeletal components can be simultaneously measured in time and space within each of many individual living cells.[7,10,11] The optical, mechanical, electronic, and digital components, are optimized for the sample chemistry and biology, and integrated into a versatile workstation. This is conceptually different from "multimodality imaging," where 3-dimensional (3-D) images obtained by very different medical imaging techniques such as computed tomography, magnetic resonance, positron emission tomography, and ultrasound, all of which are obtained at different times and locations, but can be brought together for codisplay. This new generation of light microscope workstation combines multiple methods of contrast maximization, resolution (in all four spatiotemporal dimensions), and quantitation with new methods of manipulation to explore the central challenges of biological light microscopy.[1,12,13]

The Next Step: Automated Interactive Microscopy

Although exciting results have been obtained with multimode technology, biological experiments are still limited by the speed with which multidimensional data sets can be acquired, processed, analyzed, and displayed. Processing of an N-dimensional data set (space, time, and multiple microscope modes) can take minutes to many hours. This time constraint limits biological research in three ways. First, relatively fast processes (occurring in seconds or less) usually cannot be studied using 3-D or multispectral imaging. Second, the number of trials performed for a particular experiment is often limited by the massive image processing requirement for each trial. In cell biology, where heterogeneous responses are common, multiple trials are especially important. Third, long processing times make it impossible to perform experiments in which there are conditional steps requiring interaction with the specimen in real time, dependent upon an observed condition or response in the specimen.

Our vision is to extend the power of the multimode light microscope to a dramatically new level by integrating high performance computing with high speed, high resolution optical microscopy through the construction of an Automated Interactive Microscope.[2,14] This tool will enable the biologist to perform chemical and molecular manipulations, as well as measurements in living cells and tissues. The AIM already allows acquisition and display of three-dimensional image sets in real time, as described in the application descriptions that follow. Eventually, full multimode, multicolor acquisition, processing, analysis, and display will allow the experimenter to visualize particular features of the specimen, or to detect certain structures or events in the specimen. Interventions and measurements can be controlled by the experimenter, based on results seen in the real-time display, or programmed to take place automatically when certain events are detected.

Target Biological Focus of AIM Development

The target AIM applications in our laboratories have been three biological systems: (1) cultured, fertilized mouse embryos from the single-cell stage (0.5 day postcoitum (p.c.)) to the hatched blastocyst (4.5 days p.c.); (2) organ culture of the *Drosophila* visual system; and (3) the molecular basis of glioblastoma cell motility.

Live mouse embryos have been placed in an environmental chamber on the AIM system and 3-D stacks have been acquired during different stages of development to assess the dynamic events of cell cleavage (FIG. 1) and cellular reorganization over time. Live cultured embryos can also be microinjected or stained with fluorescent probes (similar to fly tissue development studies described later, FIG. 2). Mouse embryos in culture can be either labeled and examined directly, or labeled, examined, and returned to the uterus of a pseudopregnant female. The labeled embryos can then be removed after further embryonic development *in utero,* to track the redistribution of the labeled probe at a later stage of development. *In vitro* culturing methods have enabled the embryo to progress through early organogenesis stages (7.5–10 days p.c.). During this period, we can study the early development of the nervous system as it forms from the neural plate. The rapid acquisition of 3-D stacks over time on the AIM system allows detailed 3-D analysis of the highly dynamic events, such as embryonic cell division, and the neuronal development in the early brain. Although the initial focus of AIM has been embryonic development, this experimental approach is sufficiently general to be useful in a variety of applications in the biomedical sciences.

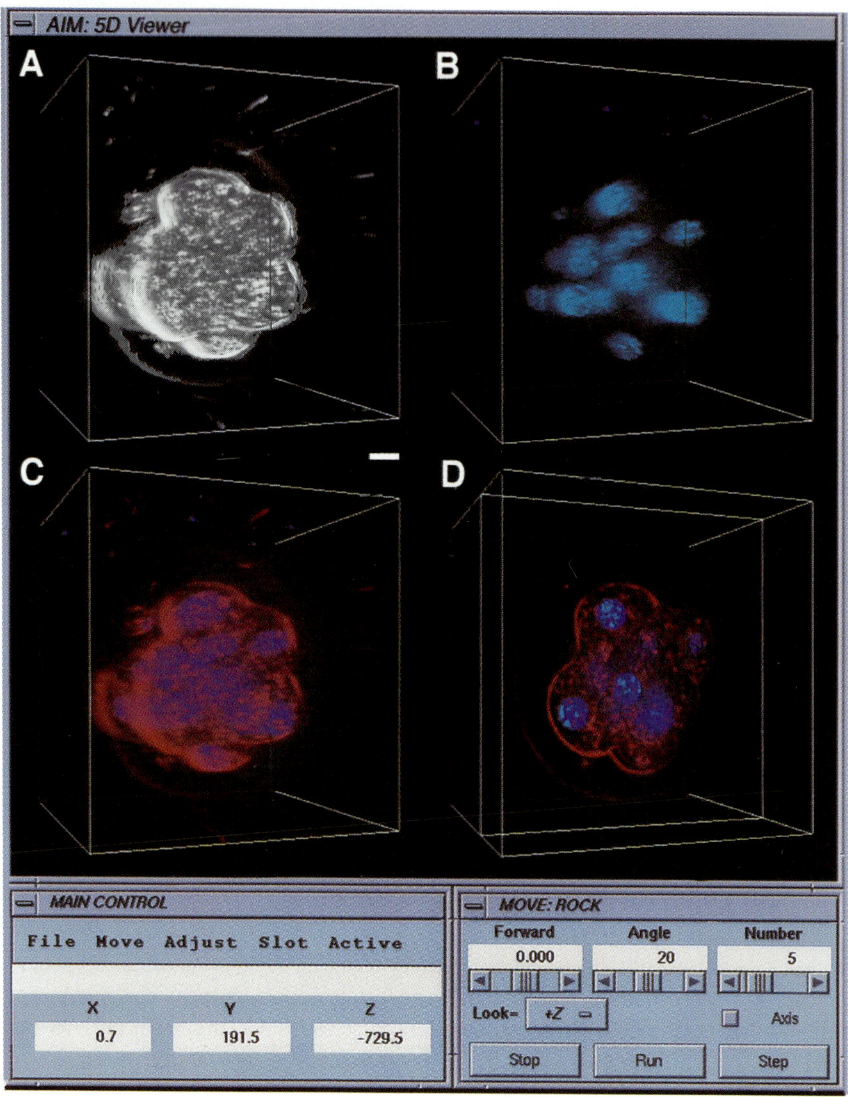

FIGURE 1. Mouse embryo displayed in the AIM 5-D Viewer. **(A)** Gray-scale maximum-pixel-value rendering of a variance-processed DIC image stack. Variance processing enhances the visibility of features in 3-D DIC data renderings.[48] (A–D: *Bar* = 10 μm). **(B)** Projection rendering of Hoechst-labeled nuclei in the same embryo as shown in (A). Prior to rendering, the image stack was deconvolved[49] by expectation maximization. **(C)** The same DIC and Hoechst data sets rendered simultaneously in red and blue, respectively, to compare the structural features visible in the DIC rendering with the features and locations of the nuclei. **(D)** A single plane from the DIC and Hoechst stacks shown in its relative position so as to reveal spatial relationships in the interior of the embryo. In the live display, the software can continuously scan through the planes in the stack to reveal the relative localization of features at different levels in the embryo.

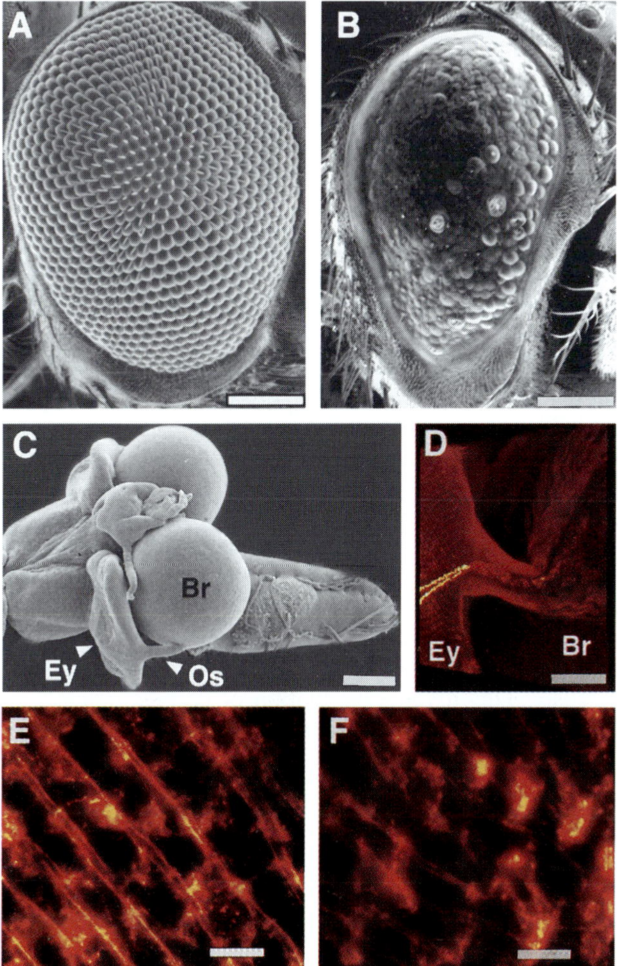

FIGURE 2. The fly eye as a model for neural development. **(A)** Scanning electron micrograph of the normal adult compound eye. Approximately 750 ommatidia or facets create a regular array of lenses. *Bar* = 100 μm. **(B)** Scanning electron micrograph of the mutant lz^{mr1} adult compound eye. Lenses are missing or highly irregular implicating defects in cone and pigment cells[20] (scaled the same as A). **(C)** Scanning electron micrograph of the normal cephalic complex dissected from a third larval instar. The eye imaginal disc is connected to the brain hemispheres via the optic stalk. *Bar* = 50 μm. **(D)** Normal eye and brain immunohistochemically stained and rendered in three dimensions reveals the developing photoreceptor array in the retina and the axons projecting down the optic stalk to fan out in the brain. MAb24B10[56] visualized with secondary Cy3. *Bar* = 25 μm. **(E)** High magnification view of a normal brain immunohistochemically stained and rendered in three dimensions to reveal the developing photoreceptor axons from cells R7 and R8 in the second optic ganglia, the medulla. Note the regular and linear paths. MAb24B10, Cy3. *Bar* = 10 μm. **(F)** Mutant lz^{mr1} brain immunohistochemically stained and rendered in three dimensions to reveal the developing photoreceptor axons from cells R7 and R8 in the second optic ganglia, the medulla. Note the mutant and irregular axon paths. *Bar* = 10 μm.

EYE DEVELOPMENT IN *DROSOPHILA MELANOGASTER:* ORGAN CULTURE WITH AUTOMATED MICROSCOPY

To investigate the development of the visual system in the fruit fly, *Drosophila melanogaster,* we are adapting and developing the AIM technology for 3-D time-lapse microscopy of organ cultured retina and brain. Ultimately, we plan to investigate photoreceptor axon pathfinding in *Drosophila* and compare growth in normal tissue to growth in genetic mutants such as *lozenge.* Three main challenges have been resolved: (1) keeping the eye/brain tissue alive and developing in culture; (2) labeling axons; and (3) acquiring and compositing images into a movie.

Pattern Formation and Cellular Differentiation in the Fly Eye

Eye development in *Drosophila* is an extremely precise and stereotyped process.[15] The compound eye of the adult fly (FIG. 2(A)) develops from an epithelial sac known as the eye-antennal imaginal disc. Each eye disc is connected to one of the hemispheres of the brain of the fly via the optic stalk (FIG. 2(C)). The third larval instar cell fates first become apparent when a wave of morphogenesis, known as the morphogenetic furrow, progresses across the eye disc from posterior to anterior. As this furrow progresses, cell fates are established, including eight types of photoreceptor neurons and supporting cells.[15] This diverse population of cells is precisely arranged in three-dimensional space to create ommatidial clusters, approximately 800 such facets constitute the adult eye.

As the photoreceptor cells differentiate, they extend axons that fasciculate with the other axons from the same cluster making a bundle of eight. The fascicles grow across the basal eye disc to the optic stalk, passing in to the brain, where they fan out (FIG. 2(D)). At a particular position in the brain each bundle of axons plunges downward and forms connections with specific interneurons.[16,17] Despite having to traverse long distances, photoreceptor axons make highly stereotyped pathfinding and target-recognition decisions to create a precise neural superposition retina.[17,18] The innervation of the retina into the brain forms a retinotopic map that oversamples the visual field. This elaborate neural network, which is necessary for the proper function of the fly's visual system, arises from the developmental program encoded by the genome. The analysis of mutants where pathfinding is aberrant may provide insights into which interactions are most critical for the development of a neural network.

Phenotype and Expression Pattern of Lozenge

As indicated in FIGURE 2(B), mutations in *lozenge* (*lz*) affect the eyes.[19,20] Mutations in *lz* can also be pleiotropic, affecting the antennae as well as other systems.[20,21] The eye defects arise because the products of the *lz* gene first influence cell survival in the developing eye. Then *lz* influences the choice of cell fate and the differentiation of photoreceptor neurons R1, R6, and R7 and the supporting cells.[20,22] Encoding a transcription factor, *lz* is expressed in the affected cells and appears to function by influencing the expression of genes such as *reaper, seven-up* and *Bar* among others.[22,23]

Axon pathfinding is defective in *lz* mutants (FIG. 2(E), (F)). This defect was revealed by immunohistochemical staining and 3-D microscopy of the medulla region of the pupal brain, allowing the specific visualization of axons R7 and R8. In normal flies these pairs of axons form a linear array as they extend through the brain. In *lz* mutants the precision of this projection pattern is lost and the growth cones appear abnormally shaped. Other studies have shown that axon fasciculation is also defective (Crew, Leonardo and Pollock, unpublished). In combination, the developmental defects in axon fasciculation, growth, and guidance result in abnormalities in the optic lobes of the adult brain.[20]

Our interests included looking at how and when pathfinding decisions are made. However, single images from fixed tissue are insufficient because axon pathfinding is a dynamic process occurring in the 3-D depth of the brain. Therefore, axon growth would best be studied with 3-D time-lapse microscopy. The examination of patterns of axon elongation rate and turning will be useful in determining if the pathfinding defects are due to misexpression of a particular signal or a result of some more general phenomenon.

Tissue Culturing

The cephalic complex (both eye-antennal discs with brains and ventral ganglion attached) is dissected from a third instar larva or early white prepupa (FIG. 2(C)). The tissue is then placed on a lysinated coverslide that serves as the bottom of a temperature regulated perfusible growth chamber and the medium is exchanged three to four times an hour. The tissue is cultured in Schneiders Insect Medium supplemented with β-ecdysone (generally 100 ng/mL) or in Sang's and Shields M3 Modified Medium supplemented with 2% fetal bovine serum and β-ecdysone. β-Ecdysone is a hormone that plays an important role in triggering developmental and behavioral changes in *Drosophila* as well as in other insects.[24]

Labeling Axons

We have investigated three approaches for labeling photoreceptor axons: (1) microinjecting rhodamine-dextran into single cells; (2) microinjecting DiI into whole-eye imaginal discs; and (3) using the molecular marker Green Fluorescent Protein (GFP) under the control of a tissue-specific promoter. Single cells and their axons can be labeled by direct microinjection with rhodamine-dextran (Pollock and DeBiasio, unpublished). Though this has the advantage of allowing individual cells to be labeled, this method is challenging and invasive. Microinjecting DiI into the whole eye imaginal disc also labeled axons, but was similarly found to be inadequate (Leonardo and Pollock, unpublished). GFP under the control of the *glass* promoter (pGMR) provides a noninvasive label for cells of the eye disc.[25,26] Although GFP is expressed in multiple cell types, this marker allowed us to detect cell differentiation in the developing eye as well as photoreceptor axons as they project into the brain.

Acquisition and Viewing of Images

For each experiment a stack of fluorescent images (generally 32–50 axial *z*-planes) is acquired through the tissue using a cooled CCD camera on the multimode inverted Zeiss microscope. Data are acquired every 15 to 30 min for up to 24 h. Video enhanced contrast (VEC) images are also typically acquired for most experiments. In some experiments the tissue is also stained with Hoechst dye, and an additional series of fluorescent images acquired (excitation wavelength 355 nm). The 3000–5000 images from a given experiment are directly saved on the Macintosh Quadra 950 and occupy 1–2 Gbytes of disk space. For some experiments initial analysis of single time points or single *z*-planes was done on the Macintosh using STC-View software. Images were transferred by FTP to the AIM host computer, a Silicon Graphics Onyx (FIG. 6). Our primary tool for viewing and analyzing our data has been the AIM 5-D Image Viewer (FIG. 3(A)). We have made time-lapse movies of several aspects of eye development,[27] including the progression of the furrow and the folding of the retina prior to disc eversion (FIG. 3(B)–(G)). The tissue also clearly grows in size (compare Fig. 3B,G). These observations suggest that development is proceeding.

Recently, similar long-term culture experiments have been carried out by Li and Meinertzhagen.[28] They tested numerous culture mediums and were able to maintain tissue alive in culture for long periods (up to 20 days with Sang's and Shields Modified Medium (MM3)). Their primary interest was in developing an optimal culture system for neurite outgrowth *in vitro,* documented by acquiring conventional still images from a limited number of time points. While some of their experiments utilized intact eye-antennal imaginal discs, most of their work was done with fragments of discs with neurites growing on to artificial substrate. Nevertheless, the still images that they acquired from developing eye tissue suggested that movement of the morphogenetic furrow may be progressing in their MM3 culture system. Our adaptation of this MM3 buffer has meet with similar success. Using our culture system, we have been able to maintain growing tissue for periods of 15 or more hours. We are making further refinements to our culture system that will extend the duration of an experiment. By using AIM software we have been able to composit thousands of images into a format that allows us to follow 3-D development over time.

DISSECTING THE MOLECULAR COMPONENTS OF PRIMARY BRAIN TUMOR CELL MOTILITY

The continual evolution of optical-based methodology, instrumentation, and reagents to measure and manipulate specific chemical and molecular processes in single cells has produced an effective approach to solving problems in cellular physiology.[1,10,29] Our use of this approach to provide molecular descriptions of normal cell functions such as locomotion,[30–33] intermediary metabolism,[34,35] signal transduction,[36–38] and cell division[39] suggests that a similar approach might be useful in dissecting the aberrant chemistry of individual cancer cells. Here, we present examples of cellular morphometry coupled with the molecular analysis of actin-cytoskeletal dynamics in single living cells[11] and the quantitation of cellular traction forces to begin to dissect, at a new level of resolution, the molecular basis of malignancy in a human primary brain-tumor model system.

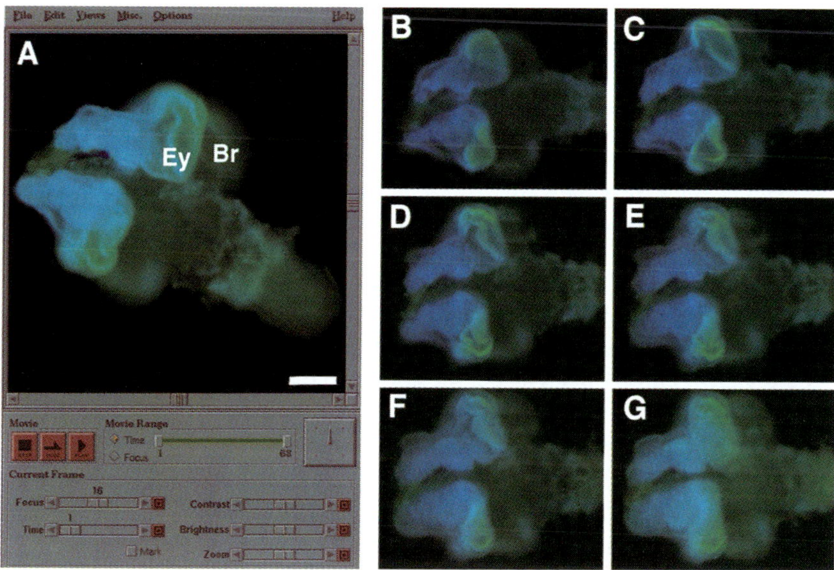

FIGURE 3. Multidimensional movie of the developing eyes and brain expressing pGMR-GFP. (**A**) AIM 5D viewer interface. *Bar* = 100 μm. (**B**)–(**G**) Six single focal-plane time points from zero h, 4 h, 6 h, 8 h, 10 h, 13 h of an 18-h organ culture stained with Hoechst to highlight nuclei *(blue)* and expressing pGMR–GFP *(green)*. Note that the tissue grows in overall size. Also note that the *bright green folds* of retina ripple and undulate with time.

The Role of the Actin-Cytoskeleton in the Malignant Cell Phenotype

Because the actin-cytoskeleton plays a major role in the regulation of cell shape, locomotion, and cell–cell interactions, an altered regulation of the actin-cytoskeleton is likely responsible for the observed morphological dynamics of tumor cells. To test this hypothesis, we have combined the dynamic morphological analysis with fluorescent analog cytochemistry[10] to measure the dynamics of the actin-cytoskeleton in brain-tumor cells.

FIGURE 4 shows an example of a multimode experiment designed to measure cell morphological and actin-cytoskeletal dynamics in a single migrating human glioblastoma multiform (SNB-19) cell. The images were taken from a time-lapse series of images and show the morphology of the cell as it migrated across the substrate. From these four image pairs alone, the tumor cell exhibited a fibroblast-like stepping mechanism of locomotion[31] rather than an epithelial-keratocyte-like gliding mechanism.[40] In the stepping mechanism of cell movement, a well-formed tail containing the nucleus first contracts and is then pulled forward after releasing cell-substrate contacts (FIG. 4(A)–(F)). Next, the leading edge of the cell spreads to make new cell-substrate attachments to stabilize the lamellipodia. The images in FIGURE 4 show the dynamic actin-cytoskeleton in the migrating brain-tumor cell. Active extension of the lamellipodia resulted in the formation of stress fibers and focal contacts immediately behind the leading-edge ruffle. The formation of stress fibers at the leading edge of this cell is consistent with the gradient of actin polymerization, highest at the leading edge and lowest in the tail, that has been measured in migrating normal fibroblasts[32] and brain-tumor cells.[7] These and other data[11] are consistent with the invasive properties of human gliomas, being dependent on an altered regulation of actin-cytoskeletal assembly and contractility. Hence, the approach of measuring and manipulating cellular processes, including the actin-cytoskeleton, in single living cells[5,29] will be valuable in diagnosing the molecular events that have transformed normal differentiated cells into malignant tissue.

TRACTION FORCES PRODUCED BY GLIOBLASTOMA CELLS IN CULTURE

Locomotion of cells through a tissue or over a substratum in culture ultimately results from the transmission of mechanical forces from the cytoskeleton to the cell's surroundings via sites of adhesion. The speed of cells strongly depends on the rapidity of cytoskeletal remodeling, as well as a balance between the formation and breaking of cell-substratum adhesions and forces applied at those sites across the cell.[41] All of these properties can change when cells are transformed, a striking example of which is the increase in motility of highly invasive glioblastoma cells relative to differentiated glial cells.[11] One approach to measuring traction forces is to seed cells onto transparent elastic substrata, so that distortions in the substratum resulting from traction forces can be imaged along with cytoskeletal structure and sites of adhesion.[42] Recent advances in this method have increased its sensitivity by over two orders of magnitude, allowing measurement of traction forces previously inaccessible to study.[43,44]

The high invasiveness of glioblastoma cells results from rapid motility

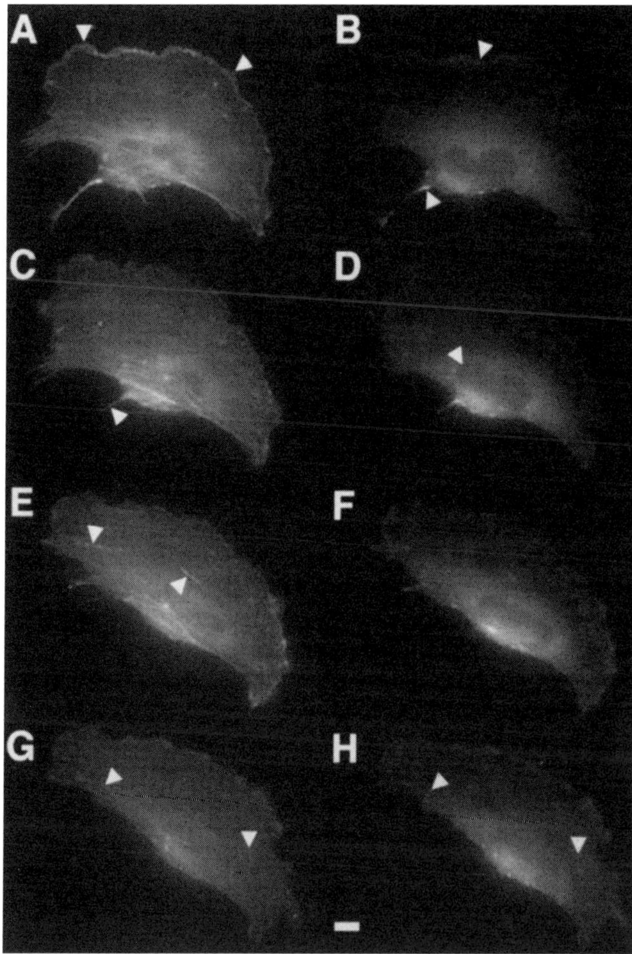

FIGURE 4. Morphological and molecular dynamics of a migrating transformed glial cell. A wound-healing model system[32] was used to generate a large number of polarized migrating SNB-19 cells. The cell depicted was microinjected with a mixture containing a tetramethylrhodamine analog of nonmuscle actin[32] **(A, C, E, G)** and a Cy5 analog of smooth muscle vinculin **(B, D, F, H)**. The cell was imaged with two modes of light microscopy[1,57] as it moved along the substrate. The entire time-lapse series comprised 60 images obtained at 1.5-min intervals. Shown here are four pairs of images from the series taken at 0 (A, B), 18 (C, D), 45 (E, F), and 82.5 (G, H) min. The dynamics of several cellular components (*arrowheads*) were measured as a function of time and include **(A)** the dynamics of leading edge ruffles; **(B)** the formation and dissolution of individual focal adhesions; **(C)** a retracting tail; **(D)** nuclear shape, size, and translocation; **(E)** the lengthening and shortening of stress fibers containing actin and an array of associated proteins; **(G)** and **(H)** the termination of stress fibers at sites of focal adhesion. *Bar* = 10 μm.

through brain tissue, which could be due to alterations in any of the properties mentioned earlier. We have studied traction forces produced by single locomoting glioblastoma cells in order to compare patterns of force generation to cytoskeletal dynamics and changes in adhesion complexes described

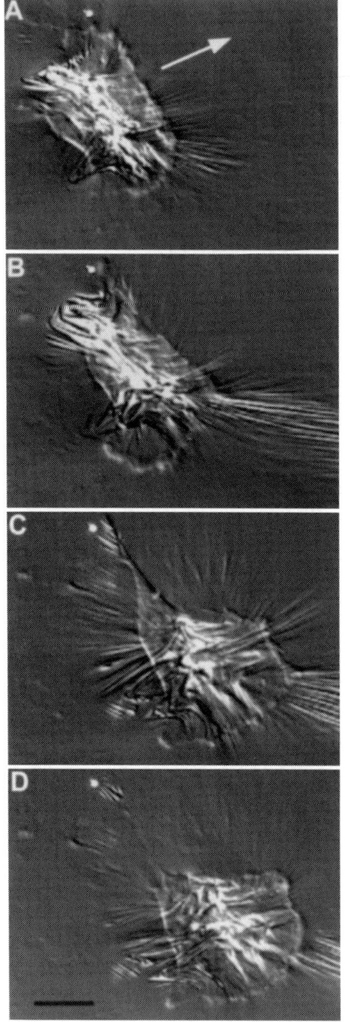

FIGURE 5. Glioblastoma cell locomoting on a silicone rubber sheet. *Wrinkles* in the sheet result from traction forces. The cell (line SNB19) was freely locomoting in the direction of the *arrow* in **(A)**, then turned to its right and started to elongate **(B)** as a "tail" adhered to the substratum, and was stretched behind the cell body **(C).** The tail lost adhesion and retracted **(D)**, at which time the cell was again freely locomoting. The *wrinkles* at the tail in (C) indicate a traction force of about 250 nN before tail retraction. (A)–(D) were taken at times 0, 16.5, 30.0, and 40.5 min. Cells were cultured in DMEM with 10% calf serum at 37°C. Nomarski DIC microscopy. *Bar* = 20 μm.

earlier, and additionally to test the possibility that forces generated by these cells are significantly different from those produced by untransformed mammalian cells in culture (e.g., fibroblasts). FIGURE 5 shows an example of a glioblastoma cell locomoting on a silicone rubber substratum. Wrinkles were produced in the silicone sheet where traction forces were applied. Cell morphology changed in a characteristic sequence during locomotion: (1) the cell initially had a large leading lamellum at the front of the rounded cell body (arrow shows the direction of movement), similar to the semilunar shape of fish keratocytes;[43,45] (2) the posterior end of the cell body was pulled out into a "tail" that slowed the cell's forward movement; and (3) the tail suddenly retracted as the cell regained its former shape and continued moving. The distribution of wrinkles shows that most areas of the cell produced traction force, including the lamellum and anterior region of the cell body. The posterior region of a rounded cell body was devoid of wrinkles, similar to observations in rapidly locomoting keratocytes,[45] and markedly different from the situation when a tail adhered to the substratum, produced wrinkles and resisted forward motion, much as observed in fibroblasts.[44] The lengths of the wrinkles indicated that the cell produced a few hundred nanonewtons of force, intermediate between those observed for fibroblasts and keratocytes. Therefore, neither the distribution of traction forces nor their magnitude was strikingly different from other locomoting cells, suggesting that glioblastoma cells produce traction forces in the normal cellular range to power their motility.

AUTOMATED IMAGING FOR BIOLOGY, BIOTECHNOLOGY, AND MEDICINE

In the history of biology, there have been a succession of technological revolutions in our ability to observe the processes and structures of life: the early light microscopes, staining techniques, electron microscopy, X-ray crystallography of biological macromolecules, radioactive labeling, and now NMR and fluorescence microscopy. Each of these new technologies, in its day, has led to a revolutionary advance in our understanding of biological systems. We believe that high-resolution, automated, interactive light microscopy will lead to another revolutionary advance in technology, allowing us to observe and interact with rapidly changing events in living cells. While we have already begun to reap the benefits of this new technology in the field of brain research, it is the unanticipated discoveries that will be most important in the long run.

AIM: Progress and Future Developments

The development of AIM has been driven by the need to define the 3-D chemical and molecular dynamics responsible for life at the cellular level. The system design requirements were determined by considering the characteristics of some fundamental biological processes of interest, described earlier. Sampling the 3-D volume of an embryo at optical resolution requires acquisition of $\geq 10^8$ voxels, while the rapid time course of some developmental processes requires the acquisition of less than 1 to more than 10 volumes per minute, continuously, for an hour or more. The variations in brightness of individual labeled embryos (interscene dynamic range) requires a detector dynamic range of at least 1000 (i.e., 10 bits). Rather than simply recording the data for subsequent analysis, however, the goal was to build a system that would allow interactive experimentation, the capability to define the course of an experiment (e.g., by the photochemical release of a reagent[5] in a particular 3-D subregion of an embryo), depending on the current state of the biological process being monitored. This imposes the additional requirement that the system be able to compute and display 3-D renderings of the processed data, in real time, as defined by the biological process. The other important advantage to on-line, high-performance computing is the ability to program the system to recognize particular features or events.[5,46] Finally, the continuous monitoring of developmental processes in 3-D requires a nonperturbing mode of microscopy, such as long-wavelength DIC,[47] and the ability to rapidly switch to other modes such as fluorescence to record an event of interest.

There are three essential components of the present AIM system (FIG. 6), a robotic light microscope, a Motion/Acquisition Processing computer, and a control, processing, and display computer. The distributed design of the AIM computing systems, along with high-speed networking, also allows access to other computing resources, such as those at the Pittsburgh Supercomputing Center, for particular computationally intensive applications. The inverted microscope is an Axiovert 135/TV (Carl Zeiss, Thornwood, N.Y.) modified for computer control. A critical element of the system is a feedback-controlled piezoelectric ring stage (Polytec PI, Auburn, Mass.) with a custom chamber holder that allows fast precision scanning of the specimen through the plane of focus. The motion of the stage is synchronized with a high-speed, cooled CCD camera (Hamamatsu, Bridgewater, N.J.) that collects 1018 × 1024 pixel images at 7 frames/s, and subregions at somewhat faster frame rates. The 10-bit images are captured by a digital frame grabber, pipeline processed, and then transferred over a high-speed DMA link from a Pentium/PCI MAP computer to an Onyx (Silicon Graphics, Mountain View, Calif.) control computer for rendering, display, and immediate storage to a hard disk array, all at >20 Mbytes/s, the maximum data rate of the camera. The hardware texture mapping in the Onyx allows real-time projection rendering of the stacks of images as they are acquired. The differential nature of the DIC images acquired in monitoring mode, however, requires an additional processing step such as integration or variance processing[48] before rendering. Fluorescence image stacks can be immediately rendered for display, or deconvolved[49,50] to enhance axial resolution before rendering.

The 5-D data sets acquired by the AIM (multiple microscope modes acquired in 3-D through time) required developing some custom display software. FIGURE 1 illustrates one of the display modes used to view multidimensional data. The AIM 5-D viewer can interactively compute projection renderings of 3-D volume data from multiple microscope modes and simultaneously display those renderings to allow comparisons of features

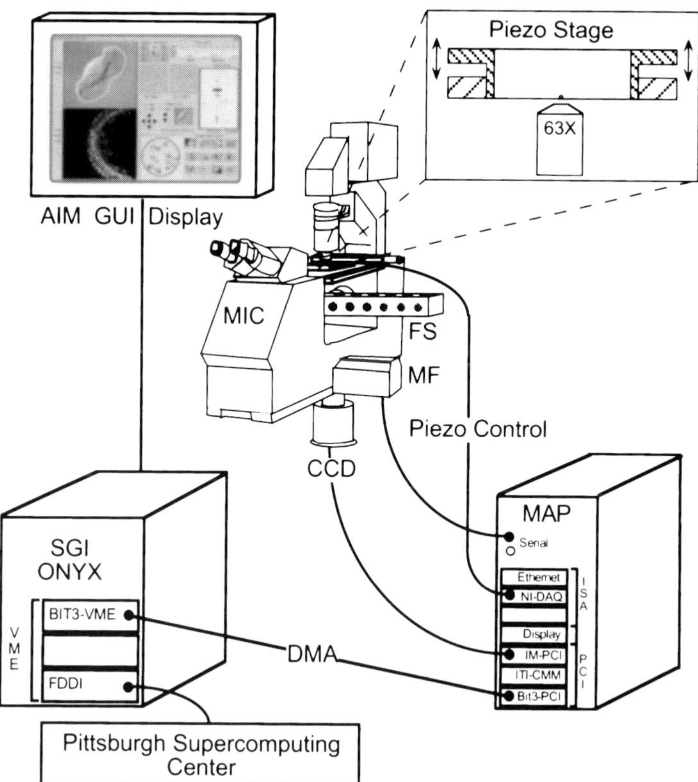

FIGURE 6. Block diagram of the AIM system. The AIM system consists of a microscope (MIC), with motorized filter slider (FS), feedback-controlled piezo stage (PS) for fast, high-precision axial positioning, motor-driven coarse focus (MF), and motorized *X, Y* stage (MS). The dual-speed (10-MHz/300-KHz) cooled CCD is used for both DIC and low-light-level fluorescence imaging. The motion/acquisition processor computer (MAP) performs three functions in response to commands from the primary AIM processing and display system, the Silicon Graphics (SGI) Onyx: (1) controls the microscope via the serial port and the NIDAQ data-acquisition and control card; (2) acquires and preprocesses the images from the camera via the IM-PCI digital frame grabber and pipeline processor; and (3) sends the images over the high-bandwidth DMA link to the Onyx for final processing and rendering in the AIM 5d-Viewer (FIGS. 1, 3A). In addition the Onyx has a fiber-optic link to additional computation resources at the Pittsburgh Supercomputing Center.

in the data acquired from the various modes. FIGURE 1 shows a set of projection renderings of AIM image data acquired from a live mouse embryo at the 16-cell stage. Alternatively, the same viewer can be used to render multiple time points simultaneously, or to render a time series in real time to view dynamic processes in the 3-D volume. What cannot be illustrated in this picture are the depth cues and other spatial relationships that are immediately obvious as these data sets are simultaneously manipulated by rotation, zooming, clipping, or contrast enhancement and rendered in real time. Other AIM viewer capabilities include viewing slices from stacks through focus or time with the ability to mix channels from multiple modes. This interactive exploration of the resulting data, while the biological specimen is still alive on the microscope, allows new kinds of experiments to be performed.

The AIM system will continue to evolve as technology advances and experimental needs arise. There are three areas in which AIM system enhancements are already planned. Smart algorithms for automated feature extraction and event detection will be developed through collaborations with researchers in computer science and robotics. Additional optical microscopy techniques, such as standing-wave fluorescence microscopy[51] and dual-view imaging[52] will be integrated to further enhance the spatial and temporal resolution of the system. Finally, the high-performance computers of today will likely be the desktop computers of tomorrow. With this in mind, the system has been designed as much as possible to be portable, in the software sense, with the ultimate goal of producing an affordable system that will be generally useful to the scientific research community. This instrument will also provide the researcher the means to directly manipulate the specimen for experimental purposes, through perfusion of biologically active agents, optical activation of caged compounds, changing the mechanical properties of the substratum, and positioning electromechanical probes.

Other Applications of AIM Technology

The importance of properly selected dyes, contrast agents, and labeling will not diminish, but rather increase as imaging technologies improve. For example, recently carbocyanine dyes and calcium-sensitive fluorescent indicators were used in combination with confocal microscopy to investigate mechanisms involved with the migration of cells in the developing cerebellum.[53] This analysis indicated that a combination of voltage and ligand activity channels work together to regulate intracellular Ca^{2+} fluxes in migrating cells. In other studies, analysis of the functional activity of two different neural networks in the intact zebrafish spinal cord have revealed a previously unknown synchrony in these networks.[54] By using optical approaches to study groups of primary and secondary motor neurons, a new understanding of the activation of the axial musculature in zebrafish escape behavior is emerging. Additionally, using acoustooptical tunable filters,[12] it should become possible to monitor (including by ratio imaging) events that are significantly faster than video rate, thus raising the possibility of following nerve impulse propagation and the related ionic changes with microscopic resolution.

The multimode and AIM microscope projects complement and extend the capabilities of researchers for investigating neural development and functional activity. Not only will we be able to investigate functional activities of cells and tissues, but the combination of noninvasive use of green fluorescent protein[55] to monitor gene expression and cellular identity can be included in the investigation. Another facet of future studies will include the analysis of genetic mutants where new, dynamic phenotypes can be quantified, such as the growth velocities and stereotypic turning angle of developing neurons. We also anticipate that by applying integrative microscopy through the continuum of NMR and fNMR imaging, to multimode and AIM light microscopy, and finally to electron microscopy, the investigator will have vast new insights into the basic function of the brain.

ACKNOWLEDGMENTS

We thank the members of the Center for Light Microscope Imaging and Biotechnology, and particularly W. Galbraith, F. Lanni, G. Larocca, and D. Pane, for their contributions to the work summarized here. J. Crew did the work on *lozenge* axon phenotypes and expression patterns, and J. Suhan assisted with the electron microscopy.

REFERENCES

1. FARKAS, D. L., G. BAXTER, R. DEBIASIO, A. GOUGH, M. A. NEDERLOF, D. PANE, J. PANE, D. R. PATEK, K. W. RYAN & D. L. TAYLOR. 1993. Multimode light microscopy and the dynamics of molecules, cells and tissues. Annu. Rev. Physiol. **55:** 785–817.
2. TAYLOR, D. L., M. A. NEDERLOF, F. LANNI & A. S. WAGGONER. 1992. The new vision of light microscopy. Am. Sci. **80:** 322–335.
3. TAYLOR, D. L. & Y.-L. WANG. 1989. Fluorescence Microscopy of Living Cells in Culture, Part B: Quantitative Fluorescence Microscopy—Imaging and Spectroscopy; Methods in Cell Biology, Vol. 30. Academic Press. New York.
4. ADAMS, S. R. & R. Y. TSIEN. 1992. Controlling cell chemistry with caged compounds. Annu. Rev. Physiol. **55:** 755–784.
5. GIULIANO, K. A. & D. L. TAYLOR. 1995a. Light-optical-based reagents for the measurement and manipulation of ions, metabolites and macromolecules in living cells. Methods Neurosci. **27:** 1–16.
6. RAMÓN Y CAJAL, S. 1937. Recollections of My Life (originally published as Recuerdos de Mi Vida, 1901–1917; English transl. by E. H. Craigie and J. Cano), in Vol. 8 of Memoirs of the American Philosophical Society, reprinted by MIT Press, Cambridge, MA (1989).
7. GIULIANO, K. A. 1997. The actin-cytoskeleton and glial cell transformation: Dissecting the molecular dynamics of tumorigenesis. *In* Advances in Neuro-Oncology, M. Walker & P. Kornblith, Eds. Futura Publishing. Armonk, N.Y. In press.
8. GALBRAITH, W., C. E. WAGNER, J. CHAO, M. ABAZA, L. A. ERNST, M. A. NEDERLOF, R. J. HARTSOCK, D. L. TAYLOR & A. S. WAGGONER. 1991. Imaging cytometry by multiparameter fluorescence. Cytometry **12:** 579–596.
9. FOCHT, D. C. & D. L. FARKAS. 1995. Mammalian live-cell microscopy environmental control. Cell Vision **2:** 450–454.
10. GIULIANO, K. A. & D. L. TAYLOR. 1995. Measurement and manipulation of cytoskeletal dynamics in living cells. Curr. Opin. Cell Biol. **7:** 4–12.
11. GIULIANO, K. A. 1996. Dissecting the individuality of cancer cells: The morphological and molecular dynamics of single human glioma cells. Cell Motil. Cytoskeleton **35:** 237–253.
12. WACHMAN, E. S., W. NIU & D. L. FARKAS. 1996. Imaging acousto-optic tunable filter with 0.35-micrometer spatial resolution. Appl. Opt., **35:** 5220–5226.

13. FARKAS, D. L., E. S. WACHMAN, L. D. HARRIS, A. H. GOUGH & D. L. TAYLOR. 1995. Digital microscope imaging of cell dynamics. Emerging applications of fluorescence technology to biophysics and cellular imaging. CLEO '95 **15:** 274.
14. TAYLOR, D. L., L. D. HARRIS, R. DEBIASIO, S. E. FAHLMAN, D. L. FARKAS, F. LANNI, M. NEDERLOF & A. H. GOUGH. 1996. Automated interactive microscopy: Measuring and manipulating the chemical and molecular dynamics of cells and tissues. SPIE Proc. **2678:** 15–27.
15. WOLFF, T. & D. F. READY. 1993. Pattern formation in the *Drosophila* retina. *In* The Development of *Drosophila melanogaster*: 1277–1326. Cold Spring Harbor Laboratory Press. Cold Spring Harbor, NY.
16. KUNES, S. & H. STELLE. 1993. Topography in the *Drosophila* visual system. Curr. Opin. Neurobiol. **3:** 53–59.
17. MEINERTZHAGEN, I. & T. E. HANSO. 1993. The development of the optic lobe. *In* The Development of *Drosophila melanogaster,* M. Bate and A. Martinex-Arias, Eds.: 1363–1491. Cold Spring Harbor Laboratory Press. New York.
18. HEISENBERG, M. & R. WOLF. 1984. Vision in Drosophila: Genetics in Microbehavior. Stud. Brain Function. Springer-Verlag. Berlin/New York.
19. CREW, J. R. 1995. A morphological and developmental analysis of the adult compound eye phenotypes caused by mutations in the *lozenge* locus of *Drosophila.* Ph.D. Thesis, Carnegie Mellon Univ., Pittsburgh.
20. BATTERHAM, P., J. R. CREW, A. M. SOKAC, J. R. ANDREWS, G. M. F. PASQUINI, A. G. DAVIES, R. F. STOCKER & J. A. POLLOCK. 1996. Genetic analysis of the *lozenge* gene complex in *Drosophila melanogaster:* Adult visual system phenotypes. J. Neurogenet. **10:** 193–220.
21. STOCKER, R., N. GENDRE & P. BATTERHAM. 1993. Analysis of the antennal phenotype in the *Drosophila* mutant *lozenge.* J. Neurogenet. **9:** 29–53.
22. CREW, J. R., P. BATTERHAM & J. A. POLLOCK. 1997. Developing compound eye in *lozenge* mutants of Drosophila: *Lozenge* expression in the R7 equivalence group. Dev. Genes. Evol. 206/8.
23. DAGA, A., C. A. KARLOVICH, K. DUMSTREI & U. BANERJEE. 1996. Patterning of cells in the Drosophila eye by Lozenge, which shares homologous domains with AML1. Genes & Dev. **10:** 1194–1205.
24. ANDRES, A. J., J. C. FLETCHER, F. D. KARIM & C. S. THUMMEL. 1993. Molecular analysis of the initiation of insect metamorphosis: A comparative study of *Drosophila* ecdysteroid-regulated transcription. Dev. Biol. **160:** 388–404.
25. MOSES, K. & G. R. RUBIN. 1991. *Glass* encodes a site-specific DNA-binding protein that is regulated in response to positional signals in the developing *Drosophila* eye. Genes & Dev. **5:** 383–393.
26. HAY, B. A., T. WOLFF & G. M. RUBIN. 1994. Expression of baculovirus P35 prevents cell death in Drosophila. Development **120:** 2121–2129.
27. LEONARDO, T. & J. A. POLLOCK. 1996. Eye development in *Drosophila melanogaster:* A study with video microscopy. 37th Annu. *Drosophila* Research Conf., p. 369.
28. LI, C. & I. A. MEINERTZHAGEN. 1995. Conditions for the primary culture of eye imaginal discs from Drosophila melanogaster. J. Neurobiol. **28:** 363–380.
29. GIULIANO, K. A., P. L. POST, K. M. HAHN & D. L. TAYLOR. 1995. Fluorescent protein biosensors: Measurement of molecular dynamics in living cells. Annu. Rev. Biophys. Biomol. Struct. **24:** 405–434.
30. DEBIASIO, R. L., L. L. WANG, G. W. FISHER & D. L. TAYLOR. 1988. The dynamic distribution of fluorescent analogues of actin and myosin in protrusions at the leading edge of migrating Swiss 3T3 fibroblasts. J. Cell Biol. **107:** 2631–2645.
31. KOLEGA, J. & D. L. TAYLOR. 1993. Gradients in the concentration and assembly of myosin II in living fibroblasts during locomotion and fiber transport. Mol. Biol. Cell **4:** 819–836.
32. GIULIANO, K. A. & D. L. TAYLOR. 1994. Fluorescent actin analogs with a high affinity for profilin in vitro exhibit an enhanced gradient of assembly in living cells. J. Cell Biol. **124:** 971–983.

33. POST, P. L., R. L. DEBIASIO & D. L. TAYLOR. 1995. A fluorescent protein biosensor of myosin II regulatory light chain phosphorylation reports a gradient of phosphorylated myosin II in migrating cells. Mol. Biol. Cell **6:** 1755–1768.
34. PAGLIARO, L. & D. L. TAYLOR. 1988. Aldolase exists in both the fluid and solid phases of cytoplasm. J. Cell Biol. **107:** 981–991.
35. PAGLIARO, L. & D. L. TAYLOR. 1992. 2-Deoxyglucose and cytochalasin D modulate aldolase mobility in living 3T3 cells. J. Cell Biol. **118:** 859–863.
36. GIULIANO, K. A. & D. L. TAYLOR. 1990. Formation, transport, contraction, and disassembly of stress fibers in fibroblasts. Cell Motil. Cytoskeleton **16:** 14–21.
37. HAHN, K., R. DEBIASIO & D. L. TAYLOR. 1992. Patterns of elevated free calcium and calmodulin activation in living cells. Nature **359:** 736–738.
38. GOUGH, A. H. & D. L. TAYLOR. 1993. Fluorescence anisotropy imaging microscopy maps calmodulin binding during cellular contraction and locomotion. J. Cell Biol. **121:** 1095–1107.
39. DEBIASIO, R. L., G. M. LAROCCA, P. L. POST & D. L. TAYLOR. 1996. Myosin II transport, organization, and phosphorylation: Evidence for cortical flow/solation-contraction coupling during cytokinesis and cell locomotion. Mol. Biol. Cell **7:** 1259–1282.
40. LEE, J., A. ISHIHARA, J. A. THERIOT & K. JACOBSON. 1993. Principles of locomotion for simple-shaped cells. Nature **362:** 167–171.
41. DIMILLA, P. A. 1994. Receptor-mediated adhesive interactions at the cytoskeleton/substratum interface during cell migration. *In* Cell Mechanics and Cellular Engineering, V. C. Mow, F. Guilak, R. T. S. Tay, and R. M. Hochmuth, Eds.: 490–514. Springer-Verlag. New York.
42. HARRIS, A. K., P. WILD & D. STOPAK. 1980. Silicone rubber substrata: A new wrinkle in the study of cell locomotion. Science **208:** 177–179.
43. OLIVER, T., M. DEMBO & K. JACOBSON. 1995. Traction forces in locomoting cells. Cell Motil. Cytoskeleton **31:** 225–240.
44. BURTON, K. & D. L. TAYLOR. 1997. Traction forces of cytokinesis measured with optically modified elastic substrata. Nature **385:** 450–454.
45. PARK, J., K. BURTON & D. L. TAYLOR. 1994. Spatial distribution of dynamic traction forces applied by keratocytes to silicone elastic substrata. Molec. Biol. Cell **5:** 170a.
46. NEDERLOF, M., A. WITKIN & D. L. TAYLOR. 1991. Knowledge driven image analysis of cell structures. Proc. SPIE **1428:** 233–241.
47. ZAND, M. S. & G. ALBRECHT-BUEHLER. 1989. Long-term observation of cultured cells by interference-reflection microscopy: Near-infrared illumination and Y-contrast image processing. Cell Motil. Cytoskeleton **13:** 94–103.
48. FEINEIGLE, P. A., A. P. WITKIN & V. L. STONICK. 1995. Processing of 3D DIC microscopy images for data visualization. Proc. Int. Conf. on Acoustics, Speech and Signal Processing, Atlanta, Ga, May 6–10.
49. AGARD, D. A. 1984. Optical sectioning microscopy: Cellular architecture in three dimensions. Annu. Rev. Biophys. Bioeng. **13:** 191–219.
50. CARRINGTON, W. A., K. E. FOGARTY & F. S. FAY. 1990. 3D fluorescence imaging of single cells using image restoration. *In* Noninvasive Techniques in Cell Biology, Foskett and Grinstein, Eds.: 53–72. Liss. New York.
51. BAILEY, B., D. L. FARKAS, D. L. TAYLOR & F. LANNI. 1993. Enhancement of axial resolution in fluorescence microscopy by standing-wave excitation. Nature **366:** 44–48.
52. KINOSITA, K., JR., H. ITOH, S. ISHIWATA, K. HIRANO, T. NISHIKAZA & T. HAYAKAWA. 1991. Dual view microscopy with a single camera: Real-time imaging of molecular orientations and calcium. J. Cell Biol. **115:** 67–73.
53. RAKIC, P. & H. KOMURO. 1995. The role of receptor/channel activity in neuronal cell migration. J. Neurobiol. **26:** 299–315.
54. FETCHO, J. R. & D. M. O'MALLEY. 1995. Visualization of active neural circuitry in the spinal cord of intact zebrafish. J. Neurophysiol. **73:** 399–406.
55. CHALFIE, M. 1995. Green fluorescent protein. Photochem. Photobiol. **62:** 651–656.
56. POLLOCK, J. A., M. H. ELLISMAN & S. BENZER. 1990. Subcellular localization of transcripts in *Drosophila* photoreceptor neurons: Chaoptic mutants have an aberrant distribution. Genes & Dev. **4:** 806–821.

57. GIULIANO, K. A., M. A. NEDERLOF, R. DEBIASIO, F. LANNI, A. S. WAGGONER & D. L. TAYLOR. 1990. Multi-mode light microscopy. *In* Optical Microscopy for Biology, B. Herman & K. Jacobson, Eds.: 543–557. Wiley-Liss. New York, NY.

DISCUSSION

QUESTION: I was just curious about the long-wavelength fluorescent label. Is that something that you prepared?

TAYLOR: Yes, Cy7 in this case was conjugated to an antibody. Its excitation peak is 750, and its emission peak is 780. When the same experiments are done with probes that excite and emit at lower wavelengths, the quality of the image is much less, because of the light-scattering properties of light. Going into it further and further at longer and longer wavelengths, we minimize that.

QUESTION: How is the solubility of these probes?

TAYLOR: One of the things that Allan Wagonner has been able to do over the last 15 years of work is to improve the solubility through sulfination and other tricks to optimize the probes.

Using Emerging Technologies such as Virtual Reality and the World Wide Web to Contribute to a Richer Understanding of the Brain

JONATHAN R. MERRIL[a]

Medical Consumer Media, and
Departments of Anatomy and Biochemistry
The George Washington University Medical Center
1709 Evelyn Drive
Rockville, Maryland 20852

THE IMPROVEMENT OF INTERFACE TECHNOLOGY

The way by which people interact with computers—computer interface technology—is undergoing rapid change. Computer input and output initially consisted of punch cards and typed correspondence. Greater spontaneity was afforded by the display and interaction with text on a computer screen. During the past 10 years, the increasing acceptance of the mouse and the Xerox-PARC 2D interface has allowed the use of spatial navigation through the computer's operating system, as well as providing greater standardization for software applications. With the advent of three-dimensional hardware acceleration, the computer's interface and applications now allow three-dimensional navigation and interaction with three-dimensional worlds. Furthermore, the explosive growth of the Internet is providing a better means of sharing and distributing information between machines, and ultimately the virtual environments that reside in those machines.

Improvement in computer interface technology has immense implications for neuroscience research. Computers, when used for quantitative and/or qualitative analysis, can aid understanding of the structure and function of the brain. However, we must also be cognizant of the fact that the strengths and weaknesses of the computer as an analytical tool can change the focus of our investigations. Sir William Osler stated, "When your only tool is a hammer, you treat everything as a nail." Because the computer is changing so quickly, recognizing its strengths and knowing its limitations, as well as identifying areas of rapid advancement will be important. So rather than limiting our investigations, as would happen with the metaphorical hammer, we need to match the computer's capabilities with our investigative and scientific reporting needs.

[a]Phone: 301/564.6100; fax: 301/564.9043; e-mail: jmerril@medcm.com

Neuroscience research involves a range of scientific endeavors: analysis of static histological images, describing electrophysiological events, tracking receptor binding, and now the arena called "functional imaging." Given our increasingly comprehensive understanding of the dynamic complexity of the brain, we require increasingly sophisticated computer hardware and software to both contribute to and communicate our understanding of the brain.

Just as scientific studies are producing massive amounts of data about the structure and function of the brain, we are seeing dramatic increases in the capabilities for the display and interaction of multi-dimensional data on the personal computer. Initially these capabilities were developed for high-end applications in computer-aided design, the military, and in flight simulation, but are now driven by the computer game industry. Virtual reality software and hardware, as well as networking applications deploying 3-D (involving virtual reality modeling language [VRML]) are trends that will contribute to a richer understanding of the brain and enable sharing and exploration of conceptual models in ways never before possible. New technology can provide more complete and concise descriptions of neuroscience models as well as capabilities that can transform the scientist's observations into models that can be explored in new ways by both the researcher and other interested scientists. The technology also offers new opportunities and challenges for collaboration and sharing of information to build increasingly comprehensive models of the brain.

Using these technologies, multi-modal data can be simultaneously displayed, enabling different types of data to be merged to create a more comprehensive understanding of the brain. For example, the dynamic processes observed by the electrophysiologist can be combined with the receptor binding studies and histological information obtained by other researchers. This capability provides an opportunity for both scientific discovery (in detecting new patterns and relationships between investigations) as well as misinterpretation (observing patterns which are artifacts of the techniques employed). Hence, an understanding of the process by which such synthetic images are created, as well as the continued development of multidisciplinary standards for data labeling, storage, normalization, and retrieval becomes increasingly critical.

COMPUTERS FOR PROFESSIONAL EDUCATION

The costs associated with providing educational courses and skill certification using traditional means continue to increase. With the growing popularity of the World Wide Web, we see significant opportunities for online training and reporting of data. Internet-based educational experiences can afford an immediacy and speed to world-wide access of data and interpretations that have never before been possible. But while this capacity for information retrieval has been increased, it is also important to maintain the standards of peer-review and the editorial functions that traditional publications have deployed; else much misinformation will be promulgated.

The World Wide Web can provide benefits beyond the unprecedented decrease in the cost and speed of the distribution of information; the technology can also display information previously unavailable in *any* format. The growth of World Wide Web–related technologies is pushing the development of other new communications technologies faster than ever. For example, three-dimensional interactive graphics have heretofore only been available on high-end workstations, such as those manufactured by Evans and Sutherland, Silicon Graphics, and others. But now we are seeing a more rapid evolution of software technologies on the network than we saw with stand-alone workstation applications. Initially, the hypertext markup language (HTML) has become a standard for displaying graphics, text, and links on the Internet. Within the past two years, technologies such as virtual reality modeling language (VRML) are providing standard methods for interacting with three-dimensional representations over the network. Personal computer manufacturers are racing to include three-dimensional graphics capabilities on the desk-top as a standard feature (just as audio capabilities are now becoming ubiquitous). Furthermore, the efforts to develop dedicated Internet boxes are under way that include advanced 3-D chip sets (developed in the game industry) and which are intended to streamline Internet connections with dedicated hardware/software solutions.

Bandwidth is also increasing with the increasing utilization of digital phone lines by modem manufacturers. In addition, several promising telecommunications technologies may increase our communications capabilities hundreds- or thousands-fold. Current contenders include asymmetrical digital subscriber lines (ADSL), which utilize current phone lines to deliver up to eight megabytes per second. Because this communication is "asymmetrical," these communication technologies allow faster communication to your computer than from your computer to the communication hubs. From the cable companies, a technology referred to as "cable modems" promises to provide a similar asymmetric communication service to your PC via the cable companies' coaxial lines. Finally, the concept of using digital satellite connections to the PC can also allow rapid download of information. With greater bandwidth, the possibility of "telementoring," or teaching scientific methods over networks, begins to come closer to a practical enterprise.

INCREASINGLY CAPABLE COMPUTERS—CAN THEY "THINK?"

These increases in technology and bandwidth afford a new paradigm for scientific reporting, training, databases, and conferences. To rephrase Osler, the tools that we have can limit or expand our understanding. The scientific models available for describing the immense number of biochemical, genetic, and environmental interrelationships in the brain are still relatively primitive.

Another of the most challenging applications of computer science has been in the construction of a financial "nervous system." Most of the large supercomputers that are sold are for calculating and verifying financial transactions. When you put your credit card through a gas pump, grocery, or retail store card reader, it requires considerable computing power to simultaneously verify, approve, register, or deny the millions of simultaneous transactions. Financial transactions are driving much computer development. Networks are facilitating an unprecedented communication between these servers. I cannot help but think that the growing capabilities of these multiprocessing environments will one day let us simulate a few moments of human nervous system activity.

EFFECT OF THE WORLD WIDE WEB ON RESEARCHERS AND LABORATORIES

In the recent past, a research laboratory's analytical capabilities were defined in part by the size and caliber of available computing resources. Now, a new model is emerging. As networks become faster, and computers become more of a commodity, we see the emergence of computers as a subscription service. As network speeds increase, computer resources such as hard drives, memory, and CPU performance all can become available by "renting" these resources from a provider on the network. Furthermore, there is strong interest in Sun Microsystems JAVA programming language, designed from the ground up to support on-demand transmission of snippets of necessary software to enable the widest possible range of customization for the software environments. Exchange of information and software tools in the scientific community will rise to new levels. In view of the inherent demands of intricacy, breadth, and constant changes that exists in neuroscience research these advances should be most welcome.

The power of one's investigative tools will be more and more dependent on the subscription databases and subscription computer resources which are available to a researcher or team of researchers. Instead of worrying about the cost of a new workstation, researchers will be more concerned whether a particular query is "computationally expensive"—taking up more of the network's resources and presumably costing more. "Agent" technology—software programs that allow an end-user to automatically search databases—will become more and more sophisticated. These agents may be built using JAVA, and additional ones can be purchased to allow increased flexibility and functionality. Ultimately, these software creations will serve the role of a librarian and research assistant, and may even have some "interpretive skills" to assess the relative significance of a particular abstract in one's field of interest. Multiple agents may be deployed to simultaneously build a highly sophisticated and interwoven computer model.

GAME MACHINES AND NEUROSCIENCE

Another area of growth in the computer science arena that will have an astonishing effect on neuroscience research is that of entertainment. Computer game development is pushing the graphics industry to achieve price/

performance ratios that were inconceivable a few years ago. This year, the fruits of a collaboration between Silicon Graphics and Nintendo will be unveiled, a game machine called the "Ultra-64." This machine, which has many of the advanced graphics features found only on $100,000-plus visualization workstations, will be available at a price of $250. Because the home-game console market represents an industry with more than a $6 billion dollar annual revenue, large research and development budgets are possible in this area.

The implications game machines have for neuroscience research are many-fold. To successfully develop a virtual environment that is realistic for an end-user, one must have an understanding of sensory physiology. The way in which the mind detects motion and perceives detail is critical in the construction of a realistic game architecture. A visualization computer (whether it is a game machine or a supercomputer) has a finite amount of graphics capabilities—usually defined as pixel-fill rates (the rapidity with which the computer can draw on a screen) and the polygon-per-second count (the speed with which the computer can represent three-dimensional geometry on the screen). As a result, many compromises must be made in order to create realistic imaging. Such compromises include representing objects with less detail when they are further from the field of view or when they are obstructed by other objects, and deploying many other tricks in both visual and behavioral representation to create an environment that can fool the eye.

One result of the increased realism of these systems is their use in psychiatry; specifically for treating agoraphobia. As the systems become more and more powerful, it may be possible to construct real-time stimulation/feedback experiments in which the interaction between subtle changes in synthetic environments will be mapped to changes in parameters derived from biophysical studies and vice-versa. The concept of using computer games to study functional plasticity of the brain has initially been attempted, and an example of how computer games are helping to understand the functional plasticity of the brain as a result of experience has recently been reported. In the studies thus far, it has been shown that after training with computer games designed to hone their temporal processing skills for acoustic stimuli, language-learning-impaired children improved their game scores and also raised their performance on standardized tests using normal unmodified speech. Thus, theirs is a demonstration that changes in processing of sensory inputs can be modified and that these disabled persons can be trained through the use of computer games.

There will almost certainly be new methods for human–computer interfaces beyond those commonly in use today. And these new interfaces may very well lead to a time in the near future in which double-blind studies will confirm the use of specialized games as accepted treatments for a wide range of neurological disorders.

Applications of Fourier Transform Infrared Imaging Microscopy in Neurotoxicity

E. NEIL LEWIS,[a,d] LINDA H. KIDDER,[a] IRA W. LEVIN,[a] VICTOR F. KALASINSKY,[b] JOSEPH P. HANIG[c] AND DAVID S. LESTER[c]

[a]*Laboratory of Chemical Physics*
National Institute of Diabetes and Digestive and Kidney Diseases
National Institutes of Health
Bethesda, Maryland 20892

[b]*Department of Environmental and Toxicologic Pathology*
Armed Forces Institute of Pathology
Washington, DC 20306

[c]*Center for Drug Evaluation and Research*
Food and Drug Administration
Laurel, Maryland 20708

INTRODUCTION

The spatial distribution of components within complex materials strongly influences both their physical and chemical properties. Thus, analytical methods that provide information on both the localization and molecular characteristics of composite materials are invaluable in disciplines as diverse as the design and fabrication of advanced materials or the chemical and biochemical elucidation of cellular systems. Spectroscopic imaging is a particularly attractive method since it can provide simultaneous information on both the spatial and chemical properties of an intact system while preserving sample integrity. In applications to biological specimens, for example, spectral imaging is also suitable for noninvasive biophysical analyses and biomedical diagnoses performed *in vivo.* Therefore, spectral imaging allows both the researcher and clinician to rapidly visualize sample "chemistry" with minimum sample preparation and disruption.

Spectral imaging extends the power of spectroscopic analysis by generating spatial information while retaining the analytical capability provided by traditional, nonimaging spectroscopies. For example, nuclear magnetic resonance techniques[1] are applied for whole-body diagnostic imaging, whereas for investigation of the microscale, fluorescence microscopy[2,3] is an effective chemical state imaging. Chemical visualization methods integrating micros-

[d]Corresponding author. Phone: 301-496-6847; fax: 301-496-0825; e-mail: neil@spy.niddk.nih.gov

copy and vibrational spectroscopic methods, including Raman,[4–6] near-infrared (NIR),[7,8] and mid-infrared (IR)[9] spectroscopies have become especially popular because of their ability to generate chemical images based on the substance's molecular vibrations, precluding the need for potentially invasive dyes or tags and extensive sample preparation.

Infrared spectroscopy, in particular, is an extremely versatile and powerful analytical method that is used extensively in research environments, general analytical laboratories, and quality-control settings. The technique is readily applied to record spectra of gases, liquids, and solids and is simple, low cost, and portable. In addition, in most cases little or no sample preparation is required before spectra can be recorded. Another advantage is that digitized spectra of a large number of materials are available in databases and, with the use of computers, can be automatically compared to newly acquired data. In many cases infrared analytical procedures can be, and are, fully automated. The utility of infrared spectroscopy originates in the wealth of compositional and quantitative information contained in a single infrared (IR) spectrum of a given sample. The spectral observables, represented by frequency, intensity, and linewidth parameters, sensitively reflect a sample's molecular structure and provide specific fingerprints for a given molecular component. In addition, infrared spectroscopy directly provides quantitative concentration data from the application of Beer's law.[10,11]

While the spectroscopic techniques and experimental conditions of spectral imaging vary widely, there are traditionally two principal methods used for image construction. The scanning approach is typically used with single-element detection and involves either (1) scanning of the sample systematically through a stationary field of view defined by the collection optics and detector or (2) scanning the imaging source (or detector) in a raster pattern across the surface of the stationary sample. For example, Fourier transform infrared (FTIR) functional group imaging utilizes an *xy* translation stage and a mid-infrared microscope to vibrationally map a sample.[12] Usable signal/noise ratios obtained by this technique require extended signal averaging at each spatial position, resulting in an inherently slow technique. Also, time constraints often allow for only crude spatial maps to be determined.

Another image-generation approach involves wide-field illumination and multichannel-detection viewing, by illuminating a stained sample with a broadband visible source and then viewing it with a color video camera. This technique is simply implemented and widely used in video microscopy of biologics and materials.[13] When greater specificity is required, optical filtering can be employed. For example, fluorescence microscopes use filters or lasers to selectively excite within the absorption band of the fluorescent label. Long-pass emission filters are used to block nonfluorescent reflected excitation energy as well as stray light prior to imaging. Multiple fluorescent labels can be used in conjunction with more than one emission filter for the simultaneous detection of several bands.[14] The bandpass filter method is satisfactory where tunability is unnecessary and relatively low spectral resolution (>5 nm) will suffice. For both spectral tunability and rapid operation, an acousto-optic-based system that has been developed for near-infrared and Raman imaging[4,6,7,15] may also be applicable to fluorescence imaging.[15,16]

We have developed a new Fourier transform infrared chemical imaging technique,[17] which, when coupled with powerful multivariate data-processing methods, allows the visualization of complex intrinsic chemical distributions in biological materials and the potential for performing rapid histological examinations. In the infrared spectral region the technique relies on the use of infrared focal-plane array detectors, a newly developed commercial technology. These array detectors are used in conjunction with standard Cassegrainian infrared microscopes and commercially available step-scan Michelson FTIR spectrometers to construct infrared imaging systems capable of collecting tens of thousands of spatially resolved infrared spectra (3 μm^2) in less than 1 minute of data-acquisition time. The data sets contain both spatial and spectral information and typically consist of hundreds of images resolved in frequency space (wave numbers, cm^{-1}), with each image comprising many tens of thousands of pixels. This novel, high-definition technique represents both a new biological imaging tool and perhaps the future of infrared chemical imaging analysis.

In order to demonstrate the capabilities of this new infrared imaging technique, we studied an established system of cellular toxicity. Standard histopathological procedures have demonstrated that the antineoplastic drug cytarabine (Ara-C) exhibits neurotoxicity at high concentrations in both human and animal models. In the rat model, this neurotoxic response has been traced to the cytotoxic action of this pharmacological agent on the cerebellar Purkinje cell layer, a single cell layer that plays a significant role in motor control and, possibly, in learning and memory. The Purkinje cells in the rat cerebellum are large in size (approx. 20 μm) and lie between the molecular and granular cell layers. Thus, cerebellar tissue is composed of cell types with the appropriate mix of diversity and size to investigate the histopathological potential of this emerging technology.

EXPERIMENTAL PROCEDURES

Infrared Step-scan Interferometric Imaging Technique

The strategy of combining an infrared detector array with an interferometer provides a spectroscopic *multiplex/multichannel* advantage. The multiple-detector elements enable spectra from all pixels to be collected simultaneously, while the modulation of infrared radiation by the interferometer allows all the spectral frequencies across the wavelength range to be measured concurrently. The step-scan imaging approach provides chemically distinct, mid-infrared images and spectra with unprecedented speed and quality. The image fidelity is limited only by the number of pixels contained on the array.

For example, we have recorded infrared chemical image data sets containing 16,384 spatially resolved FTIR spectra at 16 cm^{-1} resolution with data-acquisition times of only 12 s. That is, the detector array consists of 16,384 pixels, each of which generates a complete infrared spectrum at the end of the interferometric scan. While the spectral resolution was limited to 16 cm^{-1} in these experiments due to the complexity of handling large data sets (20 megabytes per experiment), the spectral resolution for each data set is dependent on the interferometer's mirror displacement, which may be readily extended for the acquisition of higher-spectral-resolution images.

In operation, the imaging lens system collects and collimates the light and presents it to the 50/50 beamsplitter of the FT interferometer. The two halves of light are transmitted to two plane mirrors, one of which is moveable. The light is reflected back onto the beamsplitter, where it is recombined and optically interferes either constructively or destructively. This interference image is then projected toward the multichannel detector. If the path difference between the beamsplitter and both mirrors is equivalent, the two beams recombine constructively and the detector measures the total intensity of the light through the microscope. To collect spectra, the movable mirror is stepped at small reproducible increments, with an image being recorded at each step. The optical interference is different at each retardation, and the image intensity on the detector changes as the interferometer scans. By collecting a sequence of images and performing a Fourier transform of the data at each pixel, spectral images are reconstructed corresponding to discrete wavelengths of the optical absorption or emission spectrum.

FIGURE 1 shows the high-definition step-scan FTIR microscope. The instrument comprises a commercially available mid-infrared Michelson-type step-scan interferometer (Bio-Rad FTS-6000) coupled to an IR microscope (Bio-Rad UMA 600) containing a matched 15× Cassegrainian condenser/objective pair. The detector is an indium antimonide (InSb) focal-plane array (FPA) detector (ImagIR, Santa Barbara Focalplane). The microscope optics and interferometer electronics were modified to couple efficiently with the InSb camera. Optical modifications included the addition of a CaF_2 50-mm image-formation lens placed between the microscope objective and infrared camera. Synchronization of the interferometer step sequence with the camera was performed by the addition of a counter/timer board, which, in conjunction with the computer, controlled the camera frame acquisitions.

The experiment was performed such that each time the interferometer mirror was retarded, a TTL pulse was generated by the spectrometer and recorded by the counter/timer board; this, in turn, triggered the collection of a series of image frames by the infrared camera. Each 12-bit image frame in the series was summed, averaged, and written as a 32-bit floating-point file. The final data set therefore consisted of 128 × 128 floating-point images collected at several hundred different interferometer retardations.

Although InSb detectors are sensitive from 1 to 5.5 μm, the optical bandpass for this experiment was limited to 2–4 μm (5000–2500 cm^{-1}) by an optical filter placed inside the detector cold shield. Bandpass filtering was performed for two reasons: first, by minimizing the longer-wavelength blackbody radiation emitted from all the optical surfaces in the instrument, the total signal integrated by the detector that is not related to source brightness, and therefore sample absorption, is reduced; second, reduction of the spectral bandwidth of the instrument enables a larger interferometer step size (undersampling) to be chosen between image frames. Undersampling without optical filtering can cause spectral artifacts as a consequence of frequency aliasing. The larger step size for the experiment provides higher spectral resolution with fewer data points, therefore minimizing the number of images to be collected. This, in turn, reduces the storage and processing requirements for the resulting data set.

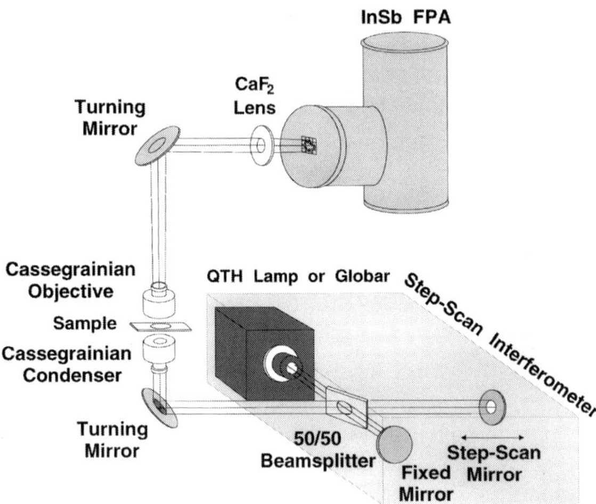

FIGURE 1. Step-scan infrared imaging system. A commercial FTIR step-scan interferometer (*shown in box*) is coupled to an IR microscope with Cassegrainian (reflective) optics and a CaF_2 image-formation lens. Samples mounted on quartz microscope slides are analyzed in transmission mode. The image is projected to a liquid-nitrogen-cooled InSb FPA detector containing 128×128 pixels. The interferometer timing and image acquisition is controlled externally via a computer (not shown).

The total data-acquisition or "staring" time for the camera for each complete data set of 16,384 spectra was approximately 16 s. To collect each image, a frame was integrated for 2 ms, with 32 frames being averaged for each interferometer mirror position. A total of 256 mirror positions were recorded for each complete spectral-image data set. After apodization, a single-sided interferogram containing 300 data points yielded a nominal spectral resolution for each image of 16 cm^{-1}.

Data collection and processing are similar to those performed for conventional FTIR studies with the exception that much larger data sets are handled.

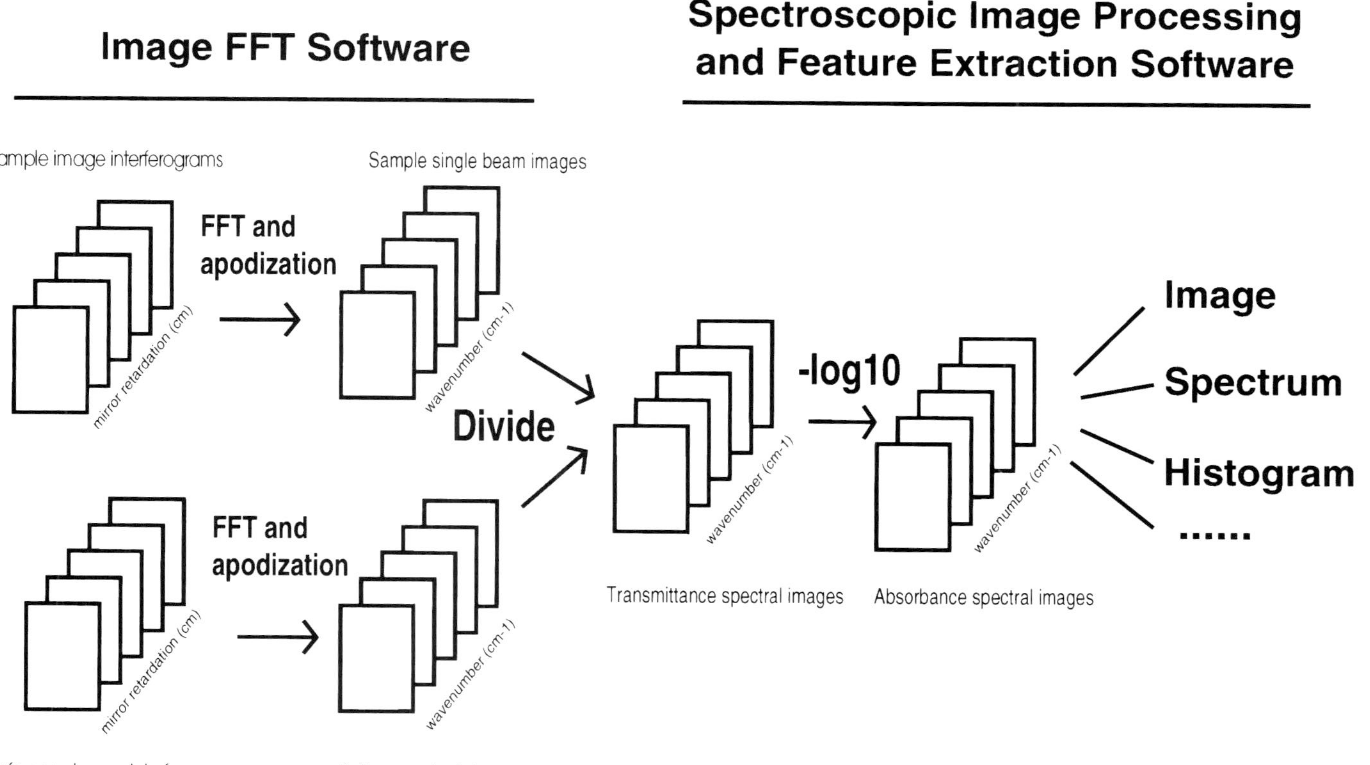

FIGURE 2. The multidimensional data sets acquired by the step-scan imaging system and the method used for data processing and feature extraction.

FIGURE 2 shows a typical data-processing sequence. Analysis involves the collection of a step-scan image sequence data set of a background, typically air. Then, using identical sampling parameters, a step-scan sequence is collected, with a sample placed under the microscope. The spatial/spectral interferometric data are organized in a 32-bit/pixel spectral image file format (SPIFF).[16] The interferograms at each pixel in the data sets are apodized and Fourier transformed with commercial software (Spectral Dimensions) to yield a total of 16,384 FTIR spectra for both the background and sample data sets. The two data sets are then ratioed to yield infrared transmittance images of the sample over the spectral range of 3950–1975 cm^{-1}. Finally, the infrared image data-set spectra are converted to absorbance.

SPIFF files are visualized with commercial spectral-image visualization software (ISIS, Spectral Dimensions) and image-processing software (*Optimas 4.02,* Optimas). For publication, digital images are printed on a dye sublimation printer (Tektronix, Phaser 440).

Infrared Imaging Detectors

High-sensitivity, cooled-silicon CCD cameras have revolutionized Raman and fluorescence spectroscopy. Analogously, multichannel IR imaging detectors, which were originally developed for military and surveillance applications[19–21] and are now commercially accessible, are expected to have a significant impact in the fields of near-infrared and infrared spectroscopy and imaging. The integration of these devices with image-quality spectral filters to perform near-infrared and infrared imaging has recently been described.[8,9]

In this study we have used an indium antimonide focal-plane array detector (InSb). InSb FPA detectors are multichannel imaging devices providing sensitive detection between 1 and 5.5 μm. One-dimensional InSb FPAs, which use line scanning to produce two-dimensional images, have been used in thermal imaging,[22] as well as in spectroscopic applications including remote sensing of earth's resources[20] and the Visible Infrared Mapping Spectrometer (VIMS) Instrument on the Mars Observer Spacecraft.[23] One-dimensional FPAs employed in night-vision applications use rapidly rotating mirrors to scan a target scene sequentially across the linear array. Scanned systems have limited sensitivity due to short dwell times of any one element of the scene on any one sensor pixel.

Two-dimensional InSb staring arrays have existed since the 1970s[19] and have been employed in the 3–5-μm range for thermal sensing and night-vision applications[24] and IR astronomy.[25] The formats of the early two-dimensional InSb FPA detectors were limited to 32 × 32 pixel architectures, but, at present, cameras having up to 256 × 256 pixels are commercially available. Two-dimensional staring FPAs have the advantage of no moving parts, and the required response time of the detector is less stringent.

InSb is not the only detector material available for imaging applications in the infrared. For example, two-dimensional FPAs based on platinum silicide

(PtSi), indium gallium arsenide (InGaAs), germanium (Ge), mercury cadmium telluride (MCT), and arsenic-doped silicon (Si:As) are available. Fundamental issues such as detector sensitivity, wavelength range, array uniformity, ease of fabrication, and detector ruggedness are determining factors that govern detector selection.

Preparation of Samples

Male adult Sprague-Dawley rats (250–275 g) were injected with either a bolus of saline or 260 mg/kg of cytarabine (Upjohn) twice a day for 5 days. The animals were then maintained under standard maintenance conditions for 20 days. Animals were sacrificed and the cerebellum rapidly removed and immediately frozen by covering with powdered dry ice. Samples were kept at −80°C until the time of sectioning. Frozen sections were cut (10 μm) on a Hacker cryostat at a temperature of −21°C. The slices were placed on calcium fluoride disks (Wilmad) and then stored in a dessicator at 4°C until the time of analysis.

RESULTS AND DISCUSSION

FIGURE 3A shows a portion of a USAF 1951 resolution target (Newport) image and a corresponding line plot drawn through group 6 (FIG. 3B). The practical spatial resolution and image quality can be quantified by the modulation transfer function (MTF). The MTF describes the image contrast of the system as a function of bar target spatial frequency (line pairs/mm), and is measured by plotting a line through the image plane in either the *x*- or *y*-dimension. The percent contrast for the target shown in FIGURE 3B, having a center-to-center spacing of 5.5 μm, is approximately 22% ± 2.0%. According to the Rayleigh criterion, features are just resolved at the 26.5% image-contrast level. Based on the MTF, it is anticipated that the practical resolution of the step-scan imaging system using the current optics will approach the diffraction limit.

FIGURE 4 shows both an infrared bright-field image (A) and infrared spectroscopic image (B) of a brain slice extracted from a cytarabine-treated rat cerebellum. Panel B has been processed by ratioing two images from the data set: one corresponding to a lipid absorption band at approximately 2927 cm^{-1} and the other corresponding to a protein absorption band at approximately 3350 cm^{-1}. The contrast in this resulting image is due entirely to differences in the lipid/protein ratio in the different cell layers. The bright yellow and red band running through the middle of the image in panel B corresponds to the molecular layer that contains a disproportinately high percentage of lipid relative to the other layers. This chemically specific contrast is intrinsic to a specific sample and is obtained without the use of dyes or stains. FIGURE 5 shows four infrared spectra extracted from the same data set corresponding to four distinct cellular regions within the section. From

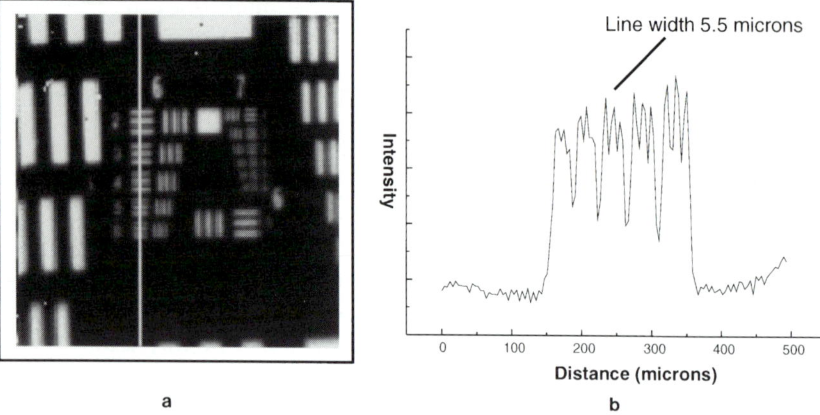

FIGURE 3. Step-scan interferometer image of a USAF 1951 resolution target. **(A)** InSb infrared image collected at interferometer zero path difference (ZPD); **(B)** line plot through group 6 of the resolution target showing the change in relative image contrast for bars of progressively higher spatial frequency.

these spectra it can be clearly seen that the signatures are different and change dramatically from one cell layer to another. The cluster of peaks centered around 2920 cm^{-1} corresponds primarily to CH stretching modes of the hydrocarbon chains of the lipids in the sample, while the broadband centered

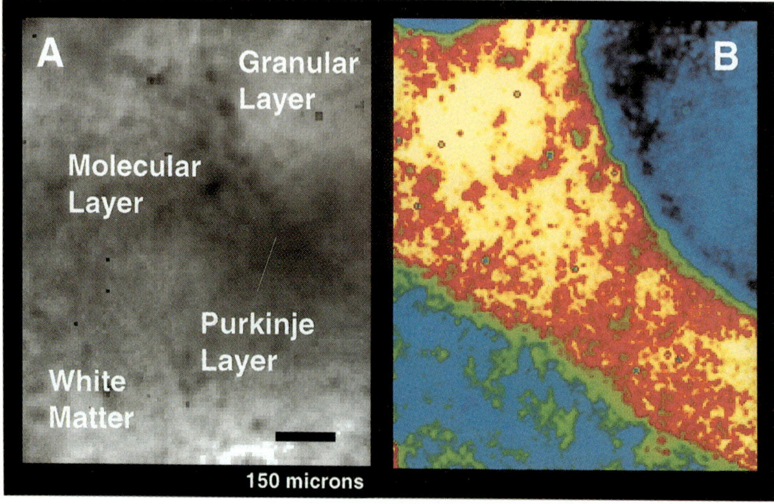

FIGURE 4. Infrared bright-field image **(A)** and spectroscopic image **(B)** of a cytarabine-treated brain slice from a rat cerebellum. The infrared spectroscopic image was created from two images that highlighted both the lipid and protein fractions of the tissue. The resulting combination image shows the variation in the lipid/protein ratio in the various cell layers.

around 3350 cm^{-1} arises from the protein species in the specimen. It is the differences in the relative intensities of these features that has been exploited to create the image in FIGURE 4B. As shown, the lipid/protein ratio varies dramatically from one cell layer to another, and is the lowest for the Purkinje cell layer (FIG. 5 panel D). This cell layer therefore appears the darkest in the spectroscopic image in FIGURE 4B. These and other differences can be used to create many different chemical images of the same sample. Thus, the wide variety of spectral signatures that occur from different chemical species can be

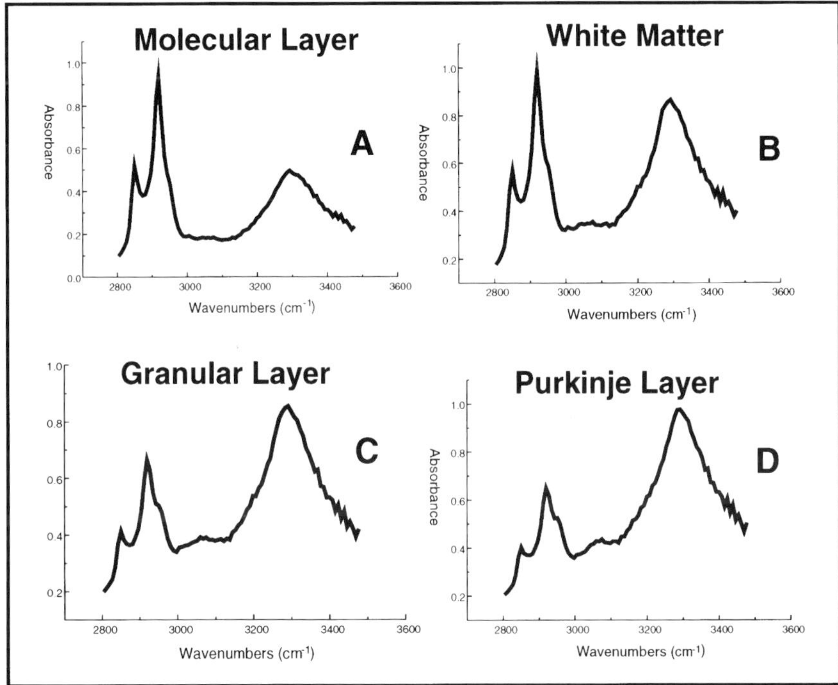

FIGURE 5. Infrared spectra extracted from the data set that provided the images for FIGURE 4. The panels show the variation of the spectral signature for each of the four distinct cellular regions in the cerebellum.

used to create images that are specific to a given chemical species. Very often, however, there are more subtle spectral changes that occur within the same chemical species or material as a result of changes in conformation or bonding within the sample. These changes can result in, for example, a line width change or a frequency shift of one of the peaks. This more subtle effect can also be exploited in creating new images. For example, FIGURE 6B shows an image created from the same sample and data set as shown in FIGURES 4 and 5. This image, however, was created by measuring the frequency of the band centered at 2850 cm^{-1}, a feature that corresponds to the CH_2 symmetric stretching mode. Using an algorithm that determines the center of gravity of this peak, each of the 16,384 spectra in the data set were measured, and a corresponding gray-scale image was created that was either brighter or darker in a continuous fashion, depending on whether the peak position for a particular pixel had shifted to a higher or lower frequency. Although there is significant noise in this image resulting from the degree of uncertainty in fitting the peak position, several interesting features can be discerned from this image. First, the individual cell layers can still be identified; and second,

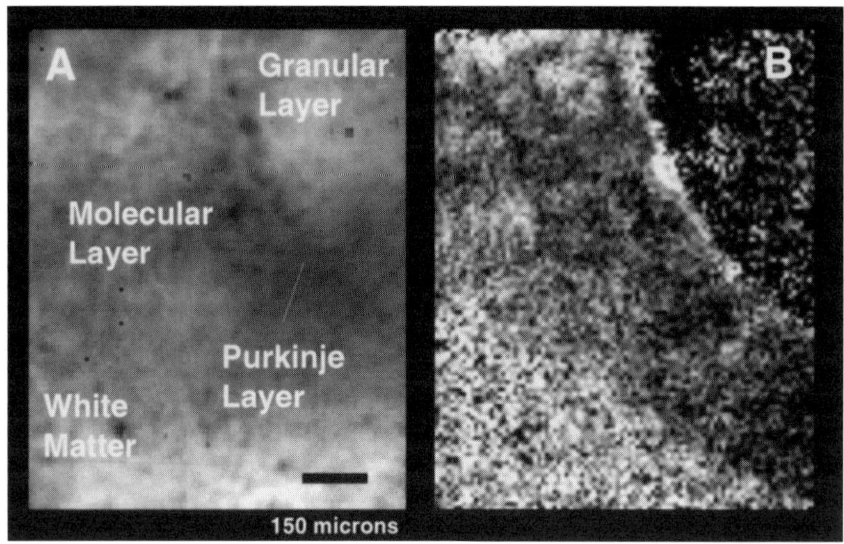

FIGURE 6. Infrared bright-field image **(A)** and spectroscopic image **(B)** of a cytarabine-treated brain slice from a rat cerebellum. The infrared spectroscopic image was created by computing the frequencies for the lipid chain CH_2 symmetric stretching modes for all 16,384 spectra and converting the results into gray-scale values. The image provides information on the spatial variation of the lipid-packing arrangements in the cell membrane for each of the layers in the sample.

the Purkinje cell layer shows up as a brighter semicircular "band" that runs from the top of the image to the center of the right-hand side. The brighter region suggests that the frequency of the CH_2 symmetric stretching mode is higher for this cell layer than for the others. This higher frequency is indicative of a greater ratio of *gauche* to *trans* isomers along the hydrocarbon chains of the lipids comprising the membranes in this cell layer. This finding is consistent with the images and spectra shown in FIGURES 4 and 5, which indicated that the cell layer has a relatively higher protein content. This elevated protein contribution results in a disordered packing arrangement for the lipid acyl chains; that is, additional *gauche* isomers were induced per chain.

CONCLUSIONS

Future developments of the technique will come from detectors with extended wavelength ranges. We are currently developing instrumentation with a new array[26] exhibiting sensitivity from 1 to 25 μm (10,000–400 cm^{-1}) that will allow one, for the first time, to image in the infrared "fingerprint" region. Since the fingerprint region of the infrared spectra represents the wavelength range that contains most of the infrared absorption bands, many more basic and subtle chemical characteristics of the sample can be imaged. Integration of conventional digital image-enhancement techniques with chemometric methods generally used for the analysis of conventional infrared spectra will provide additional power in processing the complex data sets recorded by this new imaging approach. These additional processing tools will enable both qualitative and quantitative determinations of complex samples to be made and will provide additional parameters with which to reconstruct new images for highlighting chemical properties.

The potential areas of application of this technology overlap those areas where traditional infrared spectroscopy has proved valuable. The ability to image a variety of biological or synthetic materials and products either microscopically or macroscopically, while simultaneously determining chemical composition, should be a potent tool. Applications in remote sensing or process monitoring and control in industrial environments are also possible. Specifically, for biological applications, the future should also be rich and varied. Studies underway in this laboratory include the chemical imaging of cholesterol gradients within retinal rod outer segments and neurotoxicity problems associated with other drug treatments. In addition, we are applying the technique to the histopathological characterization of tissue sections derived from human biopsies. Tissue can contain a number of different foreign inclusions originating from a variety of surgical procedures. This technique can readily visualize micron-sized particles of foreign matter in human tissue and chemically identify them. Details of these and other studies will be described in forthcoming papers.

REFERENCES

1. Kalmar, J. A., J. J. Eick, C. R. Merritt, S. E. Schuler, K. D. Miller, G. B. McFarland & J. J. Jones. 1988. Orthopedics **11:** 417.
2. Taylor, D. L. & Y. L. Wang, Eds. 1989. Methods in Cell Biology, Vol. 30. Academic Press. New York, NY.
3. Lester, D. S., D. L. Alkon & J. L. Olds. 1994. NeuroImage **1:** 264.
4. Treado, P. J., I. W. Levin & E. N. Lewis. 1992. Appl. Spectrosc. **46:** 1211–1216.
5. Puppels, G. J., M. Grond & J. Greve. 1993. Appl. Spectrosc. **47:** 1256.

6. GOLDSTEIN, S. R., L. H. KIDDER, T. M. HERNE, I. W. LEVIN & E. N. LEWIS. 1996. J. Microscopy. In press.
7. TREADO, P. J., I. W. LEVIN & E. N. LEWIS. 1992. Appl. Spectrosc. **46:** 553–559.
8. TREADO, P. J., I. W. LEVIN & E. N. LEWIS. 1994. Appl. Spectrosc. **48:** 607–615.
9. LEWIS, E. N. & I. W. LEVIN. 1995. Appl. Spectrosc. **49:** 672–678.
10. LIN-VIEN, D., N. B. COLTHUP, W. G. FATELEY & J. G. GRASSELLI. 1991. The Handbook of Infrared and Raman Characteristic Frequencies of Organic Molecules. Academic Press. New York, NY.
11. PARKER, F. S. 1983. Applications of Infrared, Raman, and Resonance Raman Spectroscopy in Biochemistry. Plenum Press. New York, NY.
12. HARTHCOCK, M. A. & S. C. ATKIN. 1988. Appl. Spectrosc. **42:** 449.
13. INOUE, S. 1986. Video Microscopy. Plenum Press. New York, NY.
14. JOHNSON, R. L. 1991. Photonics Spectra **25(10):** 126.
15. WANG, X. & E. N. LEWIS. 1996. *In* Fluorescence Imaging Spectroscopy and Microscopy. X. F. Wang & B. Herman, Eds. Wiley. New York, NY.
16. SPRING, K. R. & P. D. SMITH. 1987. J. Microscopy **147:** 265–278.
17. LEWIS, E. N., P. J. TREADO, R. C. REEDER, G. M. STORY, A. E. DOWREY, C. MARCOTT & I. W. LEVIN. 1995. Anal. Chem. **67:** 3377.
18. ChemImag Technical Reference Manual. 1995. ChemIcon. Pittsburgh, PA.
19. BAILEY, G. C. 1979. Proc. SPIE **197:** 83.
20. BAILEY, G. C., K. MATTHEWS & C. A. NIBLACK. 1983. Proc. SPIE **430:** 52.
21. BLESSINGER, M. A., R. C. FISCHER, C. J. MARTIN, C. A. NIBLACK & H. A. TIMLIN. 1990. Proc. SPIE **1235:** 204.
22. FUJISADA, H., M. NAKAYAMA & A. TANAKA. 1992. Proc. SPIE **1341:** 80.
23. DUVALL, J. 1987. Proc. SPIE **685:** 121.
24. PARRISH, W. J., J. BLACKWELL, R. PAULSON & H. ARNOLD. 1991. Proc. SPIE **1512:** 68.
25. FORREST, W. J. & J. L. PIPHER. 1986. NASA Tech. Memo. **88213:** 11.
26. ARENS, J. F., J. G. JERNIGAN, M. C. PECK, C. A. DOBSON, E. KILK, J. LACY & S. GAALEMA. 1987. Appl. Opt. **26:** 3846–3851.

DISCUSSION

QUESTION: This is a question for the forum. In general, there's been a number of talks that involved the use of infrared radiation. I wonder about the different sorts of technical constraints. I noticed that your samples are all thin sections. Can you do reflectance measurements?

LEWIS: We can do reflectance, although we haven't at this point. It's actually a little more challenging because there's less energy to work with than in transmission. But you're right, for transmission measurements you're limited to thin sections.

QUESTION: But could your technique, for example, be applied to a thicker slice of tissue or a piece of living tissue?

LEWIS: Yes. In the near-infrared you can increase the thickness of the material by a factor of 10.

QUESTION: Can you get depth-specific information, or are you basically looking at the entire light path?

LEWIS: You're looking at the entire light path the way that we did it. But you can reconstruct depth information using digital deconvolution techniques.

QUESTION: It seems to me that you have no way of doing 3D-slice selection, whereas with MRI you can. Here your wave-number axis is really not measuring a slice per se, or is it?

LEWIS: No, it's just choice of words—"frequency slice" as opposed to "sample slice." It's inherently a two-dimensional optical image where the additional dimensionality is chemical, not spatial.

QUESTION: I have a question about sensitivity. In terms of the concentration dependency, how much of a component do you need to have before you're going to see a peak above background or noise?

LEWIS: That's a tough question because different vibrational modes have different intensities, and bands overlap; so it's hard to say for a given species what's measurable and what's not. We've actually created images using very low intensity peaks. You don't have much signal to work with, so spectral noise gets translated into image noise. But you can obtain meaningful contrast. Also, you can use multivariate classification techniques and do a whole host of other analyses. We're only beginning to scratch the surface of what's possible.

QUESTION: You mentioned that the technique was both qualitative and quantitative. Do you think that you could see different degrees of lipid disposition based on drug treatment and do that in a quantitative way?

LEWIS: I don't know what the answer to that is. There are lots of variables affecting our ability to generate quantitative information—for example, uniform illumination. For the most part, we take image ratios, so we have some kind of internal standardization. But the technique is really in its infancy; I don't know what the ultimate capabilities and sensitivities are going to be.

Advances in Optical Imaging of Biomedical Media[a]

R. R. ALFANO,[b] S. G. DEMOS, AND S. K. GAYEN

Institute for Ultrafast Spectroscopy and Lasers
New York State Center for Advanced Technology for Ultrafast Photonic Materials and Applications
Physics Department
The City College of the City University of New York
New York, New York 10031

INTRODUCTION

Optical imaging of biomedical media is a rapidly growing research area that, in recent years, has attracted the concerted and coordinated efforts of researchers from diverse disciplines. The impetus for these intense research activities derives from a need for imaging modalities that are safe, noninvasive, inexpensive, and capable of monitoring body chemistry *in vivo,* preferably in real time. Although the currently available body-imaging techniques such as X-ray imaging, X-ray computed tomography (CT), magnetic resonance imaging (MRI), ultrasound, and radioisotope imaging are well developed and provide useful information,[c] there still are important limitations. For example, a major limitation of the available techniques is the inability to detect tumors in early stages, when they are most treatable. X-ray imaging, the most frequently used technique, is not suitable for imaging young dense breasts, may not distinguish between malignant and benign tumors, and may be potentially harmful if used too often for routine screening. Other limitations include (1) limited or lack of specificity to key chemicals that need to be monitored for functional body imaging, (2) potential health hazard, (3) resolution, and (4) cost.

Optical imaging modalities are sought to alleviate the majority of these limitations and to complement the existing techniques. A salient advantage of an optical imaging method is its potential for simultaneous diagnosis of disease that affects the body part to be imaged. This diagnostic ability follows from the fact that the characteristics of absorption, emission, and excitation spectra of normal tissues are often significantly different from those of infected tissues. The spectral signature of a particular lesion may thus be

[a]This work is supported in part by the New York State Technology Foundation, the Office of Naval Research, and Mediscience Technology Corporation.

[b]Corresponding author. Phone: (212) 650-5531; fax: (212) 650-5530; e-mail; alfano@scisun.sci.ccny.cuny.edu

[c]For a review of body imaging modalities, please see *The Physics of Medical Imaging,* S. Webb, Ed. Institute of Physics Publishing, Bristol (1988).

identified by wavelength-dependent measurements. In addition, even prolonged exposure to near-infrared (NIR) and visible light is not known to pose any safety problem. However, the major impediment in the development of biomedical optical imaging modalities is the strong scattering of light by tissues. Multiple-scattered light provides a noise background that deteriorates and, in extreme cases, may wash out any shadow image of structures inside the tissue that may be formed by forward-propagating light.

This article reviews some of the methods developed for shadowgram imaging by extracting image-bearing photons from the background of multiple-scattered light, and presents initial results of measurements on brain and breast tissues.

BACKGROUND

The objective of any biomedical imaging technique is to identify, locate, and diagnose an "object," such as a tumor, inside a biological tissue. In its simplest form, an optical imaging procedure would involve illuminating the part of the body to be imaged with bright light and to search for indication of pathology in the observed transillumination pattern. The physical basis of transillumination is the difference in the transmission of light through normal tissue and an object inside it. This differential transmission, in principle, should lead to the formation of a "shadow" of the tumor in transmitted light. However, a biological tissue absorbs and strongly scatters the light that passes through it. The scattered light severely degrades the quality of the shadow image, and for thick tissues, may wash it out. The key to the successful development of optical imaging techniques is to deal effectively with the problem of light scattering.

An important step in resolving the problem is to understand how light propagates through a highly scattering medium. Characteristics such as intensity, coherence, and polarization of the incident light change as it is absorbed and scattered inside the tissue. The extent of these changes depends on the wavelength of light, the type of tissue through which it propagates, and the tissue thickness. Consequently, the light that emerges from the medium has very different characteristics compared to the incident light. The transmitted light comprises three components,[1,2] commonly referred to as the *ballistic, snake,* and *diffuse* photons, as displayed[3] in FIGURE 1.

The ballistic or coherently scattered photons propagate in the incident direction, traverse the shortest path, and carry the maximum information about the interior structure of the scattering medium. The diffuse light comprises multiple-scattered photons that travel long distances within the medium, carry little information about the structures inside the medium, and emerge later in all directions. The snake photons scatter slightly in the forward direction and retain significant initial properties and information on structures inside the scattering medium.

Since the photons of an incident short pulse of light spend different times in transit through the intervening medium, the transmitted pulse becomes broadened with the ballistic photons arriving first, followed by the snake and diffusive photons, also displayed in FIGURE 1. Ballistic photons are most effective in forming a shadow image. Snake photons also generate transillumination images whose resolution depend on the temporal slice of snake photons used for imaging. The snake photons that form a well-defined shadow image arrive much earlier than the diffuse photons. The intensity of the forward-transmitted light is attenuated by absorption and scattering. The relative intensities of the three components in the transmitted beam varies, depending on the color of light and characteristics of the sample.

The optical parameters that affect the attenuation and propagation of light through a medium are absorption coefficient (μ_a), scattering coefficient (μ_s), anisotropy factor (g), and index of refraction (n). The scattering coefficient

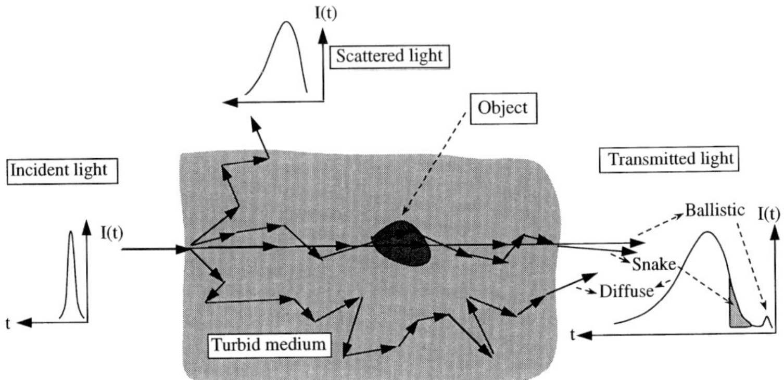

FIGURE 1. A schematic diagram of light scattering by a turbid medium showing the ballistic, snake, and diffuse photons, as well as the changes in the temporal profile of a pulse of light. (From Gayen and Alfano.[3] Reproduced by permission.)

and anisotropy factor depend strongly on the relative size of the scatterers within the medium and the wavelength of light. Accurate values of these parameters as a function of wavelength are essential for the modeling of light transport through tissues. The respective intensities of the ballistic, snake, and diffuse components of transmitted light exhibit different functional dependence on these parameters. In highly turbid media, such as biological tissues, the ballistic component is extremely weak, the snake component is somewhat stronger, while the diffusive component is the most intense. To form images of the structures inside the turbid medium using the ballistic and/or snake photons, the more numerous diffusive photons need be strongly discriminated against.

Two alternate approaches are being pursued to deal with the problem of scattered light. The first approach involves selecting the image-bearing photons from the background of multiple-scattered image-blurring photons using clever experimental techniques.[1–29] The image-bearing photons are then used to form a *shadowgram* of the object inside the scattering medium. The second approach, sometimes referred to as the *inverse problem,* is based on the detection of multiple-scattered photons at various positions around the object. The aim is to construct the image from these measured intensities, known experimental parameters, and tissue characteristics, using models of light propagation and sophisticated computer algorithms. The impetus for solving the inverse problem stems from the realization that for tissues that are more than a few centimeters thick, the only transmitted light is the diffuse light.[30,31]

Several schemes have evolved over the years to sort out the image-bearing ballistic and snake photons from the multiple-scattered diffuse photons. These schemes exploit one or more of the changes that scattering induces on the characteristics, such as directionality, polarization, coherence, and temporal duration of the incident light. Since the image-bearing photons change the least, the idea is to devise a *gate* that will let the photons with a specific initial property through but block others. There are *space, time, polarization,* and *absorption* gates. A space gate exploits the fact that the ballistic and snake photons come out of the tissue in the incident direction, while the multiple-scattered light emerges in all directions. So, a small aperture centered on the line of incidence and placed after the sample will collect the on-line-transmitted light and effectively discriminate against most of the off-axis scattered light. Similarly, a time gate capitalizes on the fact that image-bearing photons emerge from the sample sooner than the diffusive photons. To realize a time gate in practice, one then needs a shutter that will open for a short duration, typically a few picoseconds, to let the early photons through and then close in time to leave out the delayed scattered photons. Similar gating schemes based on polarization and coherence of light have also been devised. Often a single gate may not be discriminating enough. For example, a space gate cannot filter out the photons that have first been scattered out of the incident direction and then back into it. However, a time gate employed after the space gate can cut out such "on-line" scattered photons, since scattering makes them travel longer distances and emerge out of the sample later than the ballistic photons that propagate straight through.

The implementation of an optical imaging modality based on any of the gating methods mentioned earlier requires an appropriate light source and beam-delivery optics to illuminate the sample, a detection scheme to monitor the transmitted light, and a signal processing unit to construct the image from the collected data and known experimental parameters. The form in which data should be collected is a major consideration for the researchers, and three different approaches—*time resolved, frequency domain,* and *continuous wave*—are now in use.

Time-resolved methods commonly use ultrashort light pulses from an ultrafast laser to illuminate the sample. A time gate, often combined with a space gate, is then employed to measure the time evolution of emergent light. Image information is extracted by analyzing the relevant temporal slice of the data. In this article, we concentrate on the space, time, and polarization gates as well as combinations of those gates that have been demonstrated and implemented by researchers at the Institute for Ultrafast Spectroscopy and Lasers of the City College of New York.

SCOPE OF OPTICAL IMAGING OF BODY ORGANS

Before delving into specific imaging techniques, a brief overview of the scope of optical methods in probing body organs is in order. The organs of the human body with potential to be investigated by optical spectroscopic techniques include breast, brain, bladder, bone, cervix, colon, eye, digestive and gynelogical tracts, prostate, skin, and teeth. The requirements of resolution, penetration depth, diagnostic ability, and specificity to key chemicals of an optical imaging modality depend on the organ and the lesion being investigated. Breast and brain have received most attention over other organs from researchers around the world.

In breast imaging, the thrust is to detect and diagnose tumors in an early stage when they are small. The importance of early diagnosis of breast cancer is underscored by the statistic that in 1990, breast cancer accounted for 4.4% of all U.S. female deaths.[32] The efficacy of the current gold standard, X-ray mammography, is substantially reduced for premenopausal breasts. The challenge for transillumination-based optical methods is that the intensity of the ballistic and snake photons are severely attenuated in traversing the full thickness of breast tissue. Researchers in Japan have built a laser-transmission photo-scanning system for breast examination, tested its cancer diagnostic ability in comparison with X-ray mammography, and obtained promising results.[23] Different approaches for breast imaging and breast tumor characterization are being pursued by a number of researchers.[33] However, much work is needed for optical mammography to be a viable alternative to X-ray mammography.

Optical imaging of human brain activity is being actively pursued by several groups.[34–37] Imaging and spectrophotometry using NIR light offers the promise to detect hemorrhage, measure oxygenation, image stroke, and map activation of the brain during various mental tasks and stimuli. Another area of concentration has been the measurement of key optical parameters of brain tissues.[38,39] Optical parameters of neonatal and adult heads are very different. Consequently, *in vivo* optical imaging of neonatal brain shows considerable promise, but that of adult brain may be rather difficult.

An impressive development in optical imaging has been the *in vivo* measurement of human retinal structure with micrometer resolution that offers the potential for the diagnosis and monitoring of retinal diseases such as macular degeneration and macular edema.[40] Optical imaging of arteries,[41] bones and teeth,[42] gastrointestinal tissues,[43] and skin[44] has also been reported.

These developments indicate that optical imaging of body organs and functions is apt to make a transition from scientific curiosity to useful clinical technology.

PHOTON-SORTING TECHNIQUES

In this section, we first emphasize the need for selecting the proper wavelength for optical imaging, and then present a brief overview of the space, time, and polarization gating techniques that we commonly use to select out image-bearing photons for constructing shadowgrams.

Wavelength Selection

The characteristics of light to be used is perhaps the most important consideration in optical imaging of tissues. Laser beams characterized by a high degree of spectral brightness, directionality, coherence, monochromaticity, and optional short-time duration are used by most researchers these days. Several factors need to be considered to choose the optimal wavelength. First, to form a sharp image one needs light that is scattered the least. Second, the chosen wavelength should provide high spatial resolution, but should not be strongly absorbed by the tissue. Finally, the wavelength range needs to be suitable to detect the key chemicals that can indicate how the body is functioning. Unlike ultrasound and X rays, only light offers this capability of spectroscopic monitoring of body chemistry.

The importance of proper wavelength selection for shadowgram formation was underscored in a simple and revealing experiment by Dolne *et al.*[45] These authors studied the problem of imaging a grid sample through scattering media using 670, 830, and 1300 nm light from laser diodes. The scattering media were Intralipid suspensions of different concentrations. A Fourier space gate (see the following section) was used to discriminate against the diffuse light. As is evident from FIGURE 2, the best-resolved and high-contrast image of the grid was obtained using 1300 nm light. A comparison of the scattering and absorption characteristics of the Intralipid suspension at 1300 nm to that for 670 and 830 nm light provides an explanation of this result. The absorption coefficient of Intralipid suspension for 1300 nm light is much larger, and the scattering coefficient much smaller than that for the other two wavelengths. So, 1300 nm light is less scattered, making the noise problem less severe compared to that for the other wavelengths. In addition, higher absorption of 1300 nm light attenuates the multiple-scattered light more strongly than the ballistic and snake light. The reason is that the intensity of light attenuates exponentially with distance due to absorption, and scattered light travels a longer distance within the medium than the ballistic and snake light. Thus the combination of lower scattering and higher absorption favors the use of 1300 nm light for this particular case. However, it should not be

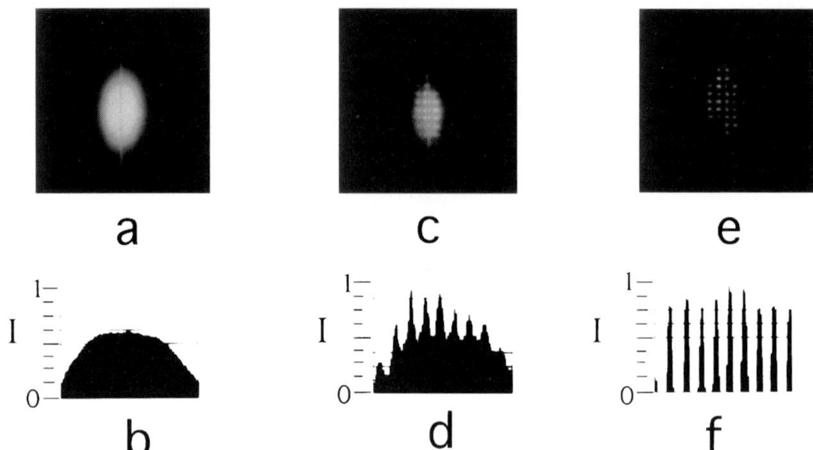

FIGURE 2. Images of a grid with 1-mm × 1-mm openings through a 1-cm glass cell containing 5.5% Intralipid suspension. Fourier spatial filtering with a 1-mm-diameter aperture was used to reduce the scattered light. The **upper frames** (**a**), (**c**), (**e**) are the transillumination images of the grid recorded by a PbS infrared camera for illumination of the grid by 670-, 830-, and 1300-nm light, respectively. The **lower frames** (**b**), (**d**), (**f**) show the intensity distribution along a line across the grid images (a), (c), (e), respectively. It is evident that the image in frame (**e**) formed by 1300-nm light is better resolved and the corresponding intensity distribution in frame (**f**) has higher contrast than those obtained for the other two wavelengths. (From Dolne *et al.*[45] Reproduced by permission.)

concluded that higher absorption, in general, would lead to better imaging. On the contrary, by reducing the intensity of the transmitted light, absorption often complicates the task of imaging. In situations where ample image-bearing light is available, absorption may improve resolution by reducing the intensity of scattered light more than that of the ballistic and snake components.

In general, near-infrared light spanning the 700–1300-nm spectral range is more suited for body imaging than light at other wavelengths. Light in this "therapeutic window" is not as strongly absorbed by tissue as the visible light, and so will have higher transmission and less likelihood of causing adverse effects. The availability of broadly wavelength-tunable solid-state lasers, such as Ti:sapphire and Cr:forsterite, that cover this spectral range is another advantage. The wavelength tunability offers the possibility of monitoring different chemical species by tuning to different wavelengths. Near-infrared light is also less scattered than visible light, and is not known to cause any tissue damage, even with prolonged exposure at intensity levels that may be needed for routine screening. However, the main problem of scattered light needs to be confronted. Some of the techniques for doing so are presented below.

Fourier Space Gate

The space gate implemented in our laboratory is a Fourier gate.[5,45] The experimental arrangement for a Fourier gate, shown schematically in FIGURE 3, uses a collimated beam of light to illuminate the object. A lens of focal length f placed at a distance f from the object focuses the photons that retain their collimation at a distance of $2f$. A small aperture placed at the focus of the lens transmits the image-bearing light and rejects most of the off-axis diffusive component. The second lens, also of focal length f, located at a distance f from the aperture forms an image of the object in the image plane located $2f$ away from the aperture. The configuration, known as the $4f$ Fourier system, serves as a focused imaging system with unity magnification.

The system is called a Fourier system since light propagation through the system may be analyzed as transmission through two Fourier-transforming subsystems.[5] The first lens performs a Fourier transform of the complex amplitude transmittance of the illuminated object, and separates the Fourier components so that each point on the Fourier plane (back focal plane of the lens) corresponds to a single spatial frequency. The spot at the center of the plane corresponds to zero spatial frequency, where most of the ballistic light is concentrated. Spots further out from the center correspond to higher spatial frequencies and receive more diffuse light. The aperture selects out the lower spatial-frequency components, that is, the ballistic and snake photons. The second lens located between the Fourier and image planes performs an inverse Fourier transform and forms an image with lower spatial frequency components.

The Fourier space gate has a high rejection efficiency for diffuse light. It has been demonstrated that by varying the aperture diameter, the Fourier spatial filter may be used as a temporal gate for selecting out the early arriving part of a light pulse transmitted through a highly scattering medium. This is illustrated in FIGURE 4 for propagation of 8-ps,

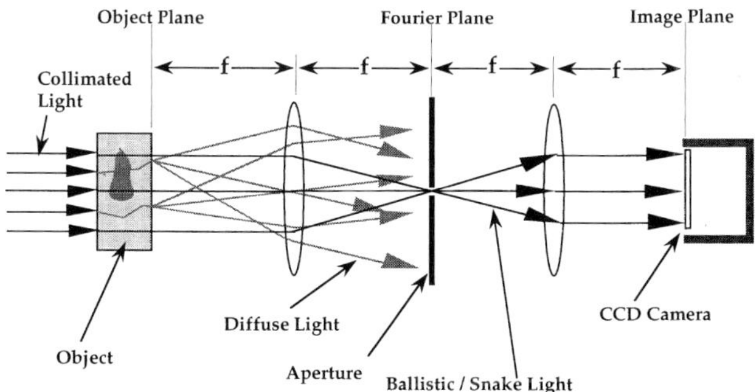

FIGURE 3. A schematic diagram of the experimental arrangement for implementing the Fourier space gate.

527-nm light pulses through an Intralipid solution, a highly scattering medium.[46]

Polarization Gating

The polarization gate makes use of the fact that scattering events depolarize an incident beam of polarized light, so that ballistic and snake photons retain their polarization memory while the multiple-scattered photons are depolarized.[6,7] In practice, a polarization gate is implemented by shining the object through a polarizer and collecting the emerging light through a second polarizer. The second polarizer is oriented to first collect the component of the transmitted light that has the same polarization state as the incident light, and then to collect the component with polarization orthogonal to the incident light. The extent of depolarization may be described in terms of the degree of polarization, D, of the transmitted light, defined as

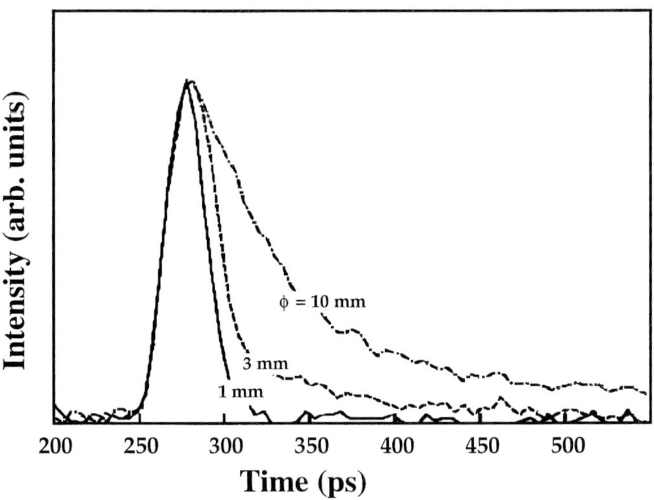

FIGURE 4. Normalized temporal intensity profiles of 1064-nm light pulses transmitted through a 50-mm glass cell filled with 0.4% Intralipid suspension. The scattered light was filtered by a Fourier space gate with an aperture diameter $\phi = 1, 3, 10$ mm as shown in the figure. (From Wang *et al.*[46] Reproduced by permission.)

$$D = (I_p - I_s)/(I_p + I_s), \qquad (1)$$

where I_p and I_s are transmitted intensities of light with the same polarization and orthogonal polarization with respect to the incident light, respectively. The degree of polarization may be used to select the image-bearing component since it is ideally expected to be unity for ballistic light, zero for completely depolarized light, and between 1 and 0 for the snake light. The snake light with higher values of D will form sharper shadowgrams than those formed by lower D-value snake light. The degree of polarization of the transmitted light depends on the characteristics of the scattering medium.[4]

For measurements using ultrashort light pulses, the parameters D, I_p, and I_s are functions of time. The temporal intensity profiles $I_p(t)$, $I_s(t)$, the difference, $\Delta I(t) = I_p(t) - I_s(t)$ between the two profiles, as well as the temporal profile of the degree of polarization $D(t)$, provide useful information for shadowgram construction. We have used the polarization gate, in combination with a space and a time gate, to examine the scattering characteristics of model media,[7] breast tissue,[47] and brain matter. The experimental arrangement and results are presented in the Applications section.

Time-resolved Methods

The time-resolved imaging methods developed to date may be broadly classified into *incoherent* and *coherent* techniques depending on how the selection of ballistic and snake photons is achieved. In incoherent techniques, these image-bearing photons are selected by opening a time gate for a short duration. A reference light pulse opens the gate and the light emerging from the sample can pass through for as long as the reference pulse is on. An optical delay line in the path of the reference pulse enables its temporal overlap with the desired part of the transmitted light. The ratio of the intensity of light that passes through when the reference pulse is on to that when it is off determines the contrast of the gate. These gates are often known as pulse gates, since the characteristics of the reference pulse play a major role in defining their properties. Examples of pulse-gating techniques are optical Kerr gate (OKG),[2,8] second-harmonic generation (SHG) gate,[9] parametric sum and difference frequency generation gates,[10] stimulated Raman scattering (SRS) gate,[11] and time-correlated single photon counting.[12] Imaging using a streak camera is an example of an incoherent electronic gate that operates by converting the temporal intensity profile of the transmitted light to a spatial one.[13] However, it has a limited dynamic range of $\sim 10^4$.

The interference between image-bearing photons and a reference beam derived from the same initial pulse of light forms the mechanism for selective detection in coherent techniques. Photons that are coherent with the reference give rise to a gated signal, while diffusive light does not. The coherence time of the reference pulse determines the duration of the gate. So, a longer-duration but broadband light pulse may be used to generate ultrafast gates. Optical coherent imaging (OCI),[14,15] holographic methods,[16–18] four-wave mixing (FWM) gate,[19] and coherent anti-Stokes Raman scattering (CARS) gate[11] are coherent techniques. In the remainder of this section, we concentrate on the optical Kerr gate (OKG) and the Streak camera method, the two techniques that we commonly use.

Optical Kerr Gate

The OKG acts as an ultrafast shutter in a camera that is triggered by an intense gating pulse to take a picture the instant the image-bearing light emerges and closed soon enough to block the diffusive light. A typical OKG experimental arrangement, shown schematically in FIGURE 5, consists of a Kerr active material such as carbon disulfide, placed between two crossed polarizers. An intense ultrashort pulse of light is split into two parts. One part illuminates the sample, the other part, known as the "reference" or "gating" pulse, is used to induce a transient birefringence in the Kerr medium. The light emerging from the sample is made to overlap spatially and temporally with

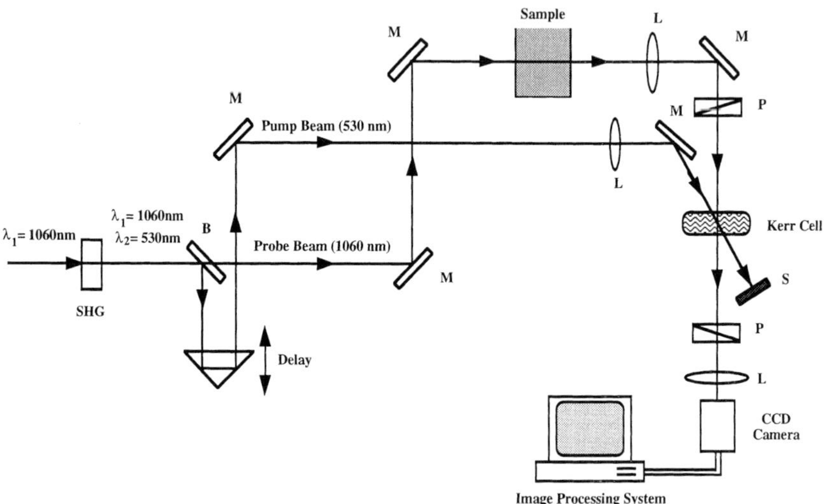

FIGURE 5. A schematic diagram of a picosecond optical Kerr gate. B: beam splitter; L: lens; M: mirror; P: polarizer; S: beam stop; SHG: second-harmonic generator. (From Gayen and Alfano,[3] modified. Reproduced by permission.)

the gating pulse inside the Kerr medium. If the reference pulse is blocked, a very small fraction of the incident light, typically less than one part in a million, may pass through the crossed polarizers. Thus, the gate is "closed." In the presence of the reference pulse, the fraction of light from the sample that is linearly polarized by the first polarizer becomes elliptically polarized as it passes through the Kerr medium while coincident with the reference pulse. A fraction of this elliptically polarized light can now pass through the analyzer. This may be looked upon as the gate being "open." Thus the light can only pass through the gate when it overlaps both temporally and spatially with the intense reference pulse.

The duration of the gating pulse or the recovery time of the Kerr medium, whichever is longer, determines how long the gate remains open. Picosecond and subpicosecond time resolutions may thus be attained using an OKG. The gate position may be varied by adjusting the arrival of the reference pulse using an optical delay line. The image-bearing early light may be extracted in a single shot by adjusting the gate position.

A picosecond OKG that uses a picosecond Nd:glass laser, a CS_2 Kerr cell, and a two-dimensional (2-D) charge-coupled device (CCD) camera has been successfully used to image test objects hidden inside human breast tissue, chicken breast tissue, and a suspension of polystyrene spheres in water.[2] While the image was completely blurred without the gate, a well-resolved image was obtained when the gate selected the initial part of the transmitted pulse.

Combined time and space gating was realized by placing the Kerr cell in the arrangement discussed earlier at the back focal plane of a lens, and an aperture at the center of the front focal plane.[8] Another lens placed at a distance equal to its focal length behind the aperture collimated the selected light and directed it to the CCD camera. Compared to simple OKG, this Kerr–Fourier gate (KFG) provided a higher dynamic range, signal-to-noise ratio, and contrast at a signal level of $\sim 10^{-10}$ of the illumination intensity. This large dynamic range enables more efficient selection of weak early light compared to other pulse-gating methods. The sensitivity of the technique to detect small changes in optical properties was underscored when it successfully imaged a pure water droplet inside a 2% Intralipid solution, as shown in FIGURE 6. In a related development, the feasibility of constructing a three-dimensional (3-D) tomographic image was demonstrated by combining 2-D shadowgrams formed with a KFG using a back projection algorithm on a personal computer.[29]

Streak-camera Method

Streak cameras have been used as fast electronic gates for early light detection by several groups.[13,48,49] A typical streak camera system comprises a streak tube, fast-sweeping electrodes, imaging optics, a video display, and a computer system. The light pulse that passes through the object impinges on the photocathode of the streak tube. The photoelectrons that are emitted throughout the duration of the pulse are multiplied and steered to form a streak on a phosphor screen, converting the temporal intensity profile to a spatial one. The video system analyzes the spatial intensity of the streak, and computer algorithms together with calibration methods can reconstruct the temporal profile. The early component of that slice can be selected and analyzed for image construction. The technique provides a temporal resolution of several picoseconds.

An important result in time-gated imaging using a streak camera has been the imaging of a 2.5-mm-thick strip of fat embedded in a 40-mm-thick

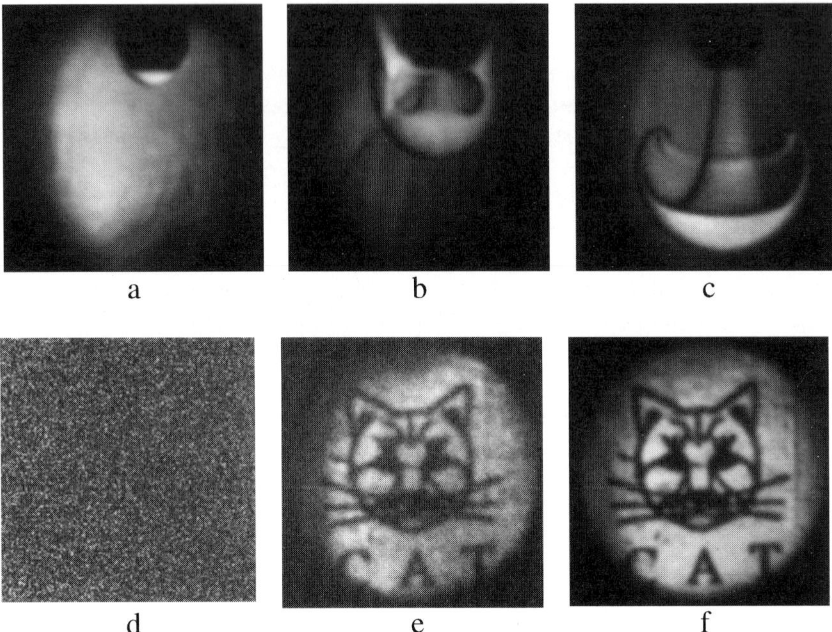

FIGURE 6. Imaging of a water droplet diffusing into a 2% Intralipid suspensions (**upper frames**), and that of a cat drawn in a transparent plastic sheet hidden inside (**lower frames**) an Intralipid solution using the optical Kerr-Fourier gate. In (**a**)–(**c**), the gate delay = 0 ps, and (**a**) $T \sim 0$ s, (**b**) $T \sim 3$ s, and (**c**) $T \sim 5$ s after the valve that releases the water droplet is opened. In (**d**) gate delay = 40 ps, (**e**) gate delay = 20 ps, (**f**) gate delay = 0 ps. (From Gayen and Alfano.[3] Reproduced by permission.)

chicken breast tissue.[48] The camera was used in the synchroscan mode and 620-nm, 100-fs, 82-MHz pulses from a colliding-pulse model-locked dye laser were used to illuminate the sample. Different temporal slices of the transmitted pulse profile were used to image the strip of fat. The location and width of the fat strip could be determined and the edges could be resolved with millimeter resolution when a 10-ps slice of the early part of the snake light was chosen.

APPLICATIONS

In this section we present a brief review of our work on demonstrating the feasibility of optical imaging of biomedical media, such as breast and brain tissue, using a combined space, time, and polarization (STP) gate. The experimental arrangements are shown schematically in FIGURE 7. The compressed fundamental (1064-nm, 6.5-ps) and second-harmonic (532-nm, 5-ps) light pulses from a mode-locked Nd:yttrium aluminum garnet (YAG) laser (Spectra Physics Model 3000) operating at 82 MHz were used in the experiments reported here. A small fraction of the laser-pulse energy was directed by a beamsplitter into a photodiode to generate the trigger pulse for the streak camera. A second beamsplitter split off another small fraction that was used as a reference pulse for the streak camera. The remaining beam illuminated the sample under investigation. The reference pulse was collected by a 110-μm single fiber, and the light emerging from the sample (signal) was collected by a 1.2-mm-diameter fiber bundle made of 110-μm single-fiber elements. The signal was accumulated both in the transmission and backscattering geometries, as illustrated in FIGURE 7 and its inset, respectively. The output ends of the fibers were coupled to the input of a streak camera system (Hamamatsu Model C1587) with S-1 spectral response, and 10-ps temporal resolution. The temporal resolution changed to approximately 14 ps when the fiber bundle-coupled input was used.

A linear polarizer (P1) placed before the sample ensured linear polarization of the incident light beam. A second linear polarizer (P2) in front of the signal-collecting fiber (F1) implemented the polarization gate. The polarizing axis of P2 could be rotated to selectively transmit the component of the signal that was polarized either parallel or perpendicular to the polarization of the incident beam. Spatial gating was accomplished by the use of the fiber bundle

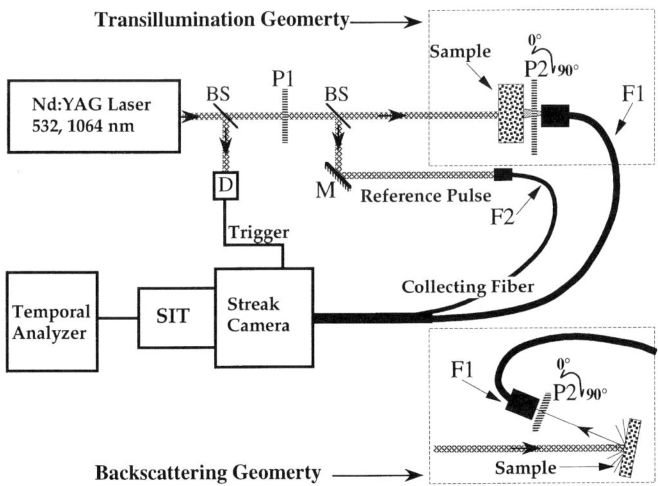

FIGURE 7. A schematic diagram of the experimental arrangement for implementing the combined space, time, and polarization gate. Both the transillumination and backscattering geometries are shown. BS: beam splitter; D: photodiode; F1: 1.2-mm-diameter signal-collecting fiber bundle; F2: 110-μm-diameter fiber to transmit the reference light pulse; M: mirror; P1, P2: linear polarizers; SIT: silicon-intensified target. (From Demos and Alfano.[7] Reproduced by permission.)

for signal collection. Since a collimated beam was used for sample illumination, the fiber bundle acted as a small aperture for the forward transmitted beam. This configuration realizes a confocal imaging arrangement with the aperture size determined by the numerical aperture of the fiber bundle. The streak camera records the temporal profile of the signal, completing the combined space, time, and polarization gate.

Experiments with Model Media

In order to test the concept of polarization gating and the overall performance of the STP gate in a controlled fashion, we first carried out a set of experiments, using suspensions of polystyrene microspheres (Duke Scientific Corporation) in water as model scattering media.[7] Microspheres of diameter 0.09, 0.2, and 1.07 μm and suspensions of different concentrations were used to vary the scattering coefficient, μ_s over the 1.0–0.1 mm^{-1} range. Measurements on these suspensions were carried out in a 5-cm × 5-cm × 5-cm glass cell.

Typical temporal profiles $I_{\|}(t)$, $I_{\perp}(t)$, $D(t)$ of light transmitted through a suspension of 0.2 μm microspheres are shown in FIGURE 8. Here, $I_{\|}(t)$ and $I_{\perp}(t)$ are temporal intensity profiles of the components of the transmitted light pulse with polarization parallel and perpendicular to the incident light polarization, respectively. It is evident that there is a distinct difference between $I_{\|}(t)$ and $I_{\perp}(t)$ up to about 100 ps, beyond which the two profiles become identical and overlap with each other. More remarkable is the time evolution of $D(t)$ that attains a distinct maximum followed by a gradual decay, reaching the minimum value of zero around 100 ps. The onset of 0 value for $D(t)$ indicates that the light that emerges after this time has no polarization memory, that is, it is diffusive. Photons exiting at earlier times (<100 ps) retain polarization memory, the extent of which depends on the details of the scattering events they have undergone. These are image-bearing snake and ballistic photons. The maximum value of degree of polarization, D_{max}, and the time, t_{max}, to attain that value were found to depend on the scattering characteristics of the medium, and the wavelength of light. These results demonstrate that polarization memory, or more specifically, $D(t)$ may indeed be used to block out image-bearing photons.

Investigation of Breast Tissue

The technique was next extended to normal and cancerous human breast tissue samples, both obtained from the same patient.[47] The samples were placed between two glass slides and were slightly compressed to a uniform thickness. Both 532- and 1064-nm pulses were used, and the signal was collected in a transmission geometry.

The temporal profiles $I_{\parallel}(t)$ and $I_{\perp}(t)$ of 1064-nm pulse transmitted through adipose (fat) and cancerous breast tissues are shown in FIGURE 9(a) and 9(b), respectively. The difference between the two profiles is much more pronounced for the adipose tissue. The value of D_{max} is 0.65 for the adipose tissue and 0.15 for tumor. Similar differences in profiles were observed for 532-nm pulses. However, the values of D_{max} for the adipose and tumor samples were 0.32 and 0.19, respectively. Histological analyses were carried out on the illuminated parts of the samples. The measurements were repeated for eight pairs of samples from different patients. Each pair, however, included an adipose and a cancerous tissue from the same patient. Similar behavior was observed for all the clinically characterized samples.

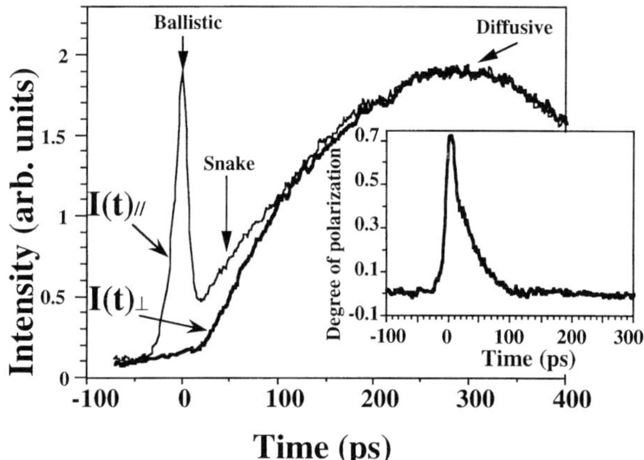

FIGURE 8. Temporal profiles of the parallel (*thin line*) and perpendicular (*thick line*) components of a 532-nm light pulse transmitted through a suspension of 0.2-μm-diameter polystyrene microspheres in water. The suspension was placed in a 5-cm-thick glass cell, and the concentration of microspheres was such that the scattering coefficient was 0.25 mm^{-1}. The *inset* shows the temporal profile of the degree of polarization. (From Demos and Alfano.[7] Reproduced by permission.)

These results demonstrate that (a) different tissues have different scattering characteristics: (b) as a consequence, the polarization characteristics of light transmitted through different types of tissues are different; and (c) the difference in polarization characteristics depends on the color of light. These results imply that these differential polarization characteristics between normal and cancerous tissues may be used as a useful signature for the diagnosis and imaging of tumors.

To explore the possibility further a sample with both normal and cancerous tissues was scanned across the illuminating 532-nm beam, and the degree of polarization was plotted as a function of the lateral position. The results are

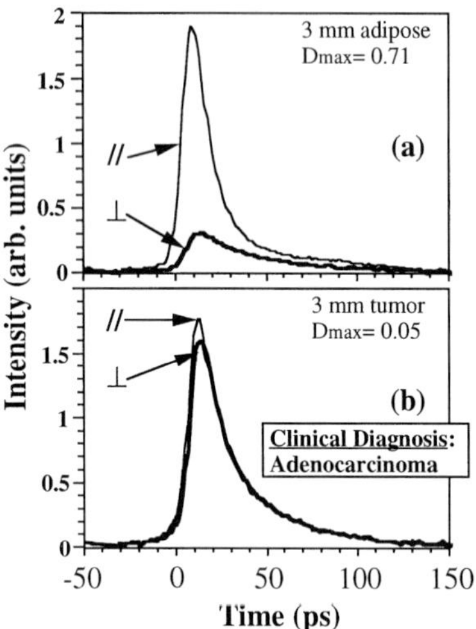

FIGURE 9. Temporal profiles of the parallel (*thin line*) and perpendicular (*thick line*) components of a 1064-nm light pulse transmitted through 3-mm-thick (**a**) adipose, and (**b**) cancerous human breast tissues taken from the same patient. Clinical diagnosis of the tumor was ductal carcinoma. (From Demos *et al.*[47] Reproduced by permission.)

shown in FIGURE 10. The sharp change in the value of D_{max} clearly distinguishes between the normal and cancerous regions.

Brain

The types of tissues encountered in the head include scalp, skull, fluid, white matter, gray matter, blood and, in ailing patients, tumor. Imaging modalities are sought to monitor tumor, detect hemorrhage, measure oxygenation, image stroke, and map activation of the brain during various mental tasks. Development of optical imaging techniques for these applications requires knowledge of key scattering parameters.

We have initiated an investigation of the light-scattering characteristics of both gray and white matters. Measurements on calf brain samples held between glass slides were carried out both in the backscattering and transmission geometries using 1064 nm light. The temporal intensity profiles transmitted through 3-mm-thick calf white and gray matters are shown in FIGURE 11. FIGURE 11(a) presents the entire profile, while the polarized profiles are displayed in FIGURE 11(b). The profiles clearly demonstrate that white matter scatters light much more strongly than the gray matter. The value of D_{max} is 0.75 for gray matter, and approximately 0 for white matter for 3-mm-thick samples.

The intensity profiles measured in the backscattering geometry are shown in FIGURE 12. The thickness of both white and gray matter samples was 5 mm.

However, the backscattered light was obtained from a smaller depth beneath the front surface of the samples. The zero time for both the transmission and back-reflection geometries was taken to be the instant when the incident light pulse hit the front surface of the sample. Both polarized and unpolarized profiles reaffirm the result of transmission measurements that white matter is a stronger light scatterer than gray matter. The value of D_{max} for backscattering geometry is 0.62 for gray matter and 0.26 for white matter.

The values of D_{max} for the gray and white matters measured in the transmission and backscattering geometries are different. More striking is the difference in the ratio of D_{max} for white matter to that of gray matter in the two geometries. These differences are believed to be due to differences in the path lengths that light actually travels inside the tissues. In transmission, early light traversing through 3 mm of white and gray matters is collected. In backscattering, the penetration of light into white and gray matter samples is different since their scattering and absorption characteristics are different. So, the early backscattered light measured within a fixed time window for the white and gray matter samples may not be arriving from the same depth range inside the respective samples.

The results presented here imply that light is almost completely depolarized in transmission through 3 mm of white matter of a calf brain. It is evident that very little image-bearing light would be available for early-light shadowgram imaging of a full-size bovine brain. The average transport length of a calf brain at 1064 nm is reported to be 1.5 mm,[50] and that for the gray and white matters of the adult human brain to be 0.59 mm and 0.13 mm, respectively.[39] So the problem of shadowgram imaging of adult human brain

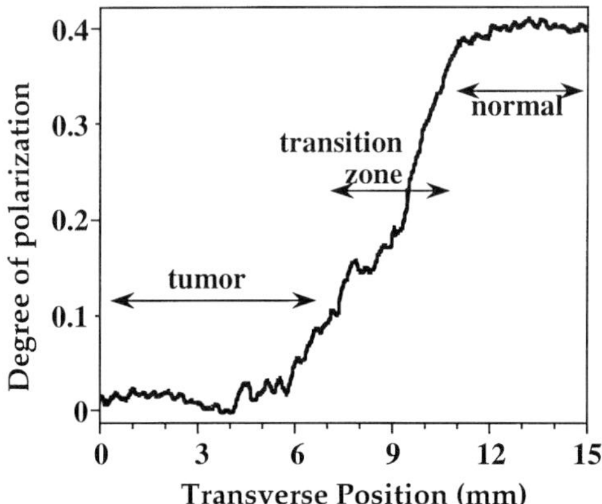

FIGURE 10. The maximum value of the degree of polarization, D_{max}, as a function of transverse position of the sample being illuminated by 532-nm laser light. The sample was a 3-mm-thick human breast tissue that had both adipose and cancerous regions. Not only are the two regions clearly delineated by the D_{max} values, but the transition region is also resolved. (From Demos *et al.*[51] Reproduced by permission.)

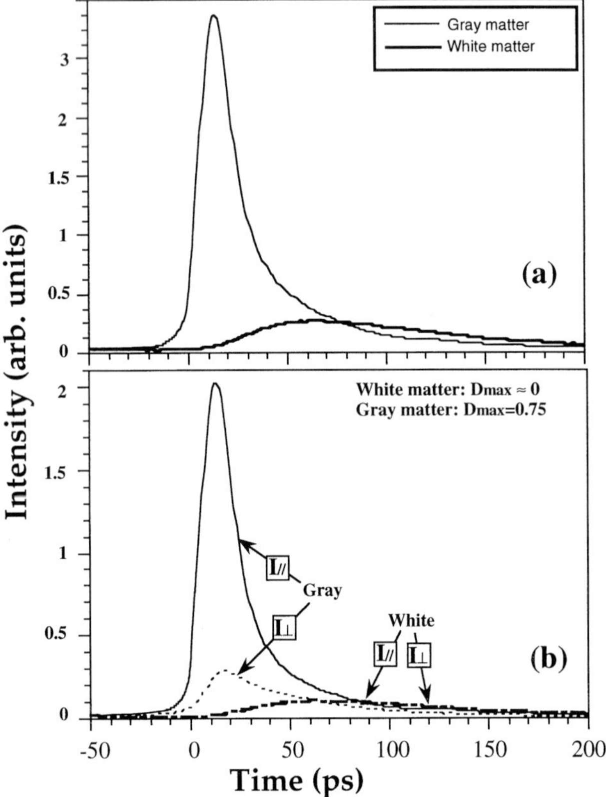

FIGURE 11. Temporal intensity profiles of a 1064-nm pulse of light transmitted through 3-mm-thick gray and white matter samples of a calf brain: (**a**) the complete profiles, and (**b**) the parallel and perpendicularly polarized components.

would be even more severe. However, for neonatal brain (40 week gestational age) the average transport lengths for gray and white matters at 1000 nm are 2.5 mm and 1.4 mm, respectively.[39] Shadowgram imaging of neonatal brains using near-infrared light around 1000 nm may thus be possible. Imaging of neonatal brains is an important application for an optical imaging modality, since X ray is an ionizing radiation that may adversely affect a growing brain. In the case of an adult brain, optical imaging in the backscattering geometry may be useful for some applications, such as, probing blood build up at small depths below the skull.

SUMMARY

In this article, we have presented an overview of fundamental issues involved in mediphotonic imaging, and reviewed some of the emerging techniques for early-light transillumination imaging of body organs. The results on human breast tissues presented here, together with the data accumulated and advances made by researchers around the globe, not only demonstrate the feasibility of optical imaging as a clinical procedure but indicate a road map to reach that goal. The milestones include evaluation of relative merits of available approaches for a particular imaging application; selection of diagnostic wavelengths, as well as sources to generate and detectors to monitor light at those wavelengths; accumulation of data on optical, spectroscopic, and transport properties of tissues and organs; *in vivo* testing; prototype instrumentation development; clinical trials; governmental approval; cost analysis and marketing; and finally system improvement based on feedback from end users.

A new era of optical clinical imaging is at the door!

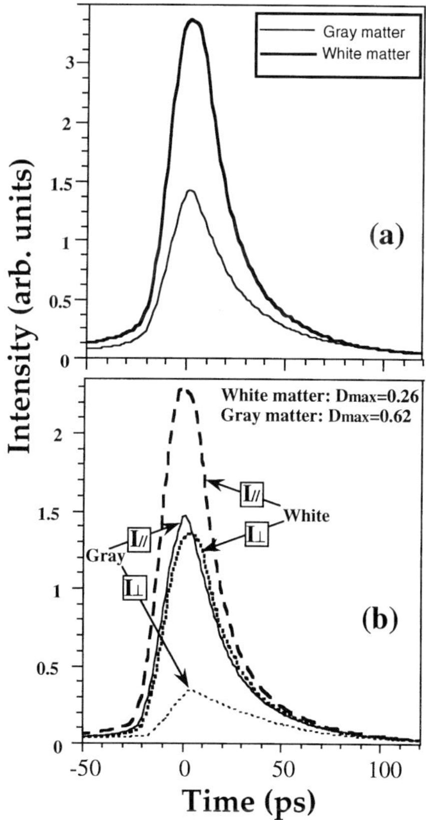

FIGURE 12. Temporal intensity profiles of a 1064-nm pulse of light backscattered from 5-mm-thick gray and white matter samples of a calf brain: (**a**) the complete profiles, and (**b**) the parallel and perpendicularly polarized components.

ACKNOWLEDGMENTS

One of the authors (R.R.A.) thanks Peter Katevates of Mediscience Technology Corp. for continued support, insight, and discussions on the terminology concerning "sorting of photons." The human breast tissue samples were obtained from our collaborators at the Memorial Sloan Kettering Cancer Center (New York, NY).[47] Calf brain samples were obtained from local butchers.

REFERENCES

1. Yoo, K. M. & R. R. Alfano. 1990. Time-resolved coherent and incoherent components of forward light scattering in random media. Opt. Lett. **15:** 320–322.
2. Wang, L., P. P. Ho, C. Liu, G. Zhang & R. R. Alfano. 1991. Ballistic 2-D imaging through scattering wall using an ultrafast Kerr gate. Science **253:** 769–771.
3. Gayen, S. K. & R. R. Alfano. 1996. Emerging optical biomedical imaging techniques. Opt. Photon. News **7**(3)**:** 17–22.
4. Dilworth, D. S., E. N. Leith & J. L. Lopez. 1991. Three-dimensional confocal imaging of objects embedded within thick diffusing media. Appl. Opt. **30:** 1796–1803.
5. Saleh, B. E. A. & M. C. Teich. 1991. Fundamentals of Photonics: 136–139. Wiley. New York.
6. Horinaka, H., K. Hashimoto, K. Wada & Y. Cho. 1995. Extraction of quasi-straightforward-propagating photons from diffused light transmitting through a scattering medium by polarization modulation. Opt. Lett. **20:** 1501–1503.
7. Demos, S. G. & R. R. Alfano. 1996. Temporal gating in highly scattering media by the degree of optical polarization. Opt. Lett. **21:** 161–163.
8. Wang, L., P. P. Ho, X. Liang, H. Dai & R. R. Alfano. 1993. Fourier-Kerr imaging in thick turbid media. Opt. Lett. **18:** 241–243.
9. Yoo, K. M., Q. Xing & R. R. Alfano. 1991. Imaging objects hidden in highly scattering media using femtosecond second-harmonic generation cross-correlation time gating. Opt. Lett. **16:** 1019–1021.
10. Faris, G. W. & M. Banks. 1994. Imaging through highly scattering media with a novel upconverting time gate. OSA Proc. on Advances in Optical Imaging and Photon Migration, Vol. 21, Ed. R. R. Alfano, 139–142. Optical Society of America. Washington, D.C.
11. Reintjes, J., M. Bashkansky, M. Duncan, R. Mahon, L. L. Tankerskley, J. A. Moon, C. L. Adler & J. M. S. Prewitt. 1993. Time-gated imaging with nonlinear optical Raman interactions. Opt. Photon. News, **4**(10)**:** 28–32.
12. Berg, R., S. Andersoson-Engels & S. Svanberg. 1993. Time-resolved transillumination imaging. *In* Medical Optical Tomography: Functional Imaging and Monitoring, G. J. Muller *et al.,* Ed: 397–424. SPIE. Bellingham, Wash.
13. Yoo, K. M., B. B. Das & R. R. Alfano. 1992. Imaging of a transluscent object hidden in a highly scattering medium from early portion of the diffuse component of a transmitted ultrafast laser pulse. Opt. Lett. **17:** 958–960.
14. Huang, D., E. A. Swanson, D. Huang, C. P. Lin, J. S. Schuman, W. G. Stinson, W. Chang, M. R. Hee, T. Flotte, K. Gregory, C. A. Puliafito & J. G. Fujimoto. 1991. Optical coherence tomography. Science **254:** 1178–1181.
15. Hee, M. R., J. A. Izzat, J. M. Jacobson, J. G. Fujimoto & E. A. Swanson. 1993. Femtosecond transillumination optical coherence tomography. Opt. Lett. **18:** 950–952.
16. Spears, K. G., J. Serafin, N. H. Abramson, X. Zhu & H. Bjelkhagen. 1989. Chronocoherent imaging for medicine. IEEE Trans. Biomed. Eng. **BME-36:** 1210–1221.
17. Leith, E., E. Arons, H. Chen, Y. Chen, D. Dilworth, J. Lopez, M. Shih, P. C. Sun & G. Vossler. 1993. Electronic holography for imaging through tissue. Opt. Photon. News **4**(10)**:** 19–23.

18. ARONS, E., H. CHEN, K. CLAY, D. DILWORTH, R. DRAPER, J. LOPEZ, E. LEITH, M. SHIH & P. C. SUN. 1994. New holographic methods for improved imagery through scattering media. *In* OSA Proc. on Advances in Optical Imaging and Photon Migration, Vol. 21, R. R. Alfano, Ed.: 239–243. Optical Society of America. Washington, D.C.
19. SAPPEY, A. D. 1994. Optical imaging through turbid media with a degenerate four wave mixing correlation time gate. Appl. Opt. **33:** 8346–8353.
20. O'LEARY, M. A., D. A. BOAS, B. CHANCE & A. G. YODH. 1995. Experimental images of heterogeneous turbid media by frequency-domain diffusing-photon tomography. Opt. Lett. **20:** 426–428, and references therein.
21. SEVICK, E. M., C. L. BURCH, J. K. FRISOLI, M. L. JOHNSON, K. NOWACZYK, H. SZMACINSKI & J. R. LAKOWICZ. 1993. The physical basis of biomedical optical imaging using time-dependent measurements of photon migration in the frequency domain. *In* Medical Optical Tomography: Functional Imaging and Monitoring, G. J. Muller *et al.,* Eds.: 485–512. SPIE. Bellingham, Wash.
22. GRATTON, E., W. W. MANTULIN, M. J. VANDE VEN, J. B. FISHKIN, M. B. MARIS & B. CHANCE. 1993. A novel approach to laser tomography. Bioimaging **1:** 40–46.
23. YAMASHITA, Y. & M. KANEKO. 1993. Visible and infrared diaphanoscopy for medical diagnosis. *In* Medical Optical Tomography: Functional Imaging and Monitoring, G. J. Muller *et al.,* Eds.: 283–316. SPIE. Bellingham, Wash.
24. BEUTHAN, J. 1993. IR-diaphanoscopy in medicine. *In* Medical Optical Tomography: Functional Imaging and Monitoring, G. J. Muller *et al.,* Eds.: 263–282. SPIE. Bellingham, Wash.
25. CHAN, K. P., M. YAMADA & H. INABA. 1995. Optical imaging through highly scattering media by use of heterodyne detection in the 1.3-μm wavelength region. Opt. Lett. **20:** 492–494.
26. INABA, H. 1993. Coherent detection imaging for medical laser tomography. *In* Medical Optical Tomography: Functional Imaging and Monitoring, G. J. Muller *et al.,* Eds. 317–347. SPIE. Bellingham, Wash.
27. SCHMIDT, A., R. COREY & P. SAULNIER. 1995. Imaging through random media by use of low-coherence optical heterodyning. Opt. Lett. **20:** 404–406.
28. FRECHER, A. F., C. K. HITZENBERGER, W. DREXLER, G. KAMP, I. STRASSER & H. C. LI. 1993. *In vivo* optical coherence tomography in opthalmology. *In* Medical Optical Tomography: Functional Imaging and Monitoring, G. J. Muller *et al.,* Eds.: 355–370. SPIE. Bellingham, Wash.
29. KALPAXIS, L., L. M. WANG, P. GALLAND, X. LIANG, P. P. HO & R. R. ALFANO. 1993. Three-dimensional temporal image reconstruction of an object hidden in highly scattering media by time-gated optical tomography. Opt. Lett. **18:** 1691–1693.
30. HIROKA, M., M. FIRBANK, M. ESSENPREIS, M. COPE, S. R. ARRIDGE, P. VAN DER ZEE & D. T. DEPLY. 1993. Monte Carlo simulation of light transport through inhomogeneous tissue. *In* Proc. Photon Migration and Imaging in Random Media and Tissues Conf., Vol. 188, B. Chance and R. R. Alfano, Eds.: 149–159. SPIE. Bellingham, Wash.
31. ARRIDGE, S. R. 1993. The forward and inverse problems in time-resolved infrared imaging. *In* Medical Optical Tomography: Functional Imaging and Monitoring, G. J. Muller *et al.,* Ed.: 35–64. SPIE. Bellingham, Wash.
32. HARPER, G. R. & B. H. ENGLISBE. 1993. Prevention and screening for breast cancer. Cancer Detect. Prev. **17:** 551.
33. KANG, K. A., B. CHANCE, S. ZHAO, S. SRINIVASAN, E. PATTERSON & R. TROUPIN. 1993. Breast tumor characterization using near-infrared spectroscopy. *In* Proc. Photon Migration and Imaging in Random Media and Tissues, Conf., Vol. 188, B. Chance and R. R. Alfano, Eds.: 487–499, and references therein. SPIE, Bellingham, Wash.
34. TAMURA, M. 1996. Multichannel near-infrared optical imaging of human brain activity. *In* Advances in Optical Imaging and Photon Migration (Tech. Dig.) 8–10. Optical Society of America. Washington D.C.
35. BENARON, D. A., J. P. VAN HOUTEN, W. F. CHEONG, E. L. KERMIT, T. R. MACHOLD & D. K. STEVENSON. 1996. *In* Advances in Optical Imaging and Photon Migration (Tech. Dig.): 275–276. Optical Society of America. Washington, D.C.

36. CHANCE, B., K. KANG & E. SEVICK. 1993. Photon diffusion in breast and brain: Spectroscopy and imaging. Opt. Photon News **3**(10)**:** 9–13, and references therein.
37. WYATT, J. S., D. T. DEPLY, M. COPE, S. WRAY & E. O. REYNOLDS. 1986. Quantification of cerebral oxygenation and haemodynamics in sick newborn infants by near-infrared spectrophotometry. Lancet **2:** 1063–1066.
38. TADDEUCCI, A., F. MARTELLI, M. BARILLI, M. FERRARI & G. ZACCANTI. 1996. Optical properties of brain tissue. J. Biomed. Opt. **1:** 117–123.
39. VAN DER ZEE, P., E. MATTHIAS & D. T. DEPLY. 1993. Optical properties of brain tissue. *In* Proc. Photon Migration and Imaging in Random Media and Tissues Conf., Vol. 1888, B. Chance, R. R. Alfano, Eds.: 454–465, and relevant references therein. SPIE. Bellingham, Wash.
40. SWANSON, E. A., J. A. IZZAT, M. R. HEE, D. HUANG, C. P. LIN, J. S. SCHUMAN, C. A. PULIAFITO & J. G. FUJIMOTO. 1993. *In vivo* retinal imaging by optical coherence tomography. Opt. Lett. **18:** 1864–1866.
41. BREZINSKI, M. E., G. J. TEARNY, S. A. BOPPART, B. BOUMA & J. G. FUJIMOTO. 1996. High resolution intra-arterial imaging with optical coherence tomography. *In* Advances in Optical Imaging and Photon Migration (Tech. Dig.): 21–23. Optical Society of America. Washington, D.C.
42. WIST, A. O., P. MOON, S. MEIKSIN, S. L. HERR & P. P. FATUOROS. 1993. High resolution light imaging system for teeth and tissues. J. Clin. Laser Med. Surg. **11:** 313–321; also DEVARAJ, B., K. FUKUCHI, H. ISHIHATA, M. KOBAYASHI, T. YUASA, M. TAKEDA, M. USA, H. HORIUCHI, T. AKATSUKA & H. INABA. 1996. Laser computed tomographic images of bones and teeth by coherent detection imaging in the visible and near-IR regions. *In* Advances in Optical Imaging and Photon Migration (Tech. Dig.): 30–32. Optical Society of America. Washington D.C.
43. IZZAT, J. A., H. WANG, M. KULKARNI, N. P. BARRY, K. KOBAYASHI, M. I. CANTO, M. V. SIVAK. 1996. Optical coherence tomography and microscopy in gastrointestinal tissues. *In* Advances in Optical Imaging and Photon Migration (Tech. Dig.): 24–26. Optical Society of America. Washington D.C.
44. SERGEEV, A. M., V. M. ZELIKONOV, G. V. GELIKONOV, F. I. FELDCHTEIN, N. D. GLADKOVA & V. A. KAMENSKY. 1996. Biomedical diagnostics using optical coherence tomography. *In* Advances in Optical Imaging and Photon Migration (Tech. Dig.): 18–20. Optical Society of America. Washington, D.C.
45. DOLNE, J. J., K. M. YOO, F. LIU & R. R. ALFANO. 1994. IR Fourier space gate and absorption imaging through random media. *Lasers Life Sci.* **6:** 131–141.
46. WANG, Q. Z., X. LIANG, L. WANG, P. P. HO & R. R. ALFANO. 1995. Fourier spatial filter acts as a temporal gate for light propagating through a turbid medium. Opt. Lett. **20:** 1498–1500.
47. DEMOS, S. G., H. SAVAGE, A. S. HEERDT, S. SCHANTZ & R. R. ALFANO. 1996. Time-resolved degree of polarization for human breast tissue. Opt. Commun. **124:** 439–442.
48. DAS, B. B., K. M. YOO & R. R. ALFANO. 1993. Ultrafast time-gated imaging in thick tissues: A step toward optical mammography. Opt. Lett. **18:** 1002–1004, and relevant references therein.
49. HEBDEN, J. C., R. A. KRUGER & K. S. WONG. 1991. Time resolved imaging through a highly scattering medium. Appl. Opt. **30:** 788–794.
50. CHEONG, W., S. A. PRAHL & A. J. WELCH. 1990. A review of the optical properties of biological tissues. IEEE J. Quantum Electron. **QE-26:** 2166–2185.
51. DEMOS, S. G., H. SAVAGE, A. S. HEERDT, S. SCHANTZ & R. R. ALFANO. 1996. Polarization imaging and characterization of human breast tissue. *In* OSA TOPS on Advances in Optical Imaging and Photon Migration, Vol. 2, R. R. Alfano & J. G. Fujimoto, Eds.: 113–115. Optical Society of America.

DISCUSSION

QUESTION: Can you use the reverse reconstruction on the backscattered light? Does it just as well?

ALFANO: Yes. Well, you have to take the scattering around the object. It's not just forward or backward. You need more data in order to reconstruct.

QUESTION: The second question concerns the polarization gate. Can that be used in the backscattering situation, too?

ALFANO: Yes. I showed data on the backscatter. It's very important also. You get rid of the front surface.

QUESTION: How do you do that?

ALFANO: Get rid of the skin. Because that comes back polarized mostly.

QUESTION: Dr. Alfano, does this mean that if you want to do the integrated reflection, you would need an array of streak cameras?

ALFANO: There are multiple fibers around the object going to one streak camera that you put on different parts of a slit. That's not the right way of doing it, but that's the way we do it right now. It's better to have a multisignal processor that has that capability. It would be expensive, too.

Ballistic-Light Imaging with Temporal Holography: Using Causality to See through a Scattering Medium[a]

JACK FEINBERG[b,c] AND ALEX REBANE[d]

[c]*Department of Physics*
University of Southern California
Los Angeles, California 90089-0484

[d]*Physical Chemistry Laboratory*
ETH-Zentrum, CH-8092
Zurich, Switzerland

INTRODUCTION

Here I review the remarkable properties of temporal holography. Ordinary holography recreates a still image, while temporal holography recreates images in time, like the frames in a movie. The images can be picoseconds apart. If the early images show light that has passed through a scattering medium without scattering, then by selectively recreating these early images one can reveal a structure hidden inside the material. Although temporal holography is attractive for medical imaging, it has limitations. In this paper we show how the principle of causality lies at the heart of temporal holography. A brief experimental account of this experimental work is found in Reference 1, which we adapt here to form the first part of this paper. A more detailed mathematical treatment can be found in Reference 2.

In a conventional hologram one records the interference pattern of two light beams arriving at the same time on a light-sensitive material, such as photographic film. In contrast, in temporal holography a molecular resonance is used to record an interference pattern between light signals that arrive at different times. This technique creates a hologram with temporal resolution. Using a timed reference pulse as a "light shutter," we can record holographic images selectively, according to the time taken by light traveling from the object to the hologram. We use this method to image an object behind a semiopaque screen, and indicate how a similar method could be used to inspect objects embedded in a dense scattering medium. In principle, such a technique might be applied to the medical imaging of tumors. (In practice, the small ratio of signal-to-noise of this technique limits its applicability to imaging through thin tissue.)

[a]One of the authors (J.F.) gratefully acknowledges support from the U.S. Air Force Office of Scientific Research.

[b]Corresponding author. Phone: (213) 740-1134; fax: (213) 740-6653; e-mail: feinberg@physics.usc.edu

PIANOS WITH STRINGS

Consider a piano with its dampers removed, so that its strings are free to vibrate. Kicking the piano will excite all of its strings. However, singing loudly near this piano will excite only some of its strings, namely those strings in resonance with notes in the music. Consider the following experiment. First sing a song to the piano, such as: "A pretty face is like a melody. . . ." Then, after a delay time, T_0, short compared to the damping time of the strings, kick the piano once. Some of the strings will now be ringing wildly, while others will be barely moving. In particular, those strings that were excited by the singing but are vibrating out of phase with the kick will have their energy diminished by the kick. Now, modify the coupling of each string according to the energy it has after the kick. (For example, cut the strings that are barely moving, so that they can move no more.) In a brief and little known paper, H. C. Longuet-Higgins[3] showed that if one now kicks the piano again, then after that same delay time, T_0, a replica of the original melody will be played by the piano's remaining strings! Even more interesting, if the first kick occurred in the middle of a phrase, then only the later parts of the phrase will emerge after the second kick. For example, if the piano is prepared by "A pretty face (*kick!*) is like a melody. . . ," then, after its strings are modified as just described, a second kick to the piano will bring forth, "   is like a melody. . . ." The kicked piano forms a "temporal shutter" that replays only the musical wave that arrived after the first kick.

PIANOS WITH MOLECULES

In this work we create a type of "optical piano" that stores and later recreates the early or the late parts of an optical wave. The 88 narrow-frequency resonators of an ordinary acoustic piano are here replaced by 20,000 narrow-frequency resonators of a hole-burning material. We create this bank of narrow-frequency resonators by doping the organic dye protoporphyrin into a solid block of polystyrene.[2,4–7] Each dye molecule acts as a lightly damped resonator, but due to inhomogeneities in the plastic matrix, each dye molecule has a slightly different resonant frequency. Cooling the polystyrene to 2 K makes the phase-relaxation time of the molecule's upper level become quite long ($T_2 \approx 1$ ns), so that each absorption has a narrow homogeneous spectral width of $\Delta\omega = 1/(\pi c T_2) \cong 0.01\ \text{cm}^{-1}$. The polystyrene matrix causes the net absorption spectrum of all of the molecules to form an inhomogeneously broadened band extending over a 200-cm^{-1}-wide range. Consequently, this material resembles a bank of 200/0.01 = 20,000 narrow resonators.

We use this doped plastic to record and store the spectral and spatial contents of an incident light beam. When illuminated by narrow-band light of frequency ω, those molecules that happen to be in resonance with the light become excited. A fraction of these excited molecules subsequently relaxes into a metastable state (which is thought to be a tautomerization of the original molecule). Once in this transformed state the molecule's absorption is shifted to a completely different spectral region, so a narrow "hole" is burned into the sample's absorption spectrum at the frequency ω. This spectral hole remains as long as the sample is kept cold.

EARLY VS. LATE

Consider two optical pulses incident on a holographic recording medium as shown in the inset of FIGURE 1. Let pulse F arrive T_0 seconds before pulse G. If we were to use photographic film as the recording medium, then an interference pattern will be recorded only if the pulses overlap with each other at least partially in time. But suppose we replace the photographic film by a bank of resonators in a spectral hole-burning material, as described earlier, with each resonator atom tuned to a slightly different optical frequency ω_j. In this case the interference pattern of the two optical pulses F and G can be recorded even if the pulses are never present in the material at the same time.[3]

If the optical pulse F is sufficiently brief, then its frequency spread will be sufficiently wide to excite all of the atoms, much like a brief kick to a piano will excite all of the piano's strings. Each atom will continue to ring at its own natural frequency ω_j. After a delay time T_0 the second light pulse G arrives, and it will transfer energy either into or out of the jth atom *depending on the relative phase* between G's optical electric field and the phase $\phi_j = \omega_j T_0$ of the still-ringing atom. Because each atom's phase depends on its own particular resonant frequency ω_j, a given time delay T_0 between the two incident light pulses will produce a unique pattern of excited and unexcited atoms in frequency space.

After interacting with both of the light pulses F and G, let the absorption of the jth atom be permanently altered by an amount proportional to the atom's final energy (much like we altered the piano's strings in the preceding example). In particular, if the material consists of a hole-burning medium, then those molecules that were excited after both pulses become removed from the absorption spectra; they leave an absorption hole behind. If the bank of now-altered resonators is illuminated by a replica of the brief pulse F, it will absorb and reradiate light, again at the frequencies ω_j appropriate to each atom. At first, the phases of the reradiated light will be incoherent, but after a time of exactly T_0, the phases of the different frequencies come together to reproduce coherently a duplicate of the pulse G.[3] It can be shown,[2] however, that application of a replica of pulse G to the altered atoms causes a reradiation of light that loses rather than gains phase coherence with the passage of time. Unlike conventional off-axis holography, where either light beam can be used to reconstruct the other, the bank of atoms here records the direction of time's arrow.

Now consider illuminating an entire scene with a pulsed laser. Record the reflected light G using a bank of tuned resonators, and let a reference pulse F also illuminate the resonators, as described before. If the reference pulse arrives at the resonators *before* any of the reflected light, then the entire scene can be recalled by simply reading with another reference pulse. However, if the initial reference pulse is delayed so that it arrives *after* some of the reflected light, then reading (with another reference pulse) will only recreate those parts of the image that arrived after that first reference pulse, that is, those parts of the scene that were located farthest from the resonators. For

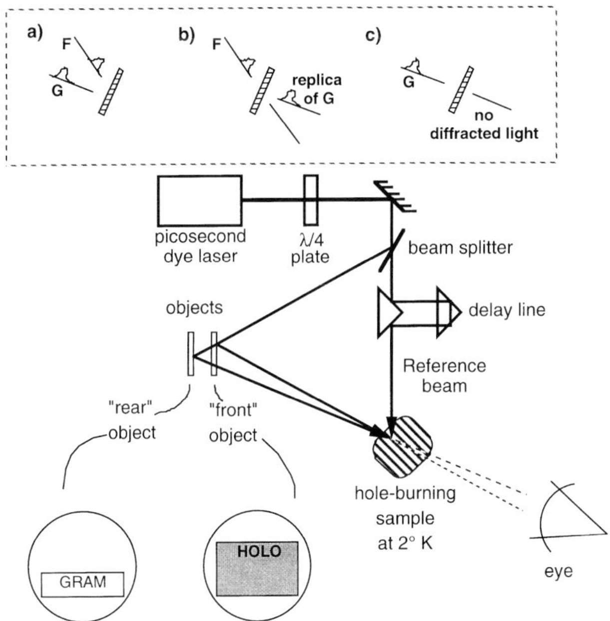

FIGURE 1. (**Inset**) (**a**) Writing the spectral hole-burning hologram with two light pulses separated in time. (**b**) Reading with the earlier pulse F recreates the later pulse G. (**c**) Reading with the later pulse G does not produce any diffracted pulse. (**Lower portion**) Experimental setup. The front object is a frosted slide with the letters "HOLO" pasted on the front. The rear object is the letters "GRAM" pasted on the back of the same slide.

example, if the scene consisted of the street view of a bookstore, then, with a suitably timed reference pulse, the reconstructed image would show the books on display deep inside the store, and would not show the reflections off of the bookstore's nearby front window.

It is also possible to reproduce the early light rather than the late light, that is, the light that strikes the hologram *before* the reference pulse arrives. To produce such an image, the hologram is read out by a replica of pulse F applied in the opposite direction to the original pulses: reversing the spatial orientation of the readout pulse reverses the relative phase relation of the reradiated light, and thereby leads to the recreation of the "early" rather than the "late" scattered light.

AN EXPERIMENTAL DEMONSTRATION

In our experiments the hole-burning medium was a 3-mm-thick block of polystyrene doped with protoporphyrin at a concentration of 10^{-3} mole/L. The useful sample area was 4 cm^2. The sample was immersed in liquid helium, and the helium vapors were pumped to reduce the temperature to 2 K. The peak of the broad absorption feature was at $\lambda = 621$ nm, at which the optical density was 1.6. The light source was a continuous-wave model-locked Nd:YAG laser (Coherent Antares 76 s) that synchronously pumped a tunable dye laser (Coherent 701) to produce pulses having an intensity temporal width of 8 ps full-width at half-maximum (FWHM). (These pulses were not transform limited; they had a coherence length of only 0.5 ps). The repetition rate of the laser pulses was 76 MHz. A beamsplitter divided the beam from the picosecond dye laser into a reference beam and a separate beam to illuminate the various objects in the scene, as shown in FIGURE 1. The reference beam was expanded by a telescope to fully illuminate the polystyrene block. Scattered light from the illuminated objects simply propagated to the polystyrene block with no intervening lens. The angle between the reference beam and the image-bearing beam was about 14°.

The recorded scene consisted of two objects. The nearby object was a 1.0-mm-thick glass slide with the letters HOLO attached to its front surface. The distant object was a white paper screen carrying the letters GRAM, which was pressed against the back of the transparent slide, so the separation between the two objects was about 1 mm. In order to increase the amount of light scattered by the slide, its front surface was sprayed with white Christmas tree flocking. The slide was then illuminated from the front. Of the scattered light from the slide reaching the polystyrene block, about 80% came from the front sprayed surface of the slide, and only 20% came from the rear surface. Viewing the laser-illuminated slide by eye from the position of the polystyrene block, one could clearly read the words HOLO, but the intense glare from the front surface almost completely obscured the letters GRAM located near the back of the slide. (This is in analogy with the glare caused by the bookseller's glass window obscuring the titles of the books located behind the window.)

Light from the laser reached the front of the slide 5 ps before it reached the back of the slide. Consequently, light from the front of the slide reached the storage medium 10 ps (twice the glass travel-through time) before light from the back of the slide. In the first experiment a hologram was recorded with the reference beam timed to arrive before both of these object waves. In the second experiment a hologram was recorded with the reference beam carefully timed to arrive within the 10 ps interval between the two object waves.

The reference beam and the object beam each had an average intensity of

0.2 mW/cm^2 at the location of the storage medium. An exposure time of 2–3 min was needed to record a hologram with a fluence of 70–100 mJ/cm^2, corresponding to 10^{10} identical pairs of laser pulses. To write the first hologram we tuned the laser wavelength to the absorption maximum of the medium at 621 nm. Because the absorption spectrum is 200 cm^{-1} wide while the dye-laser pulses have a spectral bandwidth of only ~30 cm^{-1}, we could change the wavelength of the dye laser by some 30 cm^{-1} and then record a new hologram in a fresh spectral region of the storage medium without affecting any previously stored holograms. The different holograms written at different center wavelengths were later selectively read out by simply adjusting the center wavelength of the reading dye-laser pulse. In the absence of all illumination these holograms lasted for as long as the sample was kept cold, months if desired (although liquid helium is expensive).

Readout of the holograms was performed by blocking the light coming from the objects and illuminating the hologram with only the reference beam. FIGURE 2a shows the reconstructed image when the hologram was recorded using a reference beam that arrived a few picoseconds before any of the light from the glass slide. The letters HOLO on the front of the slide are plainly visible, but the glare from the front of the slide all but obscures the letters GRAM located near the back of the slide. FIGURE 2b shows the reconstructed image when the reference beam pulse was carefully set to arrive after light from the distant object but before light from the nearby object. Now only the distant object is reconstructed, and the nearby object is eliminated. We emphasize that the light from these objects need not arrive at the polystyrene block at the same time as light in the reference pulse in order for the hologram to be recorded. In fact, because the coherence time of the light pulses was only 0.5 ps, and because we set the reference beam to arrive at the storage medium about 5 ps before the light from the back of the slide, the reference and object beams could not have produced a conventional intensity interference pattern in the storage medium. We note that the maximum time delay permitted between the object and reference beams was 10^3 ps and is set by the phase-decay time T_2 of the sample.

In the experiment reported here we were able to selectively reconstruct those objects that sent light to the hologram *after* the reference pulse had arrived, that is, the "late" light. However, for some applications it is desirable to do the opposite and recreate the light that arrived *before* the reference pulse, that is, the "early" light. For example, consider the problem of imaging an object that is embedded in a scattering medium, such as a tumor embedded in breast tissue. Illuminate the tissue from behind with a short laser pulse. Light transmitted through the tissue without any scattering will emerge before light that has been multiply scattered by the tissue.[8] Because the eye records all of this light, and because the scattered light overwhelms the unscattered light, the tumor remains unseen. However, if light that arrived earlier at the eye could be selectively enhanced, than a shadowgram of the tumor would become visible.

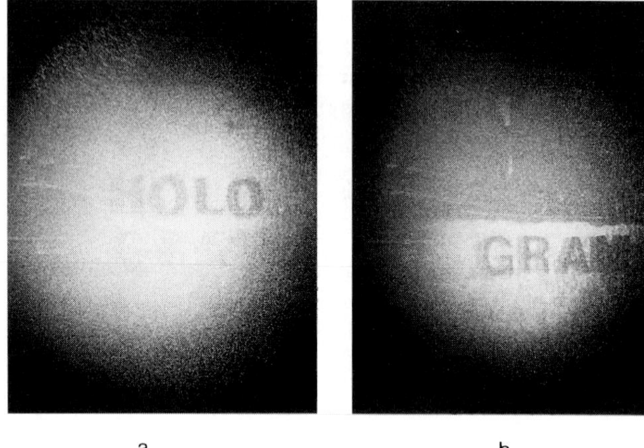

FIGURE 2. (**a**) Holographic reconstruction of both objects. The reference pulse was set to arrive before light from either of the objects. The glare from the frosted glass in front with the word HOLO obscures the object GRAM behind it. (**b**) In this hologram the reference pulse was delayed to arrive after light from the front object (frosted glass) but before light from the rear object. The front object is no longer reconstructed, while the rear object (GRAM) is now plainly visible.

This selection of early light over late light can be accomplished by simply altering the direction of the readout beam used in the preceding experiments. Instead of using a readout beam that is in the same direction as the reference beam, one should use a readout beam that is directed exactly opposite to the direction of the original reference beam. This is the "four-wave mixing" geometry of traditional phase-conjugation experiments,[9] but with a spectral hole burning material, now only the light that arrived before the reference beam is holographically reconstructed in the final image. In this way light scattered from back-lighted tissue could be eliminated, while light traveling directly through the tissue could be preserved, and would form a shadowgram of features embedded in the tissue.

Recently we achieved real-time imaging by using a different hole-burning material to speed up our writing time from 120 s to a few tens of milliseconds (personal communication). We use Zn-tetrabenzoporphin in a polymer film. This molecule does not show any permanent holes as in our previous samples, but has transient holes with a lifetime of 50 ms. Excited molecules can end up shelved in the triplet ground state for about 50 ms before they decay down to the singlet ground state. There are two advantages to this type of material. First, we can write a new hologram every 50 ms because the old one goes away. Second, the yield of the transition to the triplet state is at least ten times better than the yield of the tautomerization reaction in our previous sample. By using a bit more laser power than before we were able to write a hologram in a few tens of milliseconds, and, with the help of two mechanical shutters, we could write and then view holograms in real time. A particularly nice image was that of a wristwatch, where the seconds indicator of the reconstructed image could be clearly seen to move with time.

WHY DOES IT WORK?

Why does temporal holography work? How can the early or the late portions of a light wave be preferentially selected from a hole-burning hologram? The explanation resides with the principle of causality. A key fact is that if one writes a simple plane-wave grating in a hole-burning material using short pulses, then that grating will deflect light only in one direction (say the $+k$-direction, where k is the grating's wavevector) and not in the other direction (i.e., the $-k$-direction).

Consider a thin-phase hologram formed, not in a hole-burning material, but by two plane waves interfering in a thin piece of photographic film. As shown in FIGURE 3, when this thin, conventional hologram is read by either of the writing beams, both the $+1$ and the -1 diffraction orders appear, because the spatially periodic deformation of the film has the form $\cos(kx)$, which

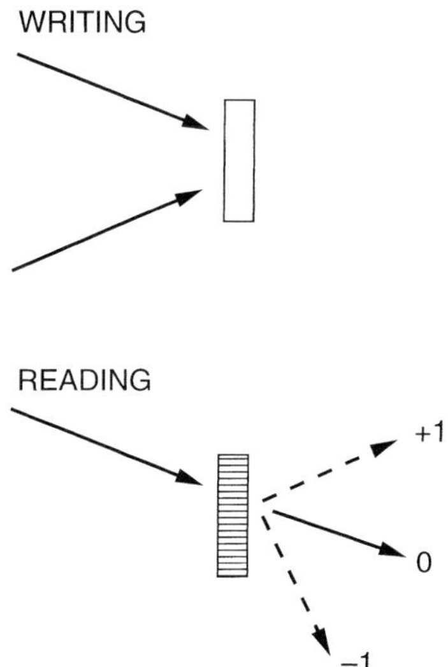

...both +1 and −1 diffracted orders appear.

FIGURE 3. Two plane waves interfere in a photographic film to make a conventional thin hologram. Reading with either wave reconstructs both the $+1$ and the -1 diffraction orders.

contains both $+k$ and $-k$ terms:

$$\cos(kx) = 1/2\,[\exp(+ikx) + \exp(-ikx)].$$

Next consider a hologram created in a thin, hole-burning material by two light pulses incident from the same side and that do not overlap in time, as shown in FIGURE 4. Now only the +1 diffracted order appears when either of the writing beams is used to read the hologram; the −1 order is mysteriously absent.

If we use thick instead of thin holograms, then the Bragg condition must also be obeyed, as shown in FIGURES 5 and 6. In the thick, ordinary hologram either reading beam yields a diffracted beam, but in the thick, hole-burning material only the early writing beam yields a diffracted beam. Reading with the late beam yields no diffracted light at all, because the $+k$ grating violates the Bragg condition, and in the thick, hole-burning hologram the $-k$ grating is

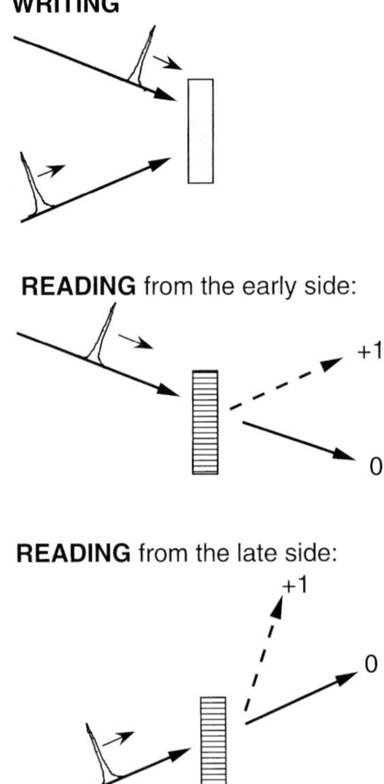

FIGURE 4. Two short pulses impinge on a thin, hole-burning medium. Reading with either of the writing beams produces only the +1 diffraction order.

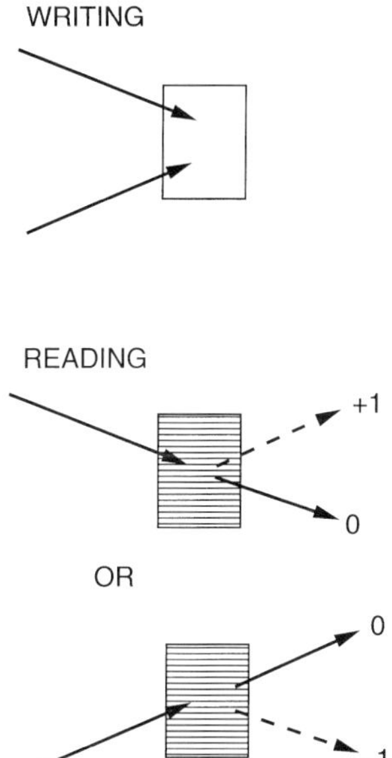

FIGURE 5. A thick ordinary hologram yields diffracted light for either reading beam.

apparently absent when read with a beam incident from the same side as the writing beams.

The reason that only the $+k$ order appears in a hole-burning medium using the geometry of FIGURES 4 and 6 is hidden in the mathematics of causality. Let the holographic material, whatever it may be, have a temporal response given by $r(x,t'', t')$ at position x and time t'' from an excitation at time t'. If the response function does not change from day to day, then it is a function only of the difference $t \equiv t'' - t'$ Causality then demands that the response function bow to the following wonderfully powerful constraint:

$$r(x, t) = r(x, t) * h(t), \tag{1}$$

where $h(t)$ is the Heaviside step function, defined as

$$h(t) \equiv 0 \quad \text{for} \quad t< 0; \qquad h(t) \equiv 1 \quad \text{for} \quad t \geq 0.$$

Equation 1 says that there is no response *before* the impulse (i.e., you can't win the lottery if you don't buy a ticket). In the frequency domain this

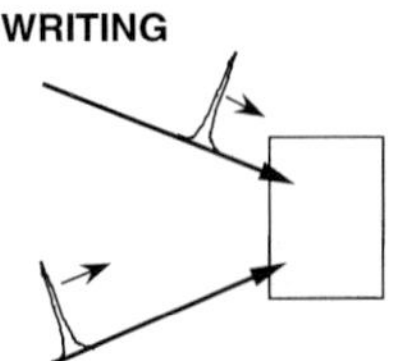

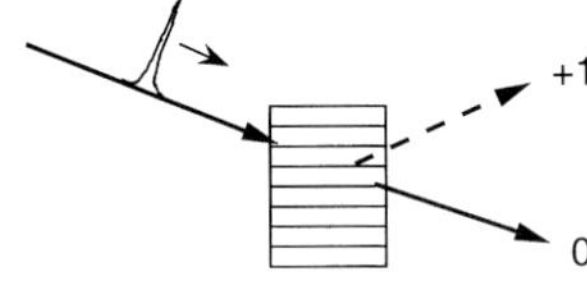

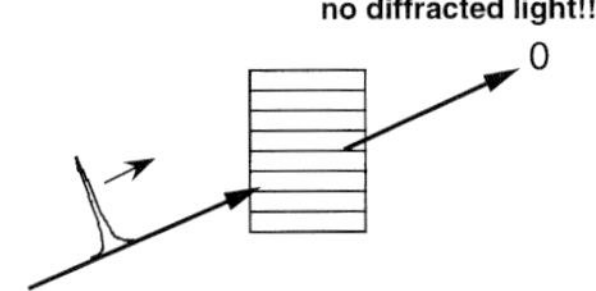

...reading from the late side gives no diffracted light for a thick, hole-burning hologram.

FIGURE 6. A thick, hole-burning hologram yields diffracted light only if read from the "early" side.

causality constraint becomes (with a bit of math)

$$R(x, \omega) = \frac{1}{\pi}\left(\frac{1}{i\omega} \otimes R(x, \omega)\right), \tag{2}$$

where the symbol $\otimes$ denotes convolution. (This convolution leads to the familiar coupling between the real and imaginary parts of the material's response function in the frequency domain, and gives the Kramers–Kronig relations, etc.)

Now, consider the following simple arrangement: two writing beams impinge on a hole-burning material from the same side, with a delay τ in one beam as shown in FIGURE 7. These light beams will create a spatially periodic grating in the material's absorption (i.e., a spatially periodic "hole") that has a different phase different for each optical frequency ω:

$$R(x, \omega)_{\text{imag}} = R_0 \cos(k \cdot x + \omega\tau). \tag{3}$$

Note that each frequency has its own phase delay $\omega\tau$. This is the key fact. One cannot write such gratings in photographic film or in a photorefractive crystal such as barium titanate, because in those materials all nearby reading frequencies ω see the *same* grating. But by using a hole-burning material, one can "burn in" different absorption gratings at different, closely spaced optical frequencies ω, with each grating having a different phase $\phi = \omega\tau$. Note that by inserting a fixed time delay τ in one of the two writing beams, one creates precisely the R_{imag} given in Eq. (3). Then causality in the form of Eq. (2) dictates that R_{real} must be of the form:

$$R(x, \omega)_{real} = -R_0 \sin(k \cdot x + \omega\tau), \tag{4}$$

and combining Eqs. (3) and (4) gives:

$$\begin{aligned} R(x, \omega) &= R(x, \omega)_{real} + iR(x, \omega)_{imag} \\ &= iR_0[\cos(kx + \omega\tau) + i \sin(kx + \omega\tau)] \\ &= iR_0 \exp[+ikx] \exp[+i\omega\tau], \end{aligned} \tag{5}$$

which is the desired result, namely, that when reading with one of the writing beams, only the exp[$+ikx$] grating is present and not the exp[$-ikx$] grating.

THE +K GRATING SLICES TIME

To see why the presence of only the +k grating allows one to preferentially select either the early or the late parts of a stream of light, consider FIGURE 8. Here a light stream and a short "marker" reference pulse expose a thick, hole-burning material. Reading the resulting hologram with a duplicate of the marker pulse itself recreates only those parts of the light stream that arrived *after* the marker pulse. That is because the early parts of the light

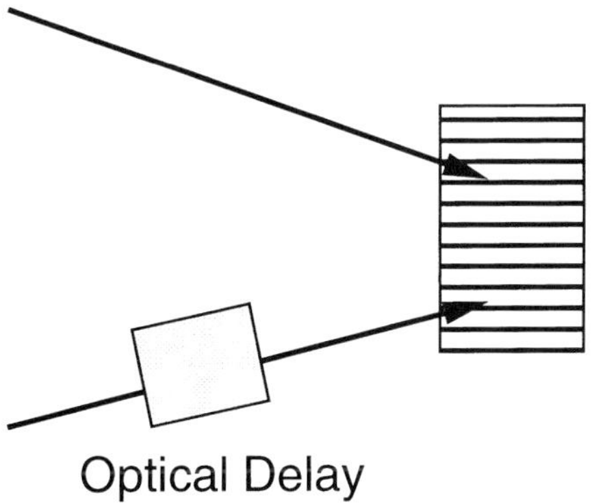

FIGURE 7. Inserting an optical delay τ in the path of one beam creates different holograms for different frequencies in a hole-burning material.

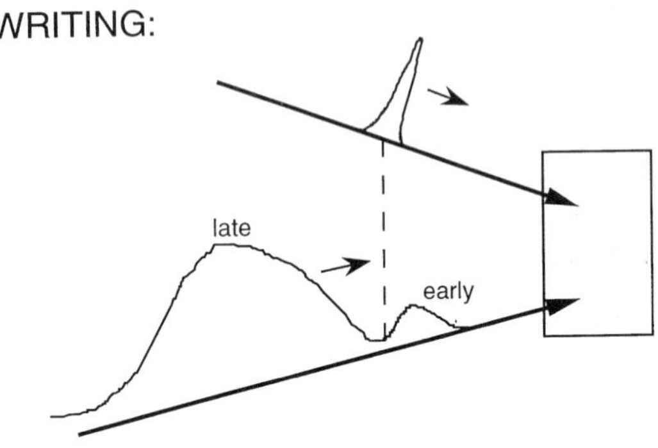

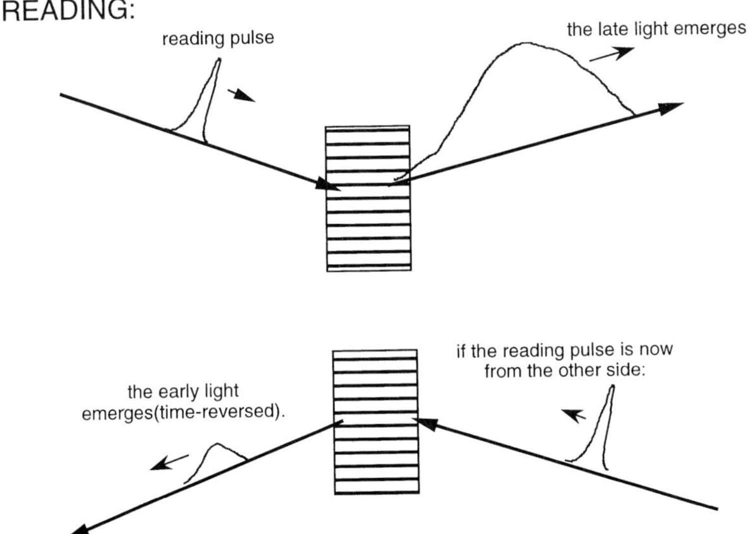

FIGURE 8. Expose a hole-burning material with a stream of light and also a short reference pulse. Reading with a duplicate of the reference pulse yields the late light. Reading with the phase-conjugate replica of the reference pulse yields the early light.

stream would make the marker pulse be reading from the late side, and that gives no diffraction according to our discussion thus far, and as seen in the bottom of FIGURE 6.

This preferential recall of late light over early light is what we demonstrated in the photographs in FIGURE 2. However, to see through a scattering material, one wants the opposite, that is, the preferential display of the early, ballistic light over the later scattered light, and for this one merely reverses the direction of the reading pulse to the phase-conjugate direction, as seen in the bottom of FIGURE 8.

We caution that for medical applications this imaging scheme requires a very large dynamic range for the hologram, because in thick tissue the scattered light can be much more intense than the unscattered light. We estimate that our present spectral hole-burning medium has a dynamic range limited to $\sim 10^3$, and so, by itself, is not particularly useful for imaging through thick tissue. However, it might prove useful for imaging through thin tissue or in conjunction with other optical shutters to improve the overall signal-to-noise ratio.

SUMMARY

It is possible to record a temporal movie of the light emerging from a scattering medium. Later, the movie can replay either the first-arriving or the last-arriving photons with picosecond temporal resolution. This temporal movie is created by directing two light beams at a hole-burning medium made from a chunk of dye-doped plastic. One light beam comes from the scattering material, while the other light beam is usually a short pump pulse. In contrast to conventional holography, here the two light beams do *not* overlap in time at the hole-burning plastic. The exposed plastic records the arrival time of *all* of the light from the scattering medium, and will store this temporal movie for months, if desired. Later one can preferentially view the early parts of the movie, and thereby see only the ballistic photons, that is, those photons that were not appreciably deflected in their passage through the scattering medium. Shining the phase-conjugate replica of the original pump pulse on the plastic medium recalls the early parts of the original scene, but not the later parts. In effect the hole-burning material creates a temporal shutter that passes the early light but blocks the later light. We presented experimental results and explained, using the principle of causality, how the plastic hole-burning medium creates this temporal shutter.

REFERENCES

1. REBANE, A. & J. FEINBERG. 1991. Nature **351:** 378–380.
2. SAARI, P., R. KAARLI & A. REBANE. 1986. J. Opt. Soc. Am. **B3:** 527–533.
3. LONGUET-HIGGINS, H. C. 1968. Nature **217:** 104.
4. MOSSBERG, T. W. 1982. Opt. Lett. **7:** 77–79.
5. REBANE, A., R. KAARLI, P. SAARI, A. ANIJALG & K. TIMPMANN. 1983. Opt. Commun. **47:** 173–176.
6. REBANE, A. 1988. Opt. Commun. **65:** 175–178.
7. MOERNER, W. E. 1988. Persistent Spectral Hole Burning: Science and Applications. Springer-Verlag. Berlin.
8. YOO, K. M. & R. R. ALFANO. 1990. Opt. Lett. **15:** 320–322.
9. HELLWARTH, R. W. 1977. J. Opt. Soc. Am. **67:** 1–3.

Noninvasive Detection of Fast Signals from the Cortex Using Frequency-Domain Optical Methods

GABRIELE GRATTON,[a] MONICA FABIANI,[b]
PAUL M. CORBALLIS,[a] AND ENRICO GRATTON[c]

[a]*Department of Psychology*
Columbia University
New York, New York 10027

[b]*Cognitive Electrophysiology Laboratory*
New York State Psychiatric Institute
New York, New York 10032

[c]*Laboratory of Fluorescence Dynamics*
University of Illinois at Urbana-Champaign
Urbana, Illinois 61801

INTRODUCTION

The study of the functioning of the human brain has recently become one of the most significant areas in science, as demonstrated by the official declaration of the 1990s as the "Decade of the Brain." A considerable amount of research has focused on the study of physiological phenomena associated with sensory, cognitive, and motor functions. Theories in these areas emphasize that these functions depend on the dynamic interaction of different brain areas.[1,2]

The last few years have also seen a considerable expansion in the physiological methods used to examine the functioning of the human brain. By and large, two major classes of techniques have evolved: techniques measuring the electromagnetic fields produced by active neurons (such as event-related potentials—ERPs—and magnetoencephalography—MEG), and techniques measuring hemodynamic or metabolic changes that are associated with neuronal activity (such as positron emission tomography—PET—and functional magnetic resonance imaging—fMRI). The types of information that are derived from these two classes of techniques are basically different. Electrophysiological techniques provide a direct, on-line window on the functioning of the brain, with excellent temporal resolution. Hemodynamic methods provide summaries of changes in metabolic rate in different brain areas during the performance of a task, and possess good to excellent spatial resolution.[3] Although the information provided by each of these approaches is invaluable, the study of the interactions between brain areas would clearly benefit from a method able to integrate temporal and spatial information, so that it would be possible to determine the relative timing of activation of specific brain areas. In this paper we will review recent data suggesting that noninvasive optical imaging may have the desired temporal and spatial resolution to provide this type of information and may help integrating electrophysiological and hemodynamic measures of brain function.

FUNCTIONAL CHANGES IN OPTICAL PROPERTIES OF NEURAL TISSUE

It has been known for some time that the optical properties of the cortex change when the cortex is functionally active. This has been demonstrated by measuring the reflective properties of the exposed cortex of animals.[4] Using this approach, it is possible to derive maps of functional cortical architecture that have a spatial resolution of up to 50 μm.[5] These studies have suggested that both absorption and scattering properties of neural tissue may change with activation.[6–8] Absorption changes seem to be caused predominantly by changes in the concentration of oxy- and deoxy-hemoglobin associated with metabolic and hemodynamic phenomena, although the activity of various cytochromes may also contribute. The time course of these phenomena is relatively slow, taking up to several seconds. The changes in scattering properties are less well understood. Studies on isolated neurons[9] and on the nervous systems of invertebrates[10] indicate that the scattering properties of neurons change during action potentials. This may be due to changes in the reflectivity of neuronal membranes; alternative explanations for these effects are also possible, and include volumetric changes or movements of ions across and around the membrane. Whatever the explanation for the scattering changes, it appears that they are more directly related (at least from a temporal point of view) to the activity of neurons than are the hemodynamic effects related to absorption changes.

NONINVASIVE NEAR-INFRARED OPTICAL IMAGING

The research reviewed in the previous paragraph described optical changes occurring in the brain during and after neural activity. For imaging purposes, it would be very useful to demonstrate that these phenomena could be detected noninvasively. The consideration that near-infrared light can penetrate deeply into living tissue has led various investigators to propose that this type of electromagnetic radiation might be used to image internal body structures.[11,12] The idea is that the optical properties of thick tissues with relatively high scattering and absorption coefficients (such as brain tissue) could be studied by measuring the parameters of the migration of near-infrared photons through the tissue. These parameters are differentially influenced by the scattering and absorption properties of the tissue itself.

Measurement of photon migration parameters of a particular area of the body can be done noninvasively by placing a light source (emitting light in the near-infrared range—between 700 and 1300 nm) and a detector on two points on the surface of the skin, separated by a few cm. The parameters of interest are the proportion of photons reaching the detector (i.e., attenuation, or intensity) and the time taken by the photons to travel between the source and the detector (i.e., delay, or time-of-flight). Most tissues in the human head are highly scattering. For instance, recent estimates of the scattering coefficients of gray and white matters of the brain range between 16.1 and 28.7 mm^{-1} (for the gray matter) and between 133 and 228 mm^{-1} (for the white matter).[13] Although head tissues also absorb light, the absorption coefficient is estimated to be much smaller than the scattering coefficient: the typical value of μ_a in animal tissues is on the order of 1 mm^{-1}.[14] These basic optical properties of head tissues indicate that the Boltzmann's transport equation for photons inside the head can be solved in the diffusion approximation,[15–20] and that the propagation of photons through the tissue can be described as a diffusion process.[21] This has several consequences of practical importance.

First, the trajectory followed by the photons emitted by the light source and reaching the detector will be highly variable. Therefore, the envelope of the trajectories will be an extended volume: knowledge of this volume is very important, because only modifications in the optical properties occurring within this volume will be able to influence the measures, and conversely, the size (and, in particular, the width) of the volume will determine the spatial resolution of the technique. The smaller this volume, the better will be the spatial resolution of the measurements. If we consider *all* the photons emitted by the source that reach a detector, the volume within which they travel is fairly wide, yielding a very poor spatial resolution (on the order of several cm). However, spatial resolution can be markedly improved by selecting photons that travel relatively quickly between the source and the detector. This is because these photons travel, on average, along a relatively straighter path than photons that reach the detector more slowly. For this reason, procedures that select photons with a relatively short time-of-flight or delay ("time-resolved near-infrared optical imaging") will have a better spatial resolution than procedures that pool together photons with short and long delays ("steady state near-infrared optical imaging") (see Alfano, this volume).

Second, the diffusion process implies that photons propagate in spherical waves. This, in turn, implies that, if the measures were taken in an infinite medium, the average path followed by photons between two points in the media would be rectilinear. However, the presence of a surface boundary with a nonscattering medium may induce marked distortions in the average photon path. This is because, as we have already seen, the individual photons do not travel straight through the media: some of the photons travel close to the surface and are quite likely, in their random walk, to reach the surface, and to exit from the medium. In this case, they fail to reach the detector. Only photons traveling deeply into the medium are likely to reach the detector. As a consequence, the volume explored by a source-detector pair located on the surface of the medium (head) is a curved spindle whose maximum depth is about one-half the distance between the source and the detector (in the case of dishomogenous media, this volume may be more complex). This theoretical prediction was confirmed experimentally using phantoms.[22] A practical consequence of this property of surface-bounded scattering media is that it is possible to study properties of relatively deep structures (such as the cortex) by placing a source and a detector on the surface of the head. Since the depth of the measured volume depends on the source-detector distance, the selection of the appropriate distance to be used in the measurements depends on the depth of the anatomical structure that needs to be imaged.

Third, the photon migration parameters are influenced by the source-detector distance: the number of photons reaching the detector (i.e., the attenuation) decreases exponentially with the source-detector distance, whereas the effect of source-detector distance on the delay parameter is linear. In the case of head tissues, the large attenuation of the light determined by the source-detector distance limits the maximum useful source-detector distance to less than 10 cm, and effectively limits the penetration of the technique to less than 5 cm from the surface. This has practical importance, because it makes full-head imaging of the adult human head impossible (unless the source or the detector were placed in some cavity inside the head such as the mouth).

NEAR-INFRARED EXPERIMENTAL APPARATUS

The earliest functional studies on the brain using photon migration methods were based on steady state optical systems, which involve measurements of the attenuation of light of particular wavelengths.[23–26] These systems are inexpensive and easy to use, but, as explained earlier, provide limited spatial resolution. A higher spatial resolution can be obtained with time-resolved methods, which allow the selection of fast-traveling photons. Photon delay can be estimated using "time-domain" methods[27] or "frequency-domain" methods.[28] Time-domain methods are very accurate, but have long acquisition time and are expensive. Frequency-domain methods are also quite accurate, but are less expensive and allow for fast data acquisition (up to 1 KHz). For this reason they are suited to the study of brain dynamics. The studies to be described later in this paper were based on a frequency-domain method derived from instruments developed for fluorescence decay kinetics.[29,30] It consists of a light source modulated at 112 MHz and of a heterodyned detector. The use of a heterodyning frequency (1 or 5 KHz, depending on the experiment) allows the translation of the signal into a frequency range that is appropriate for relatively inexpensive A/D converters. Phase delay is then measured using frequency-domain analysis methods. The final result is an accuracy of the phase measurement of about 0.1 degrees (out of 360 degrees). This corresponds to measurements of changes in photon delay with an accuracy of approximately 2.5 ps (10^{-12} seconds). This level of accuracy is necessary for the measurement of the delay and attenuation of the photon density wave-front in response to small variations (on the order of a few picoseconds) in the activity of the brain. In the experiments described, the light source was a light-emitting diode (LED) with a wavelength of 715 nm, and a power of less than 1 μW. The source-detector distance was fixed at 3 cm (computer simulations indicated that this distance allows for the detection of phenomena occurring at a depth of 0.5–2.5 cm).[31] Photon migration parameters were acquired using sampling rates varying between 12.5 and 50 Hz in different experiments. The measurements were obtained using a single-channel system (maps were obtained by repeating the observations at multiple locations). A multiple-channel system is presently under construction.

An important consideration in the study of optical parameters is the effect of vascular pulsation. The pulsation of the vascular system, and in particular of large and medium arteries, that is associated with systolic activity of the heart produces relatively large changes in the transmission of light through tissue.[32] This signal may, of course, be quite significant when the interest is in studying hemodynamic effects related to brain activity. However, when the interest is in visualizing directly the activity of neurons, this may produce substantial artifacts that are difficult to eliminate with simple filtering approaches. It is therefore important to estimate the contribution of this phenomenon to the observed data, in order to subtract it from the recordings or to study it separately. We have developed an algorithm for the estimation of this artifact based on a regression procedure in which the effect of systolic pulsation is estimated from the data.[33] The procedure takes into account beat-to-beat variability in pulse rate and amplitude. Our tests showed that, when used to estimate and subtract the effects of pulsation from the optical recordings, the procedure substantially reduces the impact of the pulsation artifact. This procedure is applied to all the data we have collected.

EXPERIMENTAL RESULTS OBTAINED USING NONINVASIVE NEAR-INFRARED TECHNIQUES

Path of Light and Effects of Skull

The purpose of these studies was to provide evidence that noninvasive optical imaging of deep structures enclosed in a highly scattering medium was possible,[12,22] at least for a depth of up to 4–5 cm. Our studies focused on two issues: (a) what is the volume explored using surface optical measures of photon migration? and (b) what is the influence of anatomical structures such as the skull on these measures? Some of the results of these initial studies were reported by Gratton *et al.*[22] These studies were conducted using simple phantoms simulating some of the optical properties of the human head. A semiinfinite scattering medium bounded by a nonscattering medium was simulated using a tank filled with skim milk. The path followed by photons migrating between a source and a detector located on the surface of the scattering medium was explored by observing the effects of a small absorbing sphere immersed in the tank on the measurements. The placement of the absorbing sphere was varied systematically, and photon migration parameters were measured for each sphere placement. The reasoning used in this study was that the sphere interferes with the measurements only if it intersects the path followed by the photons. The results confirmed the prediction that photons traveling between the source and the detector follow a semicircular path. In addition, the data demonstrated that the volume explored by time-resolved measures was much narrower than that explored by steady state measures (see FIGURE 1). In a different experimental setup, we showed that images of the small sphere submerged in the milk tank could be obtained from surface measures. We further showed that the images could be obtained even through bony structures. These images were obtained by placing a small absorbing sphere inside a sheep's skull. The skull was then submerged in skim milk. The surface of the milk was scanned using a source-detector pair. The image obtained with the sphere inside the skull was compared with an image obtained without the sphere. The difference between the two images indicated that structures with specific optical properties can be visualized through the skull.

Noninvasive Measurement of Functional Optical Effects: Distinction between Fast and Slow Effects

During the last few years, several studies have shown that optical methods based on measures of photon migration parameters are sensitive to functional changes of brain activity.[23–26,31,34] This research has led to the identification of two types of changes: *fast effects* (with a 50– 500-ms latency) and *slow effects* (with a 2–10-s latency). These two effects can be distinguished in a number of ways. First, the two effects have very different time courses. Second, they are measured in different ways. Slow effects are best observed by using a sustained activation task, such as a task involving repeated stimulations (or repeated movements) so that the cumulated effects of a number of individual stimuli can be observed. This approach is similar to that used for fMRI and PET. Fast effects, on the other hand, are best visualized by averaging the time course of the activity elicited by (or associated with) individual experimental events (i.e., stimulations or movements). This approach is similar to that used for ERPs and MEG. For this reason fast effects can be studied in conditions in which different types of stimuli (or responses) are intermixed, while slow effects can be studied only in conditions in which stimuli of the same kind are blocked. Fast and slow effects also differ in terms of the patterns of optical effects observed. While slow effects can be observed using both steady state and time-resolved methods,[24,26,31] it appears, at least on the basis of our own observations, that fast effects are best visualized using time-resolved methods.[31,34] This may suggest that fast effects are more localized than slow effects. In agreement with this hypothesis, Monte Carlo simulations reported

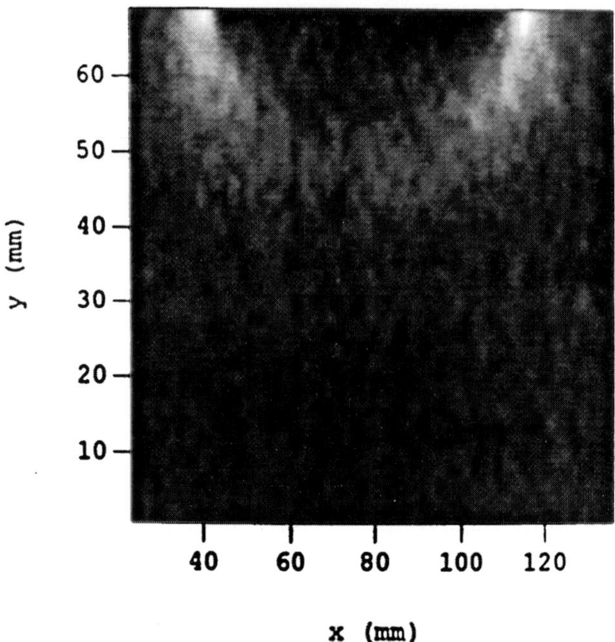

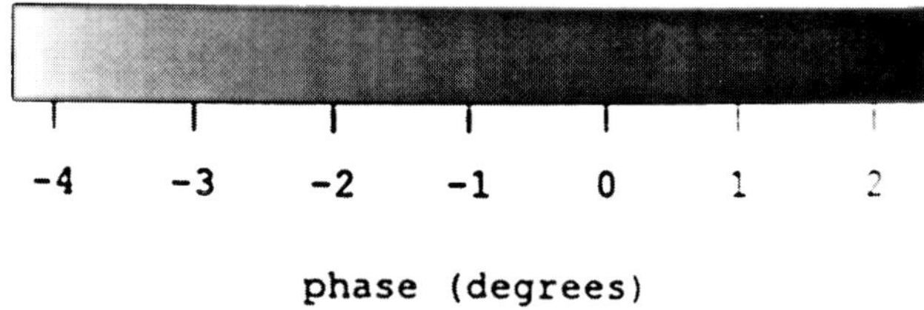

FIGURE 1. Empirical measurement of the volume influencing measurements of photon delay between two locations on the surface of an extended, surface-bound scattering medium, simulating the head. The measurements were conducted on a phantom (a tank full of skim milk). Near-infrared light was injected at the surface of the milk on the left end of the arc, and measured at the right end. The relevant volume was measured by systematically moving a small absorbing sphere in various locations within the medium. *White areas* indicate positions within the scattering medium in which the absorbing sphere will determine a reduction of the photon delay, and *black areas* indicate positions in which it will determine an increase in the photon delay. Note that the volume explored will vary if the position of the light source and/or of the detector is changed. Further details are given in Gratton *et al.*[22]

in Gratton *et al.*[31] suggested that fast effects are consistent with changes in the optical properties of relatively deep layers of the head (such as the cortex), while the slow signals are consistent with changes in deep and/or superficial layers.

To a large extent, the slow effects can be attributed to oxygenation and hemodynamic changes that occur in active areas of the brain. Therefore, these effects appear to be related to the absorption effects studied with exposed cortex reflectivity measures and with the BOLD-fMRI signal.[26,35] They may also be related with the effects observed with PET studies of blood flow, although the time course of the latter cannot be studied with the same level of detail. In the remainder of this paper we will focus on experimental results related to the fast optical signal.

The Fast Optical Signal

We have carried out several studies using the fast optical signal.[31,34,36–38] These studies indicate that the properties of the fast signal are consistent with the hypothesis that it may reflect localized neuronal activation related to specific stimulation (or preparation for movement). Using the fast signal, we have obtained maps demonstrating spatial resolution of at least 5 mm. In further studies using visual stimulation we have obtained evidence that (a) optical activity can distinguish between stimulation effects (localized to area 17) and attention effects (that are evident in extrastriate areas of the occipital cortex); (b) the fast optical signal shows spatial correspondence with fMRI data and temporal correspondence with visual evoked potential data collected in the same paradigm; and (c) in some cases the optical cortical responses may precede or occur in the absence of surface electrical activity (suggesting the presence of closed-field neuronal activity).

We will now describe in more details two of the studies we have conducted; other studies are described in other papers currently in preparation.

Tapping Task

Gratton *et al.*[31] recorded the fast optical signal (with detectors placed on the surface of the head directly above the two motor cortices, and the light source placed on the vertex) while subjects were performing a task requiring tapping with one hand or one foot at regular intervals. In this section we will review the data related to hand movements. Because of the neuroanatomical characteristics of the primary motor cortex (in which the right motor strip controls movements in the left part of the body and vice versa), differential effects were expected for hand movements that were contralateral or ipsilateral to the location of the detector. Specifically, it was hypothesized that when the detector was placed on the side contralateral to the hand movement, the photon path should cross motor areas in which neurons were active. In this study, four subjects were asked to tap with one of their hands for 10 s at a frequency of 0.8 Hz. Ten seconds of rest preceded and followed the tapping period. As hypothesized, systematic differences in the photon delay parameter emerged as a function of movement side, consisting of changes occurring at the tapping frequency (0.8 Hz) and/or its harmonics.

Quadrant Stimulation Study

The tapping experiment described in the previous paragraph had several limitations. Specifically, maps of activity could not be derived from the data because only two locations (one above each of the motor strips) were tested. In addition, the data recording was not time locked with the tapping movements of the subjects. In the study described in this section we tried to address these problems,[34] in order to determine whether fast optical signals could be used to derive a retinotopic map of the primary visual cortex. To gain more understanding of the time course of the fast optical signal, a faster sampling rate (20 Hz) was employed, and the recording of the optical parameters was time locked to the presentation of visual stimuli. The stimuli consisted of four black-and-white vertical grids, displayed in the four quadrants of a computer monitor. On each trial, one of the grids switched colors every 500 ms. The alternating grid was varied across trials. This was expected to produce systematic variations in the segment of primary visual cortex being stimulated on each trial. Photon migration parameters (light intensity and delay) were measured from 12 scalp locations over the occipital lobe, to obtain a map of the visual cortex. Average waveforms corresponding to the changes in optical parameters during the first 500 ms after stimulation were derived. The analyses identified a deflection in the delay parameter, peaking 100 msec after stimulation and reaching a maximum delay of about 10 picoseconds (see FIGURE 2). The maps obtained with these data (reported by Gratton *et al.*[34]; see also FIGURE 3) indicate that the areas of maximum response for each of the four stimulation conditions correspond to the expected retinotopic map of the visual field in primary visual cortex (i.e., the maps are inverted along both the vertical and horizontal axes). Direct data on the depth of these effects are not available. However, simulations reported by Gratton *et al.*[31] suggest that changes of about 10 ps in the delay parameter, combined with virtually no change in the intensity parameter, are consistent with variations in scattering (or absorption) of layers located at a depth of 1.5–3 cm (which corresponds to the depth of the superficial half of the primary visual cortex). The latency of the effects appear consistent with the idea that they may be due to the scattering changes ensuing in conjunction with electrical neuronal activity, as proposed by Stepnoski *et al.*[10] (see also Frostig[5]).

CONCLUSIONS

The results of the studies we have conducted using the fast optical signal (some of which were reviewed in this paper) suggest that this signal occurs simultaneously with or before the surface electrical potential (evoked potential or ERP). This makes the fast optical signal an ideal marker for indexing the occurrence of neuronal activity. The fast optical signal also appears to be

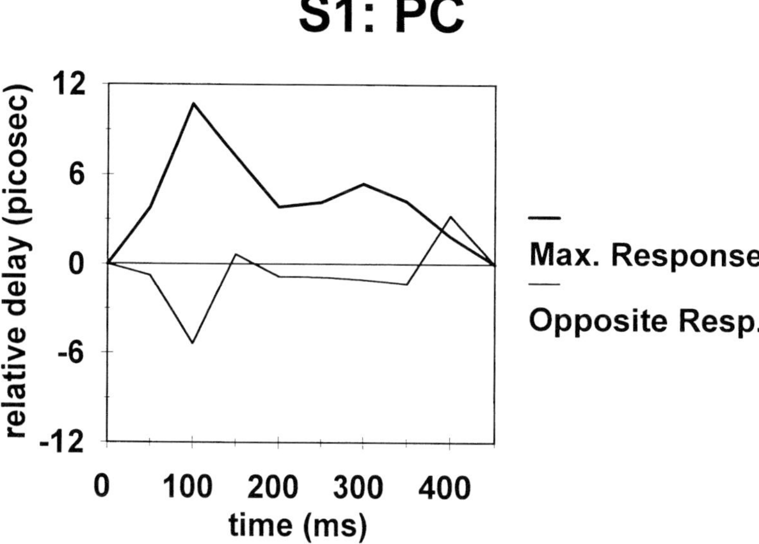

FIGURE 2. Time course of the fast optical signal elicited by grid reversals in occipital areas in a normal human subject. The measures were taken noninvasively, and indicate changes in photon delay with respect to a prestimulus baseline period. The data were averaged across four conditions in which different quadrants of the visual field were stimulated. Each condition was expected to stimulate a slightly different area of the occipital cortex. The *thick line* refers to the optical signal measured from the location at which response was maximum for each quadrant stimulation condition. The *thin line* refers to the optical signal measured from the same location when the opposite quadrant was stimulated. Note that the response peaks 100 ms after stimulation. Further details are given in Gratton *et al.*[34]

very localized, so as to allow one to distinguish between different parts of the same neuroanatomical area of the cortex (as in the case of Brodmann's area 17). Data we have recently obtained[38] indicate that this localization is consistent with that obtained using fMRI. This indicates that the fast optical signal is suited for examining the time course of neural activity in selected brain areas. This may be useful in two ways. On the one hand, it may help us study the relative timing of neuronal activity in different brain areas. This may have profound theoretical implications, since we expect most brain functions (such as vision, memory, attention, language, movement control, etc.) to depend on the dynamic interactions between different brain areas. On the other hand, the possibility of deriving data with high resolution both in the temporal and the spatial domains may help integrate various noninvasive methods for studying brain function, and in particular electrophysiological and hemodynamic techniques.

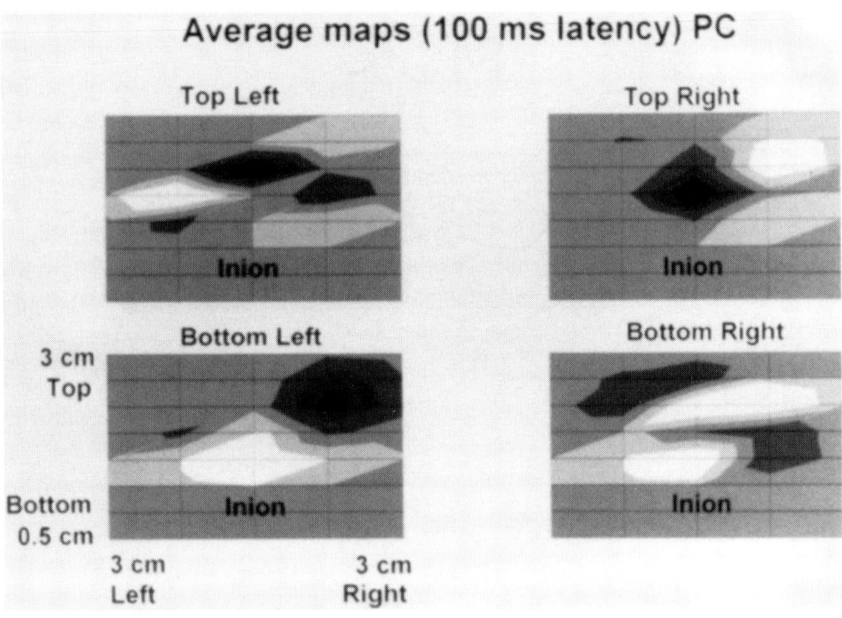

FIGURE 3. Maps of the fast optical signal elicited by each quadrant stimulation condition. The maps were obtained by scanning the surface of the occipital area of the head of a normal subject, over an area corresponding to the primary visual cortex. The *x*- and *y-axes* reflect horizontal and vertical distances from the inion, expressed in cm. *Black areas* indicate locations in which photon delay increased 100 ms after stimulation, and *white areas* indicate locations in which it decreased 100 ms after stimulation. The measurements are expected to be maximally influenced by the optical properties of brain areas with a depth varying between 0.5 and 2.5 cm from the surface of the head. The location of maximum increase in photon delay changes with the stimulation condition in a manner consistent with the contralateral, inverted representation of the visual field in primary visual cortex in humans. Further details are given in Gratton *et al.*[34]

Although noninvasive optical methods are quite promising, it is also clear that these methods are still evolving. Our data are still constrained by methodological issues. They include: (a) lack of a tridimensional reconstruction algorithm; (b) limits in the penetration into deep brain regions; and (c) limited understanding of the biophysical and physiological mechanisms responsible for the observed effects. Specific research addressing these issues may open new possibilities for the application of noninvasive optical methods to the study of brain function.

REFERENCES

1. MESULAM, M. M. 1990. Ann. Neurol. **28:** 597–613.
2. SQUIRE, L. R. 1989. *In* Molecules to Models: Advances in Neuroscience. K. L. Kelner & D. E. Koshland, Eds. American Association for the Advancement of Science. Washington, DC.
3. CHURCHLAND, P. S. & T. J. SEJNOWSKI. 1988. Science **24:** 741–745.
4. GRINVALD, A., E. LIEKE, R. D. FROSTIG, C. D. GILBERT & T. N. WIESEL. 1986. Nature **324:** 361–364.
5. FROSTIG, R. D. 1994. *In* Cerebral Cortex. A. Peters & K. S. Rockland, Eds: 331–358. Plenum. New York, NY.
6. FEDERICO, P., S. G. BORG, A. G. SALKAUSKAS & B. A. VICAR. 1994. Neuroscience **58:** 461–480.
7. FROSTIG, R. D., E. E. LIEKE, D. Y. TS'O & A. GRINVALD. 1990. Proc. Natl. Acad. Sci. USA **87:** 6082–6086.
8. HOLTHOFF, K., H. U. DODT & O. W. WITTE. 1994. Neurosci. Lett. **180:** 227–230.
9. COHEN, L. B. 1972. Physiol. Rev. **53:** 373–417.
10. STEPNOWSKI, R. A., A. LAPORTA, F. RACCUIA-BEHLING, G. E. BLONDER, R. E. SLUSHER & D. KLEINFIELD. 1991. Proc. Natl. Acad. Sci. USA **88:** 9382–9386.
11. CHANCE, B. 1989. Adv. Exp. Med. Biol. **248:** 21–31.
12. BENARON, D. A. & D. K. STEVENSON, D. K. 1993. Science **259:** 1463–1466.
13. TADDEUCCI, A., F. MARTELLI, M. BARILLI, M. FERRARI & G. ZACCANTI. 1996. J. Biomed. Opt. **1:** 117–123.
14. WILSON, B. C., M. S. PATTERSON & S. T. FLOCK. 1987. Photochem. Photobiol. **46:** 601–608.
15. CASE, K. M. & P. F. ZWEIFEL. 1967. Linear Transport Theory. Addison-Wesley. Reading, MA.
16. FISHKIN, J., E. GRATTON, M. J. VAN DE VEN & W. W. MANTULIN. 1991. *In* Time-Resolved Spectroscopy and Imaging of Tissues. B. Chance, Ed. Proc. SPIE **1431:** 122–123.
17. GRATTON, E., W. W. MANTULIN, M. J. VAN DE VEN, J. B. FISHKIN, M. B. MARIS & B. CHANCE. 1993. Bioimaging **1:** 40–46.
18. JACQUES, S. L. 1989. Appl. Opt. **28:** 2223–2229.
19. MADSEN, S. J., M. S. PATTERSON, B. C. WILSON, Y. D. PARK, J. D. MOULTON, S. L. JACQUES, M. D. ANDERSON & Y. HEFETZ. 1991. *In* Time-Resolved Spectroscopy and Imaging of Tissues. B. Chance, Ed. Proc. SPIE **1431:** 42–51.
20. SVAASAND, L. O., B. J. TROMBERG, R. C. HASKELL, T. T. TSAY & M. W. BERNS. 1993. Opt. Eng. **32:** 258–266.
21. ISHIMARU, A. 1978. Wave propagation and scattering in random media, vol. 1. Academic Press. New York, NY.
22. GRATTON, G., J. S. MAIER, M. FABIANI, W. W. MANTULIN & E. GRATTON. 1994. Psychophysiol. **31:** 211–215.
23. CHANCE, B., Z. ZHUANG, C. UNAH, C. ALTER & L. LIPTON. 1993. Proc. Natl. Acad. Sci. USA **90:** 3423–3427.
24. HOSHI, Y. & M. TAMURA. 1993. J. Appl. Physiol. **75:** 1842–1846.
25. KATO, T., A. KAMEI, S. TAKASHIMA & T. OZAKI. 1993. J. Cereb. Blood Flow Metab. **13:** 516–520.
26. OBRIG, H., T. WOLF, U. DIRNAGL & A. VILLRINGER. 1994. Paper presented at the 22nd Annual Meeting of ISOTT, Istanbul, Turkey, August 1994.
27. CHANCE, B. 1991. Optical method. Annu. Rev. Biophys. Biophys. Chem. **20:** 1–28.
28. GRATTON, E., W. W. MANTULIN, M. J. VAN DE VEN, J. B. FISHKIN, M. B. MARIS & B. CHANCE. 1990. Proceedings of the Third International Conference for Peace through Mind/Brain Science: 183–189.
29. GRATTON, E. & M. LIMKEMAN. 1983. Biophys. J. **44:** 315–324.

30. GRATTON, E., D. N. JAMESON, N. ROSATO & G. WEBER. 1984. Rev. Sci. Instrum. **55:** 486–493.
31. GRATTON, G., M. FABIANI, D. FRIEDMAN, M. A. FRANCESCHINI, S. FANTINI, P. M. CORBALLIS & E. GRATTON. 1995. J. Cogn. Neurosci. **7:** 1446–1456.
32. JENNINGS, J. R. & S. CHOI. 1983. Psychophysiol. **20:** 410–418.
33. GRATTON, G. & P. M. CORBALLIS. 1995. Psychophysiol. **32:** 292–299.
34. GRATTON, G., P. M. CORBALLIS, E. CHO, M. FABIANI & D. C. HOOD. 1995. Psychophysiol. **32:** 505–509.
35. VILLRINGER, A. & U. DIRNAGL. Cerebrovasc. Brain Metab. Rev. In press.
36. GRATTON, G. & P. M. CORBALLIS. 1996. Noninvasive optical measures reveal early attention effects in human extrastriate but not in striate cortex. To be presented at the 2nd International Conference on Functional Mapping of the Human Brain, Boston, MA.
37. GOODMAN, M. R., R. M. BAUER, P. M. CORBALLIS, D. C. HOOD & G. GRATTON. 1996. Invest. Ophtalmol. Visual Sci. **37:** S608 (Abstr.)
38. FABIANI, M., G. GRATTON, P. M. CORBALLIS, J. HIRSCH, D. FRIEDMAN. 1996. Comparison of NIR optical imaging data with fMRI and evoked potential recordings. To be presented at the 2nd Internation Conference Mapping of the Human Brain, Boston, MA.

DISCUSSION

QUESTION: What are things that you might do to improve the resolution for the brain beyond even a half centimeter, and would the modulation frequency affect that?

E. GRATTON: You can increase the frequency. There is a direct relationship between frequency and penetration. The more you increase the frequency, the less you penetrate. So actually frequency can be better used to see more deeply or superficially. In answer to the question, at least in the simulation, a resolution of half a centimeter is really the ultimate resolution that you can have at the depth of the human brain.

QUESTION: So if you get closer to the brain, then you can improve the resolution?

E. GRATTON: Of course, if you can get closer; if you can be in contact, the resolution is just the optical resolution. But at the distance of around 3 or 2.5 centimeters resolution of half a centimeter is the best you can obtain using the diffusion photons. There is no way you can improve on that. I'm talking about the resolution. That doesn't pertain to localization. Localization, of course, is much, much better.

QUESTION: Actually there was a corollary question: when you said resolution, was that two-point resolution?

E. GRATTON: Yes, resolution in the classical sense that there are two points that you can separate and see as distinct points. This is what I mean by resolution. Localization, of course, is much, much greater. And, of course, that also assumes some sort of contrast, because the larger the contrast, the better the resolution.

QUESTION: To confirm some of your ideas, have you ever thought of going to the neurosurgery room when they opened the skull?

E. GRATTON: I have not been there.

QUESTION: Could you get some results with higher resolution and accuracy without the skull there?

E. GRATTON: It should be possible practically. But with the reflectivity measurements shown today, why would you want to get anything better? Those have essentially optical resolution.

QUESTION: So you think the skull isn't really important then? What are the brain changes that take place, and are they localized in the brain as compared to the skull? So you say that there are real changes at the level of the neurons and the movement of water that changes the scattering properties of the water?

E. GRATTON: I have all the time scales. Most of the things I say are unfortunately indirect and based more on consideration of the time scale of events. The color experiments are different from the one we did before. But if you look at the time scale here, clearly you can start to see the onset of the event after 20 milliseconds, for instance. Now, to think that those things happen at different levels in the water or in the cerebral fluid or blood flow—I think that is difficult to explain. And those are scattering changes, they're not absorption changes. This is, for the moment, the information we have. So there are scattering changes; and they occur, let us say, essentially simultaneous to the electrical signals as I showed, and they are fast.

QUESTION: And if one tries your optical system on a rat brain, for example, and stimulates at various frequencies, what's the source of the scattering changes? Are there water movements within membranes associated with the action potential itself? What I'm really asking is what is the basis for the scattering change that is associated with electrical activity?

E. GRATTON: Clearly, to me, this is the most important question, so I posed the question to myself many times, and I tried to discuss it with many people. So I am not underestimating your question. The explanation that we came out with is, first of all, changes in shape. You know, changes in volume will change the scattering. Changes in reflectivity due to ions, for example, on the membrane will also change the scattering. So there are a series of processes. We cannot tell you now which one is more important than another, but those are possible sources of changes in the scattering coefficient.

STANLEY RAPOPORT (NATIONAL INSTITUTE ON AGING, BETHESDA, MD.): I know from the work of Tasaki and Saropolis from the old days that the action potential itself is associated with volumetric changes in the membrane on the time scale because the current changes are associated with ion flow changes. Is that what you're saying is occurring?

E. GRATTON: Yes, that is the best hypothesis. That doesn't mean that we proved that at all.

QUESTION: I was just going to make the point that Dr. Rapoport just made—that Dr. Tasaki several years ago was studying volume changes in the isolated nerve as the action potential moved down in there, and that very well could contribute to scattering changes.

E. GRATTON: This is the most likely explanation.

Future Directions for Neurotoxicity Testing: Towards a Unified Approach

Panel Discussion

J. P. HANIG, *Chairperson*

J. P. HANIG (*Center for Drug Evaluation and Research, FDA, Laurel, Md.*): The first thing I'd like to do, of course, is to thank the organizers for inviting me to chair this panel. It really is an honor; the quality of the presentations was outstanding as is the stature of the presenters and the members of the panel. Interestingly enough, although it wasn't planned that way, this conference represents almost 30 years of institutional history for neurotoxicology and the regulatory agency. I think that most of you will agree that we really have been exposed in the last two days to an extraordinary amount of exciting information and particularly opportunities to do the kinds of things with new technology that we probably never even dreamed of doing as recently as 10 years ago: the opportunities for doing noninvasive work in real time, real time neuropharmacology and toxicology, and so on. I think the biggest problem that we have in a regulatory agency, at least, or for anybody who is interested in discovering and documenting neurotoxicology is to try to make the applications. I don't think anybody would argue that the field of testing is different from that of research. With today's shrinking dollars, sometimes choices have to be made. Although it would be horrible if these fields were ever mutually exclusive, they ought to work a lot more closely with each other than they do most of the time. So it seems to me that the single most important issue is to determine what types of questions can we possibly address that will allow us to capture all of the important aspects of what was presented here and begin to contemplate whether or not we can go ahead and make applications to testing. For those of you who are familiar with neurotoxicology testing, you're probably aware of the fact that the Interagency Committee on Neurotoxicology has labored long and hard to develop a set of guidelines on principles of neurotoxicology as well as guidelines for risk assessment; these were published relatively recently, in the last several years, in the *Federal Register*. They serve as the very first unified background or set of guidelines for what might be considered some sort of universal approach to neurotoxicology. Whether or not there really can ever be a universal approach as was broached here remains to be seen, but I think we'd all be very interested in hearing what our panel members have to say. I'd like to begin by going around the panel table, and I would invite each of you to participate and offer your comments on what is being said. I really don't think that any of us are in a position right now to evaluate in depth the material that we were exposed to here. But we can certainly begin to ask questions.

THOMAS SOBOTKA (*Center for Food Safety and Applied Nutrition, FDA, Laurel, Md.*): I think we're all rather amazed and taken aback by the tremendous developments that have been occurring in this area of imaging. I would like to remind the investigators in this field of the realities of the regulatory agency's responsibilities and interests in the tests used to evaluate toxicologic effects. The significance of methods currently used for toxicological testing is that they are based on well-established, if not "old-fashioned," science. Toxicity is typically defined in terms of pathological changes and some evidence of clinical effects. But, with some exceptions, very little emphasis is placed on the more subtle effects of chemicals. The development of new methods for use in making regulatory decisions necessitates not only state-of-art technology, but also a rather rigorous process of validation of methodologies. The concept of validation was not mentioned or discussed in this conference. Validation implies that one must focus on replicability of effects. How well can one reproduce the effects from sample to sample and especially from animal to animal or individual to individual? Furthermore, the effects must be relevant to the functional status of the organism. This is particularly true with regard to effects on the nervous system. A subtle treatment-related metabolic change or anatomical change should be relatable to some discrete functional change. This type of detailed experimental information will be needed as the basis for validation of methods ultimately for regulatory decisions.

JOSEPH CONTRERA (*Center for Drug Evaluation and Research, FDA, Rockville, Md.*): I could amplify what Tom has said representing the Center for Drugs. One thing I want to say is that the FDA Centers differ significantly. They're different because they regulate different products. They have different statutory backgrounds, legal constraints, and benefit-risk considerations. One of the biggest differences, which is an asset for the Center of Drugs and Center for Biologics, regards the use of clinical trials, the evaluation of human efficacy and safety as part of the process of drug approval. This gives these centers an advantage in some ways over the other centers, which deal mainly with the animal portion of the equation. And that's why we have an interest in those methods that have potential clinical application. I think it's time to start thinking about perhaps picking one or two promising methods in the imaging area that have a broad application in a toxicology screening modality and focus upon their validation and regulatory acceptance as a future potential neurotoxicity screening paradigm. The power of these methods is that they allow us to evaluate interspecies extrapolation, by a direct comparison of animal findings and human findings. Adverse functional or anatomical changes in humans can be assessed in animals and vice versa. Those FDA Centers that rely upon clinical trials should be in a leadership position to advance this area.

We're at a time now when people are questioning the adequacy, the validity, the need for animal testing, and whether animals truly predict some or all of the adverse effects in humans. Powerful techniques that, like many of the imaging approaches, are noninvasive and nondestructive, and can be carried out clinically, are just what the doctor ordered in toxicology and really need to be encouraged. Even if the resolution of some of the imaging methods aren't yet adequate for a mouse or a rat, the fact that you can assess histopathological or functional neurotoxic changes in humans gives you the opportunity then to go back and develop an appropriate animal model using standard neurochemistry and neurohistopathology, which would help to validate the new method.

I think that the potential for these nondestructive approaches, the ability to use the same animal as its own control, the ability to do multiple sections—almost infinite multiple sections—using imaging techniques fill in many of the limitations that we now have in neurotoxicology. I consider the current status of the assessment of neurotoxicology totally 19th century. And I don't know how much reassurance we may have by safe passage in a functional battery and several sections through the major lobes of the brain and histopathology using H and E staining.

On the other hand, even when you get a neurochemical effect in animals that may be associated with neurotoxicity and not a pharmacological effect, such as alterations in neurotransmitter levels that persist well after a drug is removed, it's very difficult to demonstrate potential human neurotoxicological risk if you cannot demonstrate some behavioral or other potentially adverse effect in humans. And even when you get information from animal studies that there is an adverse effect, the relevance to humans is difficult to determine. Clinical manifestation of neurotoxicity by conventional approaches may not always be adequate, especially for subtle alterations in personality and mood that can result from alterations in brain function due to neurotoxicity. Imaging techniques may give better insights into such adverse events. These methods hold great promise to bridge the gap between animal and clinical safety studies. Perhaps some of them are maturing to the point where we might think about developing an industry-academia-government partnership for validating and applying them in drug development.

JENNIFER BURRIS (*Center for Veterinary Medicine, FDA, Rockville, Md.*): I represent CVM, which could, perhaps, be renamed the Center for Animal Drugs just to give you the perspective of what we do. We do review clinical trials, though we colorfully refer to them as "field tests" because they're often in large animal species. Basically we look at neurotoxicity or potential toxicities of any kind for a drug in animals for two different reasons. One is what we call "target animal safety and efficacy," which is similar to what the other centers do where the target animal is humans. Our target animal might be dogs or cows. The other aspect, though—and a very important aspect—is food safety. This concerns human safety when consuming products (meat, milk) from animals that have been given drugs. So actually these two areas (target animal safety and food safety for humans) are somewhat separate at the center because they have different requirements for testing. Neurotoxicity issues can come up in both instances. For food safety testing, we review an array of standard toxicity tests that are conducted using traditional laboratory animal species. Considering what I've heard here, the most exciting aspect is the new imaging technologies that could be used to examine whole, intact animals. True, the animals are not necessarily awake and behaving normally. They're physically restrained and probably chemically restrained, also. But even so, there is great potential for gathering much more information from any one individual animal, thereby reducing the number of animals that must be used and gaining more information. Perhaps—and again here comes the validation issue—with time and validation of some of these tests, some would be incorporated into our regulatory reviews. Many of the technologies we heard about here are only now being applied to biological systems, so it will be some time before we might be considering them in the regulatory sphere. But they're all certainly very interesting, and it will be interesting to see what effect these new methods will have on regulatory medicine.

ROBERT MUNZNER (*Center for Devices and Radiological Health, FDA, Rockville, Md.*): I come from an odd little corner of the FDA. I think our problems are probably atypical of what the rest of the agency sees. Primarily what I want to talk about is our need to assess the impact of surgical interventions and the impact of implants on the brain and in the spinal cord.

These, I think, pose some unique problems. Medical devices are, maybe, not in the mainstream today, but I think they have contributed a certain amount of success to the improvement of health care over the past 10 years or so. And I need not remind you that the imaging devices you have shown today have revolutionized the practice of neurosurgery. There's absolutely no question about that. The revolution brought about by imaging as a diagnostic tool has been so profound that we really don't need to talk about it anymore: it has altered neurosurgery of the 20th century.

We also have other interesting things. The cochlear impact has come along. The phrenic nerve stimulator is an old device and not used very widely, but it is an amazing thing that an implant can produce respiration just as a cardiac pacemaker produces cardiac pacing. Aneurysm clips are being used to treat aneurysms, which were an incurable disease 40 years ago. Shunts for hydrocephalus, after a rocky start, are now routinely used not only in infants, but in adults who have had automobile accidents. All these things are changing the practice of neuroscience and neurosurgery and the treatment of neurological patients. There are others coming on-line, too: implanted stimulators for seizure control; functional electrical stimulation as a prosthesis. These things sounded a bit bizarre 10 years ago, but they are happening today.

I came to this conference hoping to hear about some of the problems that we're facing as part of getting products on the market, where we have an interplay with the industry—where we have to ask them for information and sometimes suggest answers. There are so many questions we need to answer that I thought maybe some of them would come from this new technology we've seen here. So I made a list of questions. I'd like to make this a little more concrete, too. I'm just throwing these things out—some of them are old chestnuts—to get you thinking about what we have yet to do.

One of the primary questions is: how can we determine if a substance, an arbitrary substance, is safe for implantation in brain parenchyma? Now I'm very jealous of you people from drugs and foods. You have all these animal models. It's always presumed that a neurotoxin is either ingested or inhaled and that it gets into the bloodstream. Where is the research for direct implantation in the brain parenchyma? Point me to it. Tell me where the animal model is and who validated it.

Another problem: how can we determine that a substance is safe if it's deposited in the cerebral spinal fluid (CSF)? CSF has to depend on a pinocytotic action to leave the compartment. Anything in there—an implant or result of an accident—that ruins that mechanism causes hydrocephalus.

It's been suggested for some of these things that we do clinical trials. I would remind you that clinical trials, first of all, are terribly time-consuming. Second, they're incredibly expensive, and it's very hard for us to convince the manufacturer to do them. And worst of all, they're insensitive to detecting adverse events. When you look for an adverse event in a neurological patient, you can't separate wheat from chaff because they've got lots of "adverse events" no matter what happens. It's a poor model.

A typical problem is in the area of hemostatic agents. A surgeon wants to use something that's used elsewhere in the body to stop hemorrhage. It sounds like it should be easy enough. But how do we know, when he sprinkles that magic powder into the cerebral spinal fluid to stop flowing blood, that it is not going to cause hydrocephalus or a seizure. Where's the animal model to test for that?

Now those are two of the biggest problems. I'll give you another one: what does electric convulsive therapy do to the human brain? We have clinical evidence that it's therapeutic for severe depression. Is there a mechanism to be suggested here? Why not? The only evidence is the clinical evidence. On the other hand, we have patients complaining—another kind of evidence—of profound amnesia and loss of memory. How do you evaluate that? Have you shown us any way that we can examine the brain to see if there is really is a correlate to memory change? That's a joke, I guess—I know you can't. Our science still hasn't gone that far.

Is embolization of aneurysms curative? One of the new things we have coming along—and maybe it's not all that new—is intravascular embolization to fill aneurysms with something that will cause a clot. It is hoped that this will cause the aneurysm to resolve. Clipping aneurysms, of course, works great, if you can get the clip on the aneurysm. But in the posterior circulation, that doesn't work; so we have these attempts to treat aneurysms with embolization, but we have no way to assess the "success" on a long-term basis.

Now, in going back to some of the things that were discussed here, maybe MRI techniques will provide data from patients of the future. That's a plus, and maybe it will work.

I think you all are to be congratulated on this tremendous technology you've brought forward. It's great for understanding physiology, it's great as a diagnostic tool, and it's helping us understand the disease processes. But for the problems that I've mentioned to you here, I've tried to see if each of the things I heard here would contribute something toward these questions:

Histology is a useful tool to screen for brain injury, but it certainly is not sufficient. The brain can cease to function without losing cells. You can interfere with synaptic pathways. You're dealing with excitable tissue. You can cause seizures. We can't say that something is safe in the brain without considering how those mechanisms work.

The drug study that showed that there was impairment of function without cell destruction in the cerebellum was interesting from one point of view: could it possibly be an animal model for motor disorders to test out new therapeutic modalities? I would suggest that there might be something to be pursued in using those neurotoxic drugs to create new animal models to test for effectiveness.

MRI imaging, of course, is great for the patient, but what can it do for evaluation of medical devices? As I mentioned before, it may be just what we need to look at "treated" aneurysms to see if in fact they do resolve—as everyone hopes they will and believes they do—but for which there has been no evidence.

Ventricular volume could be studied, perhaps, as a way of assessing the effectiveness in treating hydrocephalus through an animal model in trying to understand the mechanisms of hydrocephalus or even detecting whether or not it occurs through neurotoxicity.

Is it possible that MRI, especially diffusion MRI, could show changes due to electroconvulsive therapy? I think there is work out there that somebody might do, but I don't think it will show any changes in memory.

Microscopy: maybe the meningeal cells could be studied to show what affects their uptake of fluid on a toxicity basis. Are they functioning, or are they not functioning after a treatment? One thing that wasn't mentioned was the possibility of using cell cultures, and I would suggest that someone think about using those as a way of detecting the potential for excitatory changes produced by chemical species that might be toxic.

I can't say anything about how we'll use single-cell recording in the near future. Near-infrared: there wasn't much talk about brain biopsies, but maybe there is something there.

Virtual reality: it's a great training tool; it's wonderful for information exchange; and maybe it could be used in a prosthesis. But I'm concerned about the idea of its being used in the clinic. You know: the doctor is in New York, and the patient is in Alaska, and isn't that great? After you've seen as many accidents as I have involving simple imaging devices, it would give you great pause when you consider the complexity of something like that.

You know, we used to have surgeons going in on the wrong side of the brain because they had the film upside down. Well, we kind of solved that problem, but what happens? MRI comes along, and two wires get twisted, and the image is reversed, so they go in on the wrong side of the brain. Well, what happens when we have so many reversals of phase we can't count them? Are we going to get it right? Sometimes.

In summary, I would say there is a blind spot in current clinical research, so far as the technical applications for toxicology assay methods needed in evaluating devices are concerned. The orientation is toward "the inhaled" and "the ingested," and it is away from any nonphysiological preparation. There is a good reason for this: everybody wants to work on normal physiology to show a result that no one will question, that will lead to a better understanding of physiology. However, this has biased the research community away from doing nonphysiological experiments that represent the situation we encounter with surgical intervention. So, what I want to say is: Don't let the blood-brain barrier be a barrier to information and research.

STANLEY RAPOPORT (*National Institute on Aging, NIH, Bethesda, Md.*): I think that is a good proposition. But I think there are really well-established animal models for looking at hydrocephalus and the causes of hydrocephalus that have been exploited for the last 20 years or so. And I think the effect of direct implantation is something that can be looked at specifically in an intact animal model, acutely and chronically. The methods that you have are behavior, electric recording, and metabolic *in vivo* studies—which include glucose utilization, blood flow, fatty acids, and protein synthesis; looking at structure *in vivo* as well as postmortem, and looking at differential drug sensitivity. I think those are very strong methods; for hydrocephalus, for CSF, you could look at flow rates. There's a way to look at CSF flow within the brain and the rate of disappearance of CSF as well as the volume of CSF. So there really are a lot of very powerful methods in place. The question that I have—I think hydrocephalus and direct implantation can be addressed simply by primate studies or even rat studies—is what level of toxicity are you worried about with regard to CNS active drugs beyond behavioral changes, electrical changes, structural changes, functional changes, and those other changes?

MUNZNER: I guess what I'm trying to get at is we need a validated model. When we asked the manufacturer who was to market a hemostatic agent to do the studies that were necessary to show that there was no potential for hydrocephalus, he said it's impossible. We didn't think it was impossible. The quantity was the quantity that would be used during surgery. Put it in the compartment and see what happens.

RAPOPORT: Why don't they say that would be a reasonable model and validate it? You know, hydrocephalus can be measured *in vivo* in a monkey or a squirrel monkey.

MUNZNER: Now we're getting down to the quirks of the problem. When we asked a device manufacturer to do that, he says it costs too much.

RAPOPORT: So the model exists, and now you're dealing with a cost issue. The model may exist.

MUNZNER: If the research community could go out there and produce a validated model, then we could say do it, and at least we would have an answer for that question.

RAPOPORT: I've read the literature on hydrocephalus, and that's what most neurosurgeons were doing. There's a model with hemorrhagic disease putting in various compounds and the CSF that block the arachnoid villi. There are a tremendous number of models out there on hydrocephalus that neurosurgical fellows have been working on for the last 30 years. The question I suppose for the FDA is to figure out what would be the criteria to develop hydrocephalus and say this is a model that's reasonable.

MUNZNER: Hydrocephalus is an example of what neurosurgical residents do for their year off. There's been research; there's a lot of papers out there.

HANIG: Well, I think we've picked an example where there is some sort of communication problem that may be more regulatory and financial than anything else. There is no doubt that the FDA or any other regulatory agency often runs into problems in getting the kind of work they need. But I think that the emphasis is really—and this is no criticism of what anybody said—in trying to capture some of the newer things and apply them in a way that serves the research but also gives us a new tool as far as testing is concerned. And I think that's probably what we're all going to focus on. I have been involved in both research and testing aspects; the one thing that saddens me is the fact that there isn't all that much communication between the two communities. There has to be a lot more coming together of these approaches rather than having them continue to be separate and isolated.

CONTRERA: Yes, I just wanted to add that even though the example may be a neurosurgical or implant problem, it does cut across many issues. And the issues boil down to development of new methods for assessing toxicity, and then the question of validation. But behind that, it's who is responsible for developing new methods. And it's always been my feeling that it's not enough just to tell the scientific community and say, gee, why don't you produce this validated method that we need and can't really function without? I think if it's an important parameter, I think the regulatory agencies—I'm not speaking necessarily for my center, but personally—should play a leadership role with industry as a consortium, as a collaborative undertaking to develop and validate these new models, to produce the products that we need to regulate. It's not simply enough to promulgate the standards that we currently have, but I think it's also our responsibility to assess their effectiveness and to develop new ones. Who is getting grants for developing methods anymore? Who is getting a grant in toxicology? It's now very difficult to get funding to develop these things. And so I think we have to come up with structures in which we can support that kind of work in a very focused fashion to meet these needs. You can't just wait. We're running into that right now in the carcinogenicity testing realm. We're trying to break out of those limitations by developing this type of partnership to develop alternatives to the two-year rat bioassay. I think this can be applied in many areas. We really have to come to grips with this.

HANIG: I think that's an important point. I would almost have to say jokingly that when researchers, whether they're in industry or in the academic community, take it upon themselves to become involved in validation and testing, it's almost like doing volunteer work or social work.

WILLIAM SLIKKER (*National Center for Toxicological Research, FDA, FDA, Jefferson, Ark.*): Unlike the other centers within the FDA, we're located in the pine woods of Arkansas. From that distance we look at our role and responsibility a little differently from the individual centers that are located here in the D.C. area in that we have a broader overview, look at the entire risk assessment process, and deal with agents that may be foods, chemicals, drugs, or medical devices in a more general way. One thing that I think is very important that David Lester and his colleagues Chris and Neil have done is to bring together this group of scientists to discuss these cutting-edge technologies. I believe that one of the roles of the researchers within FDA is to bring that interface to the reviewers and to the other scientists within the FDA and to make sure that we have access to the best technology and the best understanding. And I think that's been done in this particular case. I think that one of the fastest ways to move fields forward is to borrow from your colleagues, and certainly we have learned a lot here about ideas, hypotheses, and techniques that we could borrow to improve our lot in the area of neurotoxicity risk assessment in the future. So I thank them for putting together this conference.

One thing that I noted with some of these speakers is a multidisciplinary approach. I think this is very important to toxicology—neurotoxicology in particular—in that certainly we heard a lot about structure. That was one of the main themes. We heard quite a bit about neurochemistry. Dr. Taylor and Dr. Rapoport talked about neurochemical- or myelination-type situations, where we learned something about the ongoing biochemistry of the brain. And certainly we heard some about electrophysiology from Dr. Boyer's presentation. On the behavioral side we heard less, but there were some indications where we did have individuals talking about structural changes and behavioral changes. And I think those are very important. Early on, Dr. Volkow talked about those kinds of interactions. And so I would like to see more of that sort of thing occur, and I think that as this technology develops, we're going to see other end points brought to bear and compare them with those particular structural changes. I think that is an important future objective that we could look toward to.

I was thinking about the risk-assessment process during these last two days; and, because one of the major goals of the FDA is to be concerned about risk-assessment procedures, I was thinking about those steps that were outlined by the National Academy of Sciences in 1983. You probably all know them—the hazard ID, the dose-response assessment, exposure assessment, and the qualitative risk assessment as the fourth component that brings together the first three portions of the risk-assessment process. Many of these techniques that we've looked at and had the opportunity to visualize here certainly could fit in the hazard ID situation, because any sort of structural changes are oftentimes looked at as possibly a bad thing in the nervous system. What I was more concerned about and questioned during some of the presentations was whether or not the dose-response assessment could be accomplished with today's degree of development of these techniques. That is, are we able to look at quantitative changes with these particular approaches? I think this is an area that's going to undergo further development; it's going to be important to be able to look at quantitative events. Now certainly the technology itself lends itself to quantitation. There's no doubt about it that we probably saw more bits and bytes here than we're used to seeing in discussions of toxicology. So certainly it's there. It's just a matter of trying to work to a point where there is some pharmacology and toxicology involved in these processes and the dose-response curve is evaluated using these approaches. I also think that some of this technology, although not necessarily mentioned in this particular context, can be used to look at exposure assessment. As a matter of fact, there already is information out there on fluoxetine or Prozac, also d-fenfluramine, looking at levels of these particular agents in the brain. And this is done in noninvasive ways, using some of the techniques that we heard about here. I think that if some of this technology is pointed toward exposure assessment, that's a real step forward in its own right. As you understand, toxicology is really a combination of hazard or toxicity and exposure. Without exposure you don't have to worry about risk of a toxicant. So if your exposure is low, that's really a positive thing. To quantify exposure is very critical in risk assessment. I think that's one thing that this field can really add a lot to. It needs to be pointed in that direction as soon as possible.

The idea that all these techniques are noninvasive and can be used repeatedly in the same animal or in humans I think is a very critical feature. And I think this is one feature that these technologies really have a lot to offer to the area of risk assessment. Not only do they reduce the number of animals you may have to use, but longitudinal studies have much more power than the single time point studies. And, of course, the application in humans is all important. Risk assessment could be done oftentimes with human data from clinical trials. We don't want always to rely on that, of course, but in some cases it may well be the right thing to do. So that kind of approach is certainly something that this technology offers. So that is how I viewed this conference. I really feel that this area is undergoing rapid development, that we need to borrow as much as we can from it and to interact with the individuals who are bringing this technology to the front. This will allow us to move the risk-assessment process forward to better accomplish the mission of the FDA.

JAN JOHANNESSEN (*Center for Food Safety and Applied Nutrition, FDA, Laurel, Md.*): A lot of the points that I was going to make have already been made. I would just like to deviate a little bit from the issue of risk assessment in terms of looking at acute toxicology, and throw out for thought one of the things that came to my mind seeing all this. In many of the human cases that we saw where the imaging techniques were being used and disease was present or an issue—generally I think in pretty much in all cases—these are conditions that would be very apparent clinically without an MRI having to be done. In other words, stroke or brain tumors are going to be apparent from behavioral or physiological manifestations long before there is any need to bring someone into a clinic for an MRI. And one of the things that I think it would be interesting to do—and maybe someone is already doing this somewhere—is to start compiling longitudinal data from individual people over a long period of time. I'm just thinking in terms of the power of that type of approach. I think of the Harvard study in which they followed umpteen thousand physicians for years and years, and things are falling out about the use of aspirin and so forth in terms of cutting the risk of disease. I think that it may be possible with this type of approach, if the data is all compiled in one way to detect more subtle changes in retrospect, which may correlate with the development of a neurodegenerative disease, for example. I think that in some of the more obvious cases like stroke and tumors those are kinds of things that are going to be evident clinically. And what you'd like to be able to do is use imaging techniques in a more predictive way to identify some more subtle changes. This is the kind of data that, if it ever were accumulated, could be used for certain things like postmarketing surveillance, looking for developing problems before they happen. Whether or not the techniques are sensitive enough for that—I'm thinking specifically about the case of MRI—remains to be seen. But I think certainly some of the PET techniques where you're looking specifically at certain levels of receptors or uptake sites or neurons clearly have already been shown to identify lesions in certain neurodegenerative diseases like Parkinsonism. I think the other type of issue that a compilation of imaging databases might be useful for is to define population differences. One of the images that really struck me was the difference in the levels of monoamine oxidase B (MAOB) between a normal nonsmoker and a smoker. It was a tremendous difference, and it could conceivably affect the way a particular drug is metabolized. It could affect the pharmacokinetics. For many types of adverse reactions, you get a fairly wide range across a population; and the exact reason for those individual differences is not always clear. I think that in compiling a large volume of this type of data when it becomes available and again looking at these individual pieces of data retrospectively when adverse effects do occur may lead to a possible way of trying to identify certain populations that are either more susceptible, less susceptible, or may have a peculiar toxic reaction to something.

BARBARA WILCOX (*Center for Biologics Evaluation and Research, FDA, Bethesda, Md.*): My role in the CBER is as a reviewer for use of neurotrophic factors in treatment of human neurodegenerative disease. I think that we like to have a flexible approach when we are faced with a review. As the others have mentioned, we're open to looking at data from just about any approach as long as it's got a strong science base and is well validated. We encourage the development of these new imaging techniques due to their noninvasive nature. I was particularly interested in the techniques that could demonstrate potential changes before the actual behavior occurred—specifically, the

Parkinson patient in whom they were noting changes in the brain before the person knew that he was developing the disease. One of the problems that we're facing in dealing with the neurotrophic factors in the treatment of neurodegenerative disease is that biology of these molecules is not well understood at this point, and the companies are rushing to clinical trials for use of these molecules. One of the questions that always comes up every time we review an Investigational New Drug Application (IND) or speak to a sponsor is they always have a very strong rationale for a particular trophic factor in a particular disease. But the question always comes up, what else is it going to do and where else is it going to go? And we're talking about probably chronic infusion for years, possibly the rest of the patient's life. So we're interested—I personally am interested—in looking at questions of toxicology in response to long-term use of these molecules in the treatment of neurodegenerative disease; and I think that some of these whole-animal *in vivo* imaging techniques could be very helpful in identifying potential toxic effects.

HANIG: I would like to exercise my prerogative as chairman to make a couple of remarks in closing. I was very struck by the fact that these new imaging techniques offer a tremendous opportunity to look at various subtle functional changes that may not even be interpreted as being neurotoxicities per se—that might, in fact, take somebody who had the potential of being a genius and maybe turning him/her into a Fred Flintstone. Not that there's anything wrong with Fred Flinstone, a great guy; but I think that there are a lot of influences, chemical influences, that have effects that are so subtle that only computer analysis, real-time imaging, morphometric analysis, and a whole variety of other techniques can tell us that there is something wrong on a global basis with the nervous system. Maybe the ratio of one tiny brain area to another, which would not be detected visually, will, in fact, allow us in the future to deal with a variety of changes in the nervous system that may not be interpreted today as necessarily being neurotoxic because they are so subtle. There are subtle changes. In fact, the hardest thing that we ever had to do with the Interagency Committee on Neurotoxicology (ICON) Committee was to define the term *toxicity* or *neurotoxicity*.

Going on a little bit, I would say that these new techniques offer us the opportunity to examine various types of vulnerability in the nervous system that occur with age or may be part of a subtle process. The loss of neurons with age, the change in the size of ventricles, the processing of fluid are extremely important, particularly in older patients in whom there is vascular involvement. It may very well be that a whole variety of drugs that are safe and approved simply should not be used in certain contexts with patients who have vascular occlusions and have a silent intracranial pressure lesion of one sort or another, wherein the use of some sort of vasodilator is going to precipitate a Cushing's reflex or something like that. I just throw that out as one example. I think the one thing that wasn't mentioned here was the use of structure-activity relationship techniques. Very impressive computer programs are required, and also it is very expensive to screen a variety of drugs to create what is now known as toxicophores or pharmacophores, which are theoretical composite compounds that represent a variety of individual compounds that all have the same action in the same area. We can now interface that with all of our computer technology against a variety of databases so that we don't have to just screen senselessly but may, in fact, come up with two or three compounds that by virtue of structure or by class really ought to be looked at. I'm hoping that all of the techniques that we saw here will help us make the transition into doing proactive testing of one sort or another. This will give us a better predictive ability, so that we are not always caught in the reactive mode, where some sort of toxicity is reported and then, in the regulatory sense, we've got to scramble around, create an animal model, and generally produce data long after the issue has been settled in the press and so on. You're all aware of catastrophes like that.

I think, in conclusion, that it may, in fact, be possible to come up with some sort of unified approach—an approach that would allow us not to use just one single animal model but to use a variety of these techniques in combination to create something more than just the tier testing that we've relied on in the past—an approach that at least would give us correlations or p values or tell us that we're heading off in a direction that diverges from normality towards the realm of neurotoxicity. I certainly think that there were enough exciting things presented here to make us feel that we've entered into a new era. There has been a change. I think this meeting has been extraordinary in terms of being an inflection point in neurotoxicology. I'm just hoping that we all have the wherewithal and the desire to follow up on it and that the questions that we're asking today we can continue to discuss among our neurotoxicology interest groups within the Agency and across federal agencies. It is extremely important to perfect the testing aspects as an application of all of these wonderful research findings in order to truly deliver drugs and technologies to the public in a way that ensures their safety and allows them to get their full benefit.

FRANK VOCCI (*National Institute on Drug Abuse, NIH, Rockville, Md.*): Some drugs of abuse appear to have subtle toxic effects besides the ibogaine example I showed you earlier. The methylenedioxymethamphetamine (MDMA) is another one which apparently has effects on serotinergic neurons; and yet it's been studied clinically, and there's no apparent toxicity. Fenfluramine is something that the FDA has been dealing with, and again there are effects on animals that may or may not be relevant in humans. The differentiation of this is very difficult, expensive, and time-consuming. The nice thing that I think these imaging techniques allow you is that they have such power that you can see things that you've never been able to see before. Really, I think this sets the tone for the conference. You know that these techniques will make the invisible visible. The question is, in a sense, if it happens in every individual, you should be able to see it fairly rapidly. If it's a rare event that doesn't occur in everyone, it's going to take a lot of people to be able to see it. So that's another potential limitation of looking at some of these techniques. I think, for example, Nora Volkow showed you data where she said she's looked at 50 cocaine abusers and sees a pattern. Well, she's collected those data over years and years and years. If you have something that occurs in one percent of the population—we know this from statistics—you actually have to look at 300 individuals in a test to actually have the detection of that one-percent rate. So when you have low event rates for things, that seems to be the main problem. That's the problem that that FDA has always faced in safety evaluation and looking at adverse reaction rates. It isn't the common adverse reaction rates, it's the low event rates that are difficult to pick up. And if you have a low-event neurotoxicity, you're going to have a devil of a time picking it up.

SOBOTKA: I just want to underscore something. The challenge to the people that are developing these new methodologies is not only to develop something that is exquisitely sensitive, that would be able to pick up minute change. The challenge is also to make that interpretable. And I think the onus is on the people who are developing these methodologies. As Bill Slikker was saying, you have to utilize whatever interdisciplinary approaches you can muster to try to make the findings that you're coming up with interpretable. That's what the FDA and all the other regulatory agencies need to do. It's not enough just to say that I can find a spot in the brain that's glowing three or four months before any overt symptoms occur. You have to make it very clear what that particular glowing spot means and how to translate it into terms of safety and toxicity—for efficacy as well as for drug evaluation.

J. P. O'CALLAGHAN (*Environmental Protection Agency, Research Triangle, N.C.*): The EPA is another regulatory agency that is concerned with this problem. I want to underscore what Tom said, if perhaps in a little different way. Like the FDA, we're really called upon to say, is this condition, this treatment, the chemicals in the environment good or bad? So that gets into the risk-assessment process of hazard identification. Then you have to have validated methods. To underscore what Tom says, you have to have something of a consensus on what validation means and whether a given change observed can give you the answer of good or bad. The state of business at least in neurotoxicity assessment from a global testing standpoint is that we are still locked in to hazard identification. I think the benefit of this conference is that it points us in the direction of taking advantage of new and emerging technologies. But we still have to be mindful that the bottom line to all this is, How can we use these in a validated manner to make that judgment of good or bad for the benefit of human health?

DAVID LESTER (*Center for Drug Evaluation and Research, FDA, Laurel, Md.*): I'd like to thank the panel for their insightful comments and for bringing us back down to reality. I'd like to thank you all very much for your participation.

Index of Contributors

(Page numbers in italics indicate discussions.)